Computers in Health Care

Kathryn J. Hannah   Marion J. Ball
Series Editors

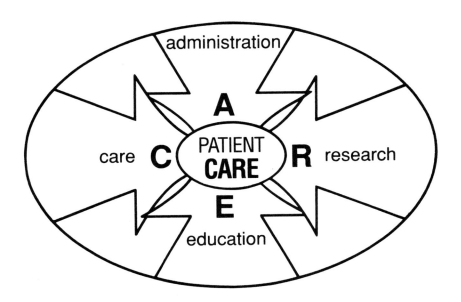

Computers in Health Care

Series Editors:
Kathryn J. Hannah   Marion J. Ball

Marion J. Ball   Morris F. Collen
Editors

Aspects of the Computer-based Patient Record

With 18 Illustrations

Springer-Verlag
New York Berlin Heidelberg London Paris
Tokyo Hong Kong Barcelona Budapest

Marion J. Ball, Ed.D.
Associate Vice President
Information Resources
University of Maryland at Baltimore
610 West Lombard St.
Baltimore, MD 21201, USA

Morris F. Collen
Director Emeritus
Kaiser Permanente Medical Care Program
3451 Piedmont Ave.
Oakland, CA 94611, USA

Cover illustration: The illumination on the cover is from a medieval manuscript found in the National Library of Medicine collection. This manuscript, by Hunain Ibn Ishaq, El Abadiis, is from the 13th century. This is the oldest book in the National Library of Medicine's collection.

Library of Congress Cataloging-in-Publication Data
Aspects of the computer-based patient record / Marion J. Ball, Morris
    F. Collen, editors.
        p.   cm. " (Computers in health care)
    Includes bibliographical references and index.
    ISBN 0-387-97723-6.
        1. Medical records—Data processing. I. Ball, Marion J.
II. Collen, Morris F. (Morris Frank), 1913-   . II. Series:
Computers in health care (New York, N.Y.)
R864.A87 1992
651.5′04261′0285″dc20   91-33021

Printed on acid-free paper.

Production managed by Christin R. Ciresi; Manufacturing supervised by Jacqui Ashri.
Typeset by Princeton Editorial Associates, Princeton, NJ.
Printed and bound by R. R. Donnelly and Sons, Harrisonburg, VA.
Printed in the United States of America.

9 8 7 6 5 4 3 2 1

ISBN 0-387-97723-6 Springer-Verlag New York Berlin Heidelberg
ISBN 3-540-97723-6 Springer-Verlag Berlin Heidelberg New York

The book is dedicated to Judith Vetter Douglas in grateful recognition of her diligence and devotion to making the series entitled "Computers in Health Care" the success it is today. Her dedication to working with the contributing authors has earned her the respect of the international informatics field. It is individuals such as Judith Vetter Douglas who make it possible to continually produce such high quality manuscripts. It is with grateful appreciation that I wish to acknowledge the continuing invaluable support that I receive from Judith.

Marion J. Ball, Ed.D.

Foreword

Don E. Detmer

Health care is experiencing an information explosion in the form of knowledge and data. Medical knowledge is increasing virtually on a daily basis. The questions that we are asking about the appropriateness and effectiveness of clinical treatments will provide even more information for practitioners to consider in providing patient care. We have more data and more complex data to track for patients over the course of their lives.

At the same time as the quantity and complexity of patient data are increasing, there is greater demand for data to support activities other than direct patient care. Health services researchers, managers of provider institutions, third party payers, and others seek access to patient care to evaluate, manage, and reimburse health care services. We do not, however, have a means of managing all of this knowledge and these data, and this lack of information management capability is adding stress to the already burdened U.S. health care system.

In April 1991, the Institute of Medicine (IOM) of the National Academy of Sciences completed an 18-month study on improving patient records in response to the need for better information management and increasing technological advances. The study was conducted by a multidisciplinary committee of experts and was funded by a diverse set of public and private sector organizations. The study committee was charged to do the following:

- Examine the current state of medical record systems
- Identify impediments to the development and use of improved record systems
- Identify ways to overcome impediments to improved medical records
- Develop a research agenda to advance medical record systems
- Recommend policies or other strategies to achieve these improvements

The conclusions and recommendations of this study are described in *The Computer-Based Patient Record: An Essential Technology for Health Care* (National Academy Press 1991).

As a means of accomplishing its work and achieving broader representation in the study process, the committee established subcommittees to explore three major dimensions of patient record improvement. Donald Berwick, M.D., and Carmi

Margolis, M.D., chaired the *Users and Uses Subcommittee*, which was charged with identifying the users of patient records, the uses of patient records, and the functional characteristics of records that would meet user needs. The *Technology Subcommittee* was chaired by Morris Collen, M.D., and Marion J. Ball, Ed.D., the editors of this volume. Their task was to examine the current state of technology available to support patient records and to identify the areas where patient record technology could not yet meet the needs of users. The third subcommittee, *Strategy and Implementation*, was chaired by Edward Shortliffe, M.D., and Paul Tang, M.D. This subcommittee was charged with defining a strategy to overcome the technical, logistical, sociopolitical, and financial impediments to timely phased improvements in the patient record.

The detailed work of the three subcommittees contributed significantly to the committee's deliberations, as did several background papers that were prepared on specific issues for the committee. One of the challenges faced by the committee in preparing its report was to provide a thorough yet concise description of what patient records should be and why computer-based patient records are essential to health care. As a result, all of the detailed papers that were considered by the committee were not included in its final report. This volume complements the study committee's report by presenting the subcommittee reports, as well as discussion papers and background papers. The volume thus provides a valuable service by enabling us to share those contributions with a broader audience.

I offer a brief discussion of the study committee's recommendations below to provide a framework within which the contents of this volume can be better understood. For a more detailed explanation of the recommendations and the rationale underlying the recommendations, I refer you to the committee's report.

The first and primary recommendation of the committee is that *health care practitioners should adopt the computer-based patient record (CPR) as the standard for medical and all other records related to patient care*. The future patient record envisioned by the IOM committee is not simply a digitized version of the current paper record; rather, it provides broader functions to practitioners, is used actively by practitioners in the delivery of care, and serves as a resource in the evaluation and management of patient care.

The committee developed a very specific definition of what a CPR is and identified basic attributes of CPRs and CPR systems. CPRs should contain a problem list, health status and functional level, and clinician rationale for patient care decisions. They should be able to be linked with other clinical records to provide a longitudinal patient record. CPR systems must protect patient confidentiality. They must also provide convenient access to authorized users at all times, support direct data entry by practitioners, and allow custom-tailored views of the data. CPR systems should be able to be linked to knowledge, literature, and bibliographic databases. They must be flexible and expandable to support the evolving needs of users. Such CPRs and CPR systems will assist the process of clinical problem solving and enable practitioners and institutions to evaluate and manage the quality and costs of care.

The committee concluded that the CPR is an essential technology for health care for three key reasons. First, the uses and demands of patient data are increasing. Second, the increasing complexity of treatment, the growing numbers of elderly patients with chronic illnesses, and a continually mobile population are generating more data to be tracked and greater difficulty in tracking them. Third, achieving the goals of improving the quality and managing the costs of health care requires improved information management capabilities.

The committee also concluded that widespread implementation of CPRs can be achieved within a relatively short time frame (i.e., 10 years) *if* adequate resources and coordination are devoted to the effort. The committee based this conclusion on the increasing prevalence of computers in everyday life and the advances achieved to date in computer and networking technologies. Thus, the committee's second recommendation is that *the public and private sectors should join in establishing an institute to promote and facilitate the development and implementation of CPRs.* Such an institute would be involved in a range of activities including standards setting, demonstration projects, and educational programs on CPRs. The committee proposed an organizational structure for such an institute in its report, but emphasized that the means used to achieve widespread implementation of CPRs are less important than achieving that end.

The committee's four remaining recommendations identify ways to *overcome specific barriers to CPR development and implementation.* The committee recognized that, although a great deal of progress has been made in computer technology, more work is needed for CPRs to meet the functional requirements of users. Thus, the committee recommended that both the public and private sectors expand support for CPR research and development, and the committee provided an agenda to guide that research. The committee emphasized the need for and importance of both data and security standards in its recommendation that the CPR institute should promulgate such standards.

Legal issues surrounding CPRs need attention. Many states do not recognize computer-based records as a legitimate means of storing patient data. There is no consistency among state laws on patient record form, access to records, and protection of patient records. Thus, the committee recommended that the CPR institute *conduct a review of state and federal laws and regulations and propose model legislation and regulations to facilitate implementation of the CPR.* Such a review should include an examination of unnecessary regulations that add waste and redundancy to patient records so that future records can be streamlined.

Obviously, there are costs associated with developing, acquiring, and operating CPR systems. The committee believed that those *costs should be shared by those who benefit from the CPR* and recommended that such costs be *factored into reimbursement levels or payment schedules of both public and private sector third party payers.* Users of secondary databases created from CPRs should also support the costs of creating such databases.

Success in CPR implementation requires that users have adequate computer skills and that there be more individuals with training in medical informatics to support the development of CPRs. The IOM committee recommended that health care professional schools and organizations enhance their educational programs for students and practitioners. *This educational effort should address the use of computers, CPRs, and CPR systems for patient care, education, and research.*

It is interesting to note that when the committee began its deliberations, we identified two possible outcomes that might result from our study. First, it was possible that little would result from our effort since the concept of linking computers and patient records was not a new one and progress in that area had been slow. Second, it was possible that the conditions were right for us to make a contribution toward advancing computer-based patient records by making a strong case for the value of such records and identifying the potential to achieve them. All of the committee completed the project with a great deal of *optimism and enthusiasm for a future vision of computer-based patient records—a vision that we strongly believe can become a reality.*

The committee concluded its work with the hope that its report would generate increased commitment to and resources for patient record development. On the day that the report was released, my testimony before the Health Subcommittee of the Ways and Means Committee in the U.S. House of Representatives on behalf of the IOM study committee received a very receptive hearing. Congressional interest in this issue is evident in the form of H.R. 1565 (102d Congress, first session, 1991)—which would provide a strong impetus to achieving our CPR agenda.

Within a week of the report release, we also had the opportunity to share the results of the study directly with the American Medical Association Council on Scientific Affairs, the American Medical Record Association, and the New England Healthcare Assembly. Additional briefings and presentations have been given to a variety of groups since then.

At the time of this writing, it is impossible to judge how successful the committee and its subcommittees will prove to be in advancing CPR development and implementation and, in so doing, influencing the shape of the health care system of tomorrow. We certainly were successful in learning from one another and we share a common sense of what the future can hold.

I am confident that you will both enjoy and benefit from the various contributions in this volume. The IOM patient record study brought together people with the greatest experience and interest in this subject; more than 200 individuals from across the nation were involved with this effort. The project proved to be consistently challenging, illuminating, and entertaining.

A final word of appreciation is offered to all of the committee members, subcommittee members, and subcommittee advisors who contributed to the study. As chair of the study committee, I am personally grateful to the individuals whose work appears in this volume for their contributions not only to the study but also to my own understanding of the issues surrounding computer-based patient records. I would also like to acknowledge the study staff, Elaine Steen and Richard Dick, for their continuing expertise and efforts to bring the report to a timely and successful conclusion. Cliff Goodman deserves mention for helping start the study, as do Dick Rettig, Queta Bond, and Sam Thier. Completion of the study also is a result of the efforts of Kathy Lohr and Karl Yordy.

Preface

The increasing need of patients for better access to good quality care, the great mobility of people in this nation and their quest for care from a variety of health care professionals, the need for clinicians to have online decision making support and readily transferrable patient records, the continuing increase in the costs of medical care with frustrated health policy makers searching for adequate databases to better analyze complex health care delivery problems, the need for faster and lower cost electronic claims reimbursement processes all have made it very clear that it has become essential—indeed, have made it *imperative*—that throughout this country the current obsolescent paper-based medical records must be replaced as soon as possible by *computer-based patient records (CPRs)*.

Medical informatics—the application of computers and communications to medicine—has sufficiently advanced to permit a realistic vision of a new and improved patient record. Informatics technology will not only replace the traditional documentation functions of paper based records, but can provide through computer-based patient records a new dimension of support for patient care, administration, policy making, and research.

In recognition of this high priority need, the Institute of Medicine (IOM) formed the Committee on Improving the Patient Record. The result was the publication of *The Computer-Based Patient Record: An Essential Technology for Health Care*, edited by Richard S. Dick and Elaine B. Steen, and published by the National Academy Press, Washington, D.C., in 1991. As stated Dick and Steen state in the preface of their book,

> This report advocates the prompt development and implementation of computer-based patient records (CPRs). Put simply, this Institute of Medicine committee believes that CPRs and CPR systems have a unique potential to improve the care of both individual patients and populations and, concurrently, to reduce waste through continuous quality improvement.

The enthusiastic support of this IOM project by members of its committee and subcommittees resulted in the preparation of such a large number of worthy supporting papers that it was not possible to include them in the IOM publication. Accordingly, the IOM authorized the editors of this book to publish separately some papers that fit appropriately into this more technology-oriented book. We hope that this collection of papers will be useful as a supplement to the IOM report for those who want to read more of the detailed texts that were available to the writers of that report.

Marion J. Ball
Morris F. Collen

Acknowledgments

The authorization by the Institute of Medicine (IOM) for the separate publication of these papers, arranged by Kathleen N. Lohr, is gratefully acknowledged. We are indebted to the subcommittee members and the many authors of these papers for all the time they volunteered to prepare the manuscripts and for their willingness to have their papers included in this book.

The chairs and assistant chairs of the three subcommittees, responsible for the preparation of these papers, were as follows:

Users and Uses Subcommittee, Donald M. Berwick, Chair, and Carmi Margolis, Assistant Chair

Technology Subcommittee, Morris F. Collen, Chair, and Marion J. Ball, Assistant Chair

Strategy and Implementation Subcommittee, Edward H. Shortliffe, Chair, and Paul C. Tang, Assistant Chair

We acknowledge the help of Richard S. Dick, IOM Study Director, and Elaine B. Steen, IOM Staff Officer, in collecting and providing copies of the papers included in this book. We thank the Institute of Medicine for providing the following list of professionals who contributed their time and energy to the Committee to Improve the Patient Record and its deliberations:

Denise L. Allec, Ray Aller, Terry Alley, Stuart H. Altman, Margret Amatayakul, Kathleen G. Andreoli, James N. Applebaum, Howard L. Bailit, Landon Bain, Ruth E. Baldwin, John Ball, Marion J. Ball, Steven Bandian, G. Octo Barnett, William Barrick, Kenneth Bartholemew, Paul B. Batalden, Eric Batson, J. Robert Beck, Donald M. Berwick, Brian Biles, Jay C. Bisgard, Gordon C. Black, Jeff Blair, E.F. Blasser, Merryl Bloomrosen, M. A. Bobenrieth, Sal Bognanni, Enriqueta Bond, A. Peter Bouxsein, Vincent M. Brannigan, William Bria, Karen Brigham, Karen Berg Brigham, Judith Brinkerhoff, Melanie Brodnik, Robert H. Brook, Maria T. Brooks, Michael H. Brown, Lynda S. Browne, Michael Buckley, William H. Buckley, John M. Burns, Henry N. Camp, Paul C. Carpenter, Eugene Santa Cattarina, Jean Chenoweth, Arnold Cherdak, Stephan E. Chertoff, Paul D. Clayton, Clifton R. Cleaveland, J. Jarrett Clinton, Jerry Cohen, Morris F. Collen, Michael Congleton,

Donald P. Conway, Dick Corley, Jerome R. Cox, Jr., Harold D. Cross, Glenn
Crowe, Clayton Curtis, Frank Davidoff, Allyson Ross Davies, Nicholas E. Davies,
Holly V. Dawkins, Jim Demetriades, Michael Denny, Don E. Detmer, Richard S.
Dick, Kenneth Dickie, Susan Dowell, Paul Dragsten, Paul M. Ellwood, Mark H.
Epstein, Paul Y. Ertel, Robert J. Esterhay, Jr., Betty Falter, John Farrer, Daniel D.
Federman, William R. Felts, John H. Ferguson, David M. Ferris, Rita Finnegan,
Craig Fisher, J. Michael Fitzmaurice, Suzanne W. Fletcher, Nathaniel Folster,
Sandra Forquer, Arden W. Forrey, John L. Foy, Richard B. Friedman, Barbara
Fuller, Hugh S. Fulmer, Elmer R. Gabrieli, John S. Gage, Elizabeth M. Gallup,
Wilbur H. Gantz, Donna Ganzer, Elizabeth Gardner, Andrew Garling, Leland E.
Garrett, Jr., Gwen Gengler, Paul M. Gertman, Diane Gianelli, Ann C. Giese, Paul
Ginsburg, John P. Glaser, Jerome C. Goldstein, Paul F. Griner, Susan Grobe, Nancy
Guadagno, David H. Gustafson, Glenn M. Hackbarth, Ethan Halm, William E.
Hammond, Kathryn Hannah, Jack Harrington, Randall Harris, Gary Hassalblad,
Robert R. Hausam, Alice Hersch, Guy Hess, Barry R. Hieb, Thomas Higgins, Ane
F. Higley, Mary M. Hill, John Holbrook, Benjamin L. Holmes, Gary Hong, Susan
D. Horn, Robert Hoyer, Michael R. Huber, G.M.K. Hughes, Robert G. Hughes,
Betsy L. Humphreys, Robert W. Hungate, James C. Hunt, Karen Hunt, Karen
Ignani, John L. Indermuehle, Stephen F. Jencks, Richard Johannes, Judith Jones,
Judy Miller Jones, DeSoto Jordan, Joseph Jorgens, Evanson Joseph, Linda S.
Joseph, Charles N. Kahn III, Douglas B. Kamerow, Arthur Kaufman, Alan C. Kay,
Hazel K. Keimowitz, Samuel H. Kiehl, Steven King, Larry Kingsland, Deborah
Kohn, Ralph Korpman, Henry J. Krakauer, Hans Kuttner, Ann LaBelle, Richard
Landen, John Landon, Maria Elena Lara, Richard Leadem, Pepper Leeper, Allan
H. Levy, Thomas Lewis, Donald A.B. Lindberg, Orley Lindgren, Kathy Lohr,
Gwilyn S. Lodwick, Harold S. Luft, Alice Lusk, Walter B. Maher, Jane Majcher,
Sandra A. Mamrak, Carmi Margolis, Albert Martin, William Mason, Katie
Massuckelli, R. Masys, Patrick Mattingly, Michael G. Mayberry, Leah Mazade,
Kathleen A. McCormick, Thomas F. McCoy, Clement J. McDonald, James Mc-
Donald, Mary McHugh, Sean McLinden, Barbara J. McNeil, Bruce McPherson,
Regina McPhillips, Paul Mehne, Kenneth L. Melmon, Albert I. Mendeloff, Enrique
Mendez, Jr., Marianne Miller, Randy Miller, Charles E. Molnar, John Morgan,
Thomas Q. Morris, Thomas Morrison, Jennysue D. Mott, Gretchen Murphy, Jack
Myers, Richard Nani, John Napoli, Nicholas Negroponte, Alan R. Nelson, John C.
Nemiah, Joseph P. Newhouse, Donald R. Newkirk, Jeremy Nobel, Lowell Noble,
Nanci Noie, John Norris, Deborah G. Novak, Ellie N. Oakley, Karen J. O'Connor,
Patrick O'Keeffe, Dennis O'Leary, Helmuth F. Orthner, Judy Ozbolt, Walter
Parrin, Ramesh Patil, Robert Patricelli, Stanley B. Peck, H. Ross Perot, Gilles
Pigeon, Jesse M. Polansky, Samuel Porter, Fred Prior, David B. Pryor, T. Allan
Pryor, Robert B. Ramsey, James Reinertsen, Stanley Reiser, Kathy Renz, Peter
Rheinstein, Joe Ribatto, Del Richmond, James S. Roberts, Fredrick Robins,
Noralou P. Roos, William L. Roper, Harold P. Roth, John Rother, Virginia K. Saba,
Damaian M. Saccocio, John Salley, Jerome H. Saltzer, Cecil O. Samuelson, Ralph
Schaffarzick, Donald Schiffman, Peter Schipma, Robert S. Schlotman, Martin L.
Schneider, Paul Schoemaker, Stephen C. Schoenbaum, Dale N. Schumacher,

Harvey Schwartz, Michael Scotti, Cary Sennett, Gerard E. Seufert, Jr., J. Christopher Shank, Roger H. Shannon, Richard S. Sharpe, Barclay M. Shepard, Gregory I. Shorr, Edward H. Shortliffe, Eliot Siegel, John Silva, Herbert Simon, Dee Simons, John D. Simpkins, Roy L. Simpson, Warner V. Slack, Scott Slivka, Dale P. Smith, Peter Spitzer, Eugene A. Stead, Jr., William W. Stead, Elaine B. Steen, Donald M. Steinwachs, Michael Stoto, MaryAnn Stump, Richard Suddick, James Summe, John P. Sulima, Paul C. Tang, Jack R. Taub, Zachary Taylor, Francis A. Testa, Samuel Thier, B.G. Thompson, Paul Tibbits, Sheldon Tobin, Elaine Ullian, Carlos Vallbona, Elaine Viseltear, Peggy Vollstedt, Adele Waller, Peter Walton, John E. Ware, Jr., Homer R. Warner, Lawrence L. Weed, Kathi Weis, Leonard Weiss, Norman W. Weissman, Rebecca J. Welty, Elizabeth West, Sue West, Jeff White, John Whiteman, Gio Wiederhold, Gail R. Wilensky, Albert P. Williams, Willis H. Williams, Mary Joan Wogan, Steven H. Woolf, Alfred Yankauer, Eli Yecheskel, Karl Yordy, Donald Young, Steven Zatz.

We also thank Joann Sommers, who contacted the authors of the papers included in this volume; Charles Baker, a college student who spent a good part of his summer retyping manuscripts not available in electronic form; and Judith Douglas, who oversaw the editorial process and helped bring this book to print.

Contents

Section 2   Technologies for Computer-based Patient Records (CPRs)

Section 3 The Future of the Computer-based Patient Record (CPR)

Contributors

MARGRET K. AMATAYAKUL, R.R.A.
Associate Executive Director, American Medical Record Association,
Chicago, IL, USA

MARION J. BALL, Ed.D.
Vice President of Information Services, University of Maryland at Baltimore,
Baltimore, MD, USA

G. OCTO BARNETT, M.D.
Professor of Medicine, Harvard University, Boston, MA, USA

J. ROBERT BECK, M.D.
Professor, Department of Pathology, Oregon Health Sciences University,
Portland, OR, USA

WILLIAM H. BUCKLEY
Director of Patient Care Representatives, Massachusetts General Hospital,
Boston, MA, USA

IFAY F. CHANG, Ph.D.
Manager of Application Solutions Institute, IBM T.J. Watson Research Center,
Yorktown Heights, NY, USA

PAUL D. CLAYTON, Ph.D.
Professor and Director, Center for Medical Informatics, Columbia Presbyterian
Medical Center, New York, NY, USA

MORRIS F. COLLEN, M.D.
Director Emeritus, Division of Research, Kaiser Permanente Medical Care
Program, Oakland, CA, USA

ERIC COTTINGTON, Ph.D.
Director of Research Support, Allegheny Singer Research, Pittsburgh, PA, USA

JEROME R. COX, Sc.D.
Welge Professor of Computer Science and Director, Applied Research Laboratory, Washington University, St. Louis, MO, USA

GREGORY C. CRITCHFIELD, M.D.
Associate Professor of Microbiology, Brigham Young University, Provo, UT, USA

ALLYSON ROSS DAVIES, Ph.D.
Director of Quality Assessment, New England Medical Center Hospitals, Boston, MA, USA

DON E. DETMER, M.D.
Vice President for Health Sciences, University of Virginia Health Sciences Center, Charlottesville, VA, USA

RICHARD S. DICK, Ph.D.
Executive Director for the Coalition for the Computer-Based Patient Record Institute, Washington, DC, USA

CAROL FRIEDMAN, Ph.D.
Assistant Professor, Computer Science, Queens College of the City University of New York, NY, USA

REED GARDNER, Ph.D.
Professor of Biophysics, University of Utah, Salt Lake City, UT, USA

W. EDWARD HAMMOND, Ph.D.
Professor, Biometry and Medical Informatics, Duke University, Durham, NC, USA

GEORGE H. HRIPCSAK, M.D.
Assistant Professor, Center for Medical Informatics, Columbia Presbyterian Medical Center, New York, NY, USA

BETSY L. HUMPHREYS, M.L.S.
Deputy Associate Director, Library Operations, National Library of Medicine, Bethesda, MD, USA

STEPHEN F. JENCKS, M.D.
Chief Scientist, Office of Research, Office of Research and Demonstrations, Health Care Financing Administration, Baltimore, MD, USA

STEPHEN B. JOHNSON, Ph.D.
Assistant Professor, Center for Medical Informatics, Columbia University,
New York, NY, USA

DAVID P. LAWRANCE, M.D.
Assistant Professor, University of Illinois, College of Medicine and Visiting
Assistant Professor, National Center for Super Computing Applications, University of Illinois at Urbana-Champaign, Urbana, IL, USA

ALLAN H. LEVY, M.D.
Professor and Head, Department of Medical Information Science, University of
Illinois Medical Center, Urbana, IL, USA

DONALD A.B. LINDBERG, M.D.
Director, National Library of Medicine, Bethesda, MD, USA

ROBIN MACDONALD, R.N.
Senior Consultant, Booze, Allen & Hamilton, Inc., Bethesda, MD, USA

DAVID MARGOLIES, M.D.
Associate in Medicine, Children's Hospital, Boston, MA, USA

CARMI Z. MARGOLIS, M.D., M.A.
Hersch Professor of Community Health and Primary Care and Vice Dean for
Medical Education, Ben Gurion University, Beer-Sheva, Israel

ALBERT MARTIN, M.D.
President and Chief Executive Officer, InterPractice Systems, Inc.,
San Francisco, CA, USA

CLEMENT J. McDONALD, M.D.
Professor of Medicine, Regenstrief Institute for Health Care, Indianapolis, IN, USA

MARY L. McHUGH, Ph.D., R.N.
Director of Nursing Research and Development, St. Francis Regional Medical
Center, Wichita, KS, USA

THOMAS Q. MORRIS, M.D.
President and Chief Executive Officer, Columbia Presbyterian Hospital,
New York, NY, USA

GRETCHEN MURPHY
Director of C/RIS, Group Health Cooperative of Puget Sound, Seattle, WA, USA

JEREMY J. NOBEL, M.D., M.P.H.
Lecturer in Health Policy, Department of Health Policy and Management, Harvard School of Public Health, Boston, MA, USA

JOHN A. NORRIS, J.D., M.B.A.
Corporate Executive Vice President, Hill and Knowlton, Inc., Walpham, Massachusetts and Lecturer in Health Law, Harvard School of Public Health, Boston, MA, USA

HELMUTH F. ORTHNER, Ph.D.
Director of Division of Academic Computer Services, Department of Computer Services and Professor of Computer Medicine, George Washington University Medical Center, Washington, DC, USA

ALLAN T. PRYOR, Ph.D.
Professor of Medical Informatics, University of Utah, Salt Lake City, UT, USA

CARY SENNETT, M.D.
Medical Director and Director, Clinical Quality, Aetna Life Insurance Company, Hartford, CT, USA

EDWARD H. SHORTLIFFE, M.D., Ph.D.
Professor of Medicine and Computer Science, Stanford University Medical School, Stanford, CA, USA

JOHN S. SILVA, M.D.
Assistant Professor of Surgery, Department of Surgery, Uniformed Services University of the Health Sciences, USAF, Bethesda, MD, USA

WILLIAM W. STEAD, M.D.
Associate Vice Chancellor for Health Affairs and Professor of Medicine, Vanderbilt University, Nashville, TN, USA

ELAINE B. STEEN, M.A.
Assistant to the Vice President, University of Virginia, Health Sciences Center, Office of the Vice President, Charlottesville, VA, USA

PAUL C. TANG., M.D.
Program Manager, HP Laboratories, Palo Alto, CA, USA

ELAINE ULLIAN, M.P.H.
President and Chief Executive Officer, Faulkner Hospital, Boston, MA, USA

GIO WIEDERHOLD, Ph.D.
Research Professor, Computer Science Department, Stanford University,
Stanford, CA, USA

MARY JOAN WOGAN, R.R.A.
Director of the Washington Office, American Medical Record Association,
Washington, DC, USA

ANTHONY J. ZAWILSKI, M.E.E.
Technical Program Manager, MITRE Institute, The MITRE Corporation,
McLean, VA, USA

Section 1
User Needs for Computer-based Patient Records (CPRs)

1
Physicians' Needs for Computer-based Patient Records

Clement J. McDonald

Background

Machine Ready versus Not

Much of clinical data are already stored somewhere in machine-readable form. Examples are:

- Lab results in lab computers
- Discharge summaries on a word processor
- Prescription records stored in a local pharmacy computer hospital
- Case abstracts generated and stored out of medical record systems

Other clinical data are not, for example, handwritten chart notes and bedside laboratory test results.

In developing computer-based patient records (CPRs), the place to start in any environment is with machine-ready data.

Free Form versus Structured Information

Machine-ready information comes in two categories—that which is structured (e.g., case abstracts) and that which is free form (e.g., radiology dictation). There are also hybrids (e.g., a laboratory result is usually stored in a structured record, but some of the information about the result may be stored as a text comment).

Machine-stored free text has genuine value to the direct care of patients, because it can be easily retrieved and displayed for patient care. However, such information has little value to the higher-level functions of a medical record such as research retrievals and decision support, because the computer has difficulty understanding free text.

The kinds of information that are currently stored as free text (e.g., radiology reports) have not generally evolved to as mature a state of evolution as that which is currently stored as structured formats (e.g., laboratory reports). Time and some large scale experience will be necessary before the latter will reach the evolutionary stage of the former.

The Difference between Earning and Spending

The hard part about maintaining a bank account is obtaining the money. The easy part is spending it. Similarly, it is easy to develop ways to use the information in a medical record system, much more difficult to obtain it. Yet, groups such as the IOM subcommittee on technology spend most their time deciding how to use the data within a computer-based patient record and almost no time on how to obtain it in the first place.

Our experience and that of others is that all the barriers to the development of medical record systems are on the input side and none on the output side. Almost all proposed uses for medical record systems have already been accomplished within circumscribed areas of application. Most outputs from CPR have already been accomplished within the confines of special applications. Computerized electrocardiogram (EKG) systems are perfect examples. They now can retrieve, display, transmit, summarize, and provide interpretations of EKG tracings. The focus of the IOM committee on how to use the medical record content will be moot if we do not concentrate most of our efforts on how to obtain that data.

Standards, an Overreaching Need

Numerous sources of machine-ready medical information already exist. However, the information is located on separate machines within hospitals, medical practice offices, pharmacies, commercial laboratories, and nursing homes. Despite the fact that these sources of machine-ready data exist, hospitals and clinics use the paper record to do case abstracts, discharge summaries, quality assurance reviews, and utilization reviews, and must then enter the abstracted information into yet another machine. The only solution to this fragmentation and redundancy is standards: standard formats for transmitting information from one machine to another, standard codes for representing the contents of categorical fields. The chapter on data exchange standards for CPRs provides details about the current progress toward standards for exchanging clinical data and medical knowledge.

Functional Requirements

What Physicians Really Want

(I think it is the same for inpatient as for outpatient care.) What they say they want day in and day out is:

To obtain patient information when they need it, where they need it (Gardner 1982). At LDS (Latter Day Saints) Hospital, laboratory results were the most frequently sought after piece of information in an intensive care setting (Gardner 1982). In general, physicians want to know: What drugs have been prescribed? What happened during the last hospitalization? As soon as they are produced, what are the laboratory test results? What was the patient's state during care by the previous physician?

Less intensively, but explicitly expressed, physicians also want

1. Clear displays of information (if only typewritten instead of handwritten)
2. Clear and appropriate organization of information
3. Display of trends and patterns
4. Selection and organization of subsets of information (e.g., evidence supporting diagnosis of vertebral disk disease). (Physicians do not want to trudge through all the information to see some of it.)
5. Help with the process of obtaining and reporting information needed by special reporting services

   - Pre-approval forms
   - Nursing home admission forms
   - Patient insurance forms
   - School physical forms
   - Free from disease forms
   - Marriage certificates

Research

Medical staff members need to be able to retrieve the records of patients with specified characteristics from a medical record system and compare them statistically with those of other populations. Retrievals are motivated by business, management, and research needs, as well as by efforts to continually improve quality. Users wish to ask questions such as How many referrals did doctor Y provide to me in the last year? What is the average postoperative time in surgical intensive care for my patients compared to patients of other physicians in my hospital? What is the infection rate for one knee prothesis compared to another in our HMO? How many patients had repeated treatments for urinary tract infections in one year? How many patients given Cimetidine in an ICU developed pseudomonas pneumonia compared with patients not given an H_2 blocker?

The more coding and structure contained in the computer-stored record, the easier it is to answer these kinds of questions.

Decision Support

Medical records provide great opportunities for decision support. Automatic decision support in the form of reminders has had important influences on physicians (McDonald 1976, 1984; Tierney 1988, 1990; Barnett 1978, 1984; Evans 1986; Hulse 1976; Pestotnik 1988). A computer-stored medical record provides the ideal context for automatic application of logic. Physicians are not demanding decision support systems at the present time. Yet, I expect they will come to appreciate them over time. Health care managers may need such capabilities even more than physicians to assure uniform quality of care at reasonable expense.

Broad Information Needs

In addition to patient-related information, clinicians need access to general medical information such as that found in textbooks, books, and the medical literature. Fast medical education might best be delivered continuously in small doses, as part of the order entry process (McDonald 1983). They want rapid answers to such questions as: What is the proper dose of vancomycin for a patient with moderate renal failure? What is the current therapy for coccidiomycosis? What are the indications for treating HIV-positive patients with AZT? The computer-based patient record could provide rich troves of medical information, including the contents of the entire National Library of Medicine, at exactly the point in the decision process that it was needed.

Administrative information may be required even more frequently than medical information, as suggested by Covell and others (1985). Clinicians ask questions such as: What is the closest alcohol rehabilitation center? Is this patient eligible for Medicaid? How much blood is needed to determine a serum theophylline level? Does the patient's insurance cover birth control pills? And so on. This suggests the need for electronic links to sources of such information.

Order Entry

Physicians are not seeking such systems at the present time, but their use could substantially improve the efficiency, economy, uniformity, and quality of medical care in large care systems (Tierney 1988, 1990).

Results of Subcommittee Survey

We solicited the opinion of all twenty-eight attendees of the last users committee. The requirements fall roughly into three categories:

- The content of the record: That is, what kind of data it should contain?
- The function of the record: Once data are in, what kinds of things should it do?
- Performance characteristics of the system: How available should it be? How fast should it be? How much training should it require?

Record Content

Data Elements. Specific data elements were suggested for inclusion in the record. These include such items as

- The problem list
- Medication profile

- Lists of acute and minor problems, long-term and major problems
- Social and functional measurements such as daily activities, meals, kind of work done, home setting, job satisfaction, social community, etc.
- Manifestations, studies and test orders, results, and clinical course
- Psychosocial values, including information about family situation, patient expectations, and so on

The requests for data elements come from two quite different sources:

- Clinicians who want the information needed for clinical care, that is, information about medications, recent test results, and problem lists
- Policymakers, managers, and researchers who want the information needed to satisfy regulatory and quality assurance requirements (management)

Policymakers and researchers want information that will help them assess illness severity and judge outcomes. This would include a minimum of information about the patient's mental and functional status, as well as disease and/or procedure-specific information to characterize severity before and after the procedure.

We must acknowledge, however, that the goals of managers and policymakers for complete information may conflict with the goals of professional users for systems that do not cost them time. Compromise will have to be made in terms of the number of required data elements and the time required to capture them. A larger minimum set could be expected from hospital stays and surgical procedures than from outpatient visits.

Scope and Comprehensiveness. Another dimension of the record's content is the scope of the data collected. The most strongly stated physician requirement was for comprehensive records. This can best be stated in the words of participants:

- Relevant data, accessible regardless of the site of care, the source of care, or the time of care
- Long-term information
- Comprehensive care
- System links to other clinical data bases for the possibility of comparing outcomes in different institutions
- Ability to merge data collected from multiple sites, multiple types of users, and different points in time
- Consolidation of one record for one patient covering multiple visits to multiple institutions
- Ability to form linkages between databases of individual physician offices and hospitals
- Lifetime medical record essential for good preventive care
- Built-in, standardized measures to allow ongoing evaluation of effectiveness and usefulness

- Minimal data set containing lifelong data concerning the patient's dates of immunizations, pregnancies, and the like

Implicit in these requirements is the need to capture information from many different kinds of providers—for example, laboratories, physicians, radiologists, nurses—and from many different kinds of sites—physicians' offices, hospitals, surgical recovery rooms. There is also the explicit need to merge information from independent organizations.

The need to capture and merge information from many kinds of providers and from different institutions over time can only be met if we have data transfer standards.

The clinical world is ripe for such standards because so much clinical information is already being stored in computers. Discharge summaries are in dictation systems within hospitals. Radiologist's notes are within computerized radiology systems or word processors. Vital signs and blood pressures appear in intensive care and nursing unit systems. Hospitals capture a variety of clinical information. There are quality assurance, utilization review, and case abstract systems. Laboratory systems and pharmacy systems contain laboratory and pharmacy information, respectively. These issues are described more fully in the chapter on data exchange standards.

Performance Requirements

Users specified a number of things they want the computer record to do. The first is to display the information in a flexible format. A frequently repeated request was for a medical record abstract: a subset of the medical record information for quick assimilation. One specific suggestion was to present the problem list, medication list, and recent laboratory requests as the abstract at the beginning of the record, allowing users to quickly search the medical content further as required. This specification is principally a problem of retrieval and/or formatting, so it is easy to recommend that sophisticated retrieval and formatting subsetting capabilities be built into the system. I would go further and suggest that a general structured query language (SQL) capability be available so that knowledgeable users could define very complex patterns of retrievals and/or displays. On the other hand, simple menu options should permit access to standard kinds of report formats by naive users.

A second requirement is for intelligent analysis by the computer so that it can react to its own contents. This could be described as reminders, alerts, and/or decision support for care providers and/or the enterprise at large (McDonald 1976, 1984; Tierney 1988, 1990; Barnett 1978, 1984; Evans 1986; Hulse 1976; Pestotnik 1988). Users should be able to write the rules that specify the remainders or alerts. The computer would be able to interpret and execute such rules. With the capability, the computer could automatically check to see if the patient obtains the necessary follow-up or a particular diagnosis, treatment, or test result.

A third category of retrieval capability would be that required by administrators, managers, and clinical researchers. At the very minimum, an SQL level capability should be available. Higher level primitives should make it easier for users to find what they want. This would imply the ability to define sets of variables that users can manipulate as a unit.

Operational Requirements

The requirements that appeared repeatedly in the users' wish lists were speed and ease of use. Users want all computer-related processes to be fast, preferably as fast as the manual procedures, but at least not much slower. One suggestion was that data input by professionals should be no slower than 50 percent of the speed of comparable manual processing. One participant suggested that the physician should not be required to enter any information into the computer, that it all should be done by secondary personnel. I disagree. Rather, the system should permit entry of physician data by physicians or indirect entry by support personnel according to local requirements. Another contributor suggested that the system should be easy to use. One took the position that no training should be needed to use the CPR system.

We should make distinction between professionals' use of computer systems to retrieve patient information versus their use of the system to enter patient information. Finding patient data in a computer almost always saves time, compared with manual alternatives, as long as the user spends enough time in an institution to become familiar with the system. The question of the professional entry of orders and/or clinical data into the computer is a more difficult one. It is our experience that physicians are eager to take information directly from the computer but less eager to provide it directly to the computer. In this context, we must distinguish between the free text and structured entry. Free text information can easily be captured from physicians via dictation transcription. All that is needed is a program to transfer transcribed text to the medical record system. With slight additional effort, physicians might structure their dictation in such a fashion that separate chunks of the information could be accessed individually. For example, each of the components of the review of systems might be a separately accessible result. Direct entry of free text by professionals into the medical record should become easier as voice input technology improves.

Structured information is another matter. Whether entered by voice or by menu selection, by keyboard or by mouse, it is likely to take extra time compared with free form entry. To satisfy the requirements of users that the system be fast, we will have to be careful about the amounts of required structured data. A minimum data set should not be so large that it would impede the acceptance of such a system. On the other hand, the minimum should not be the maximum. The system should be able to take most information in a fully structured form and permit users to migrate as they are comfortable from less to more structured data entry once technology eliminates the time penalties.

Because the capture of information from physicians is more difficult than the capture of information from existing data sources such as clinical laboratory systems or pharmacy systems, high priority should be given to the transfer of such information from existing computer sources to initial computer-stored medical record systems. This returns us to the need for standards.

References

Hammond, W.E. 1991. Health level 7: An application standard for electronic medical data exchange. *Topics in Health Record Management* 11:59–66.

ASTM E1238.88. 1988. Standard specification for transferring clinical laboratory data messages between independent computer systems. ASTM Subcommittee E31.11. Philadelphia: American Society for Testing Materials.

ASTM E1239.88. 1988. Standard guide for description of reservation/registration-admission, discharge, transfer (R-ADT) systems for automated patient care information systems. ASTM Subcommittee E31.12. Philadelphia: American Society for Testing Materials.

ASTM E1381.90. 1990. Low-level protocol to transfer messages between clinical laboratory instruments and computer systems. ASTM Subcommittee E31.14. Philadelphia: American Society for Testing Materials.

ASTM E1384. 1991. Standard guide for description for content and structure of an automated patient health record. ASTM Subcommittee E31.12. Philadelphia: American Society for Testing Materials.

ASTM E1394.91. 1991. A standard specification for transferring information between clinical instruments and computer systems. ASTM Subcommittee E31.14. Philadelphia: American Society for Testing Materials.

Barnett, G.O. 1984. The application of computer-based medical-record systems in ambulatory practice. *New England Journal of Medicine* 310:1643–1650.

Barnett, G.O., R. Winickoff, J.L. Dorsey, M.M. Morgan, and R.S. Lurie. 1978. Quality assurance through automated monitoring system and concurrent feedback using a computer-based medical information system. *Med Care* 16:962–970.

Covell, D.G., G.C. Unman, and P.R. Manning. 1985. Information needs in office practice: are they being met? *Annals of Internal Medicine* 103:596–599.

Evans, R.S., R.A. Larsen, J.P. Burke, R.M. Gardner, F.A. Meier, J.A. Jacobson, M.T. Conti, J.T. Jacobson, and R.K. Hulse. 1986. Computer surveillance of hospital-acquired infections and antibiotic use. *JAMA* 256:1007–1011.

Gardner, R.M., B.J. West, T.A. Pryor, K.G. Larsen, H.R. Warner, T.P. Clemmer, and J.F. Ortner Jr. 1982. Computer-based ICU data acquisition as an aid to clinical decision-making. *Critical Care Medicine* 110:8223–30.

Hulse, R.K., S.J. Clark, J.C. Jackson, et al. 1976. Computerized medication monitoring system. *American Journal of Hospital Pharmacy* 33:1061–1064.

McDonald, C.J. 1976. Protocol-based computer reminders, the quality of care and the non-perfectability of man. *New England Journal of Medicine* 295:1351–1355.

McDonald, C.J., S.L. Hui, D.M. Smith, W.M. Tierney, S.J. Cohen, M. Weinberger, and G.P. McCabe. 1984. Reminders to physicians from an introspective computer medical record. A two-year randomized trial. *Annals of Internal Medicine* 100:130–138.

McDonald, C.J., W.M. Tierney, S.L. Hui, M.L.V. French, D.S. Leland, and R.B. Jones. 1985. A controlled trial of erythromycin in adults with nonstreptococcal pharyngitis. *Journal of Infectious Disease* 152:1093–1094.

McDonald, C.J., and W.M. Tierney. 1988. Computer-stored medical records. *JAMA* 259:3433–3440.

McDonald, C.J. 1983. Computer technology and continuing medical education: a scenario for the future. *Mobius* 3:7–12.

Pestotnik, S.L., R.S. Evans, J.P. Burke, R.M. Gardner, and D.C. Classen. 1990. Therapeutic antibiotic monitoring: surveillance using a computerized expert system. *Am J Med* 88:43–48.

Tierney, W.M., C.J. McDonald, S.L. Hui, and D.K. Martin. 1988. Computer predictions of abnormal test results: effects on outpatient testing. *JAMA* 259:1194–98.

Tierney, W.M., M.E. Miller, and C.J. McDonald. 1990. The effect on test ordering of informing physicians of the charges for outpatient diagnostic tests. *New England Journal of Medicine* 322:1499–1504.

2
Clinicians' Needs for Office Computer-based Patient Records

Carmi Z. Margolis

My charge is to discuss what physicians in office settings

- Use the medical record for
- Consider to be the most significant functional requirements
- Require as data elements
- Consider to be the strengths and weaknesses of the record

However, I must clarify at the outset that my perspective on physicians in office settings with regard to the medical record is different from that of other clinicians only in how they use two functional elements of the record, namely, the clinical data base and progress notes. In other respects, the key need in improving the clinical part of medical record is not to define problems it poses for any specific group of clinician users, but rather to first adopt an operational analysis of how the record works for all clinicians. Only then can the needs of specific users be defined.

Functional Analysis of the Clinical Record

At the risk of being misunderstood, I would like to suggest that the best operational analysis of how the clinical record works was that first published by Weed (1969). I am referring neither to the PROMIS system, nor to Weed's claims regarding how the problem-oriented medical record can improve health services, nor to how much of the record should belong to the patient. Rather I am referring to the functional analysis of how the record should be used as the clinician thinks through and records the clinical management of a patient's problems. This analysis, as many of you are aware, defines four basic functions:

- Clinical data collection
- Problem definition
- Systematic clinical planning
- Followup

Although various peripheral elements of the problem-oriented medical record, related to computerization and implementation, have been called into question, over the past 25 years the above four elements of clinical thinking and recording have been refined and internalized by those of us who teach clinical problem solving and practice. I maintain that in those teaching facilities I have visited where these principles have been forgotten, no better systematic approach to clinical thinking and recording or occasionally none at all has been introduced.

Two Key Structural Differences Between Office and Hospital Records

If we accept the problem-oriented analysis of clinical thinking at least operationally, then there are two record functions that are different for physicians and other clinical practitioners in offices compared with their counterparts in hospitals. First, the office clinical database is both substantively different and may be collected over time rather than all at once, as is convenient in hospital. Substantive differences include a tracking system for data relevant to preventive practice and a record of past acute self-limited illnesses. Data collection over time requires that retrieval be maximally flexible and clinically modular (i.e., the modules should make sense to a clinician) so that the clinician can instantly call up only that part of the record into which entries need to be made at a particular time. Second, office records may not be accessed at all during follow-up visits for acute illnesses. Some years ago, we demonstrated that the likelihood an experienced clinician will consult the record for background on an acute problem is significantly less than that for a chronic problem. Therefore, in keeping with the need for flexible and clinically modular retrieval, an office record must be so designed that the clinician can consult its problem list or updated summary without accessing the record at all.

Use of the Clinical Problem List

The office problem list is defined no differently from the hospital problem list. In both settings, there are basically six categories of problems, in roughly increasing levels of sophistication:

* Symptoms
* Signs
* Abnormal laboratory data
* Pathophysiologic states
* Diagnoses
* Psychosocial problems

However, an office problem list is conveniently divided into an acute and a chronic or recurrent problem list; in addition, a summary list of major problems, current medications, and recent visits is useful.

From the perspective of the practitioner, his or her need at the end of a hospitalization is for a complete problem list accompanied by discharge recommendations and medications. Lengthy discharge summaries are not generally used, but the details of problem management for any problem should be accessible. An operational paper hospital summary would therefore have a detailed problem and drug list on the front page, with details of problem management accessible on later pages or elsewhere. An electronic hospital summary might thus benefit from being arranged according to hypertext principles, so that deeper layers of a problem could be accessed from the problem list as needed. From the hospital physician's perspective, at that critical moment when the patient first arrives from his or her primary care colleague's office, the record most needed is the problem list/medications summary and a detailed history of the present illness.

Current Strengths and Weaknesses

Common weaknesses of office records include fragmentation and user inability to quickly access relevant data, missing or incomplete clinical data, lack of transfer of relevant hospital problems or data to the office record, missing data to the office record, missing data on psychosocial problems specifically, illegibility, and lack of linkage with medical knowledge. It has been demonstrated repeatedly that systematic use of the principles of problem-oriented medical recording can correct many of these problems. Three important problems, however, illegibility, fragmentation, and linkage to medical knowledge, will not be solved until interactive records are operational. Only an electronic record has clinical reminder potential that can improve considerably the problem of missing data while also changing patterns of care and providing hooks into the medical literature. However, I cannot insist strongly enough that no record system will ever take the place of training clinician users at whatever clinical level and whether hospital or office based in principles of clinical problem solving and recording.

Summary

From a functional clinical perspective, an operational office record should contain four basic elements:

- A defined data base tailored to a geographic community location
- Acute and chronic or recurrent problem lists that are also available as a summary containing a medications list
- Defined problem-oriented planning
- Problem-oriented progress notes

These clinical modules or their clinically functional submodules should be accessible directly, and updating of any submodules should necessitate updating of the same data element elsewhere in the record. In an electronic record, clinical reminder systems and links to the medical literature should be integral parts of the system.

It should be emphasized that the above discussion is by no means comprehensive, but only a selection of what I believe are critical elements of the office record. I strongly agree with almost all of the criteria proposed, that is, the importance of specifying a clinical database suitable for a particular environment, the importance of including already available electronic clinical data, and the importance of data interchange standards for users.

Reference

Weed, L.L. 1969. *Medical Records, Medical Education, and Patient Care*. Chicago: Year Book Medical Publishers, Inc.

3
Nurses' Needs for Computer-based Patient Records

Mary L. McHugh

Functional Specifications for an Automated Nursing Record

Considerations of System Design

The system must fully accommodate the range and complexity of clinical nursing data.

- Nurses collect a large number of distinct data items.
- Many of the data items collected must permit multiple repeat entry of the same data item type (e.g., multiple measurements of a patient's vital signs).
- In many cases, repeat measures are performed in an essentially random fashion. That is, nurses may collect not only the routinely scheduled measures, but may also collect additional instances of the data item based upon clinical judgment. For example, values for vital signs may be scheduled to be taken every 4 hours, but the nurse may need to obtain extra, unscheduled measures if changes in the patient's warrant them.
- The format of the data items varies widely. For example, some of the items are numeric, some are non-numeric characters, some items may be represented by a single character-type entry (e.g., patient's gender = M or F), and some require multiple characters or the combination of two distinct measures into one (e.g., systolic and diastolic blood pressure).
- The system should permit new data item types (e.g., new patient care variables) to be added to the database as needed and obsolete data items to be purged as necessary.

Rationale: It is essential that the system be a full and complete automated charting system so that nurses are not forced to use multiple systems—some automated and some paper based—to be able to document patient care. It would be useful for the system designers to consider the possibility of a true paperless chart in order to meet the changing documentation requirements throughout the health care delivery system.

The system must offer the advantages and power inherent in relational database management system (DBMS) technology (whether or not the system actually uses a DBMS).

- Elimination of data redundancy. Data entered once should be available for a variety of uses so that redundant data entry is unnecessary.
- Multiplicity of retrieval keys. The system should permit virtually every data item in the system to be used as a key for retrieval.
- English-like retrieval language. The system should permit users to retrieve charts and specific information easily and directly. That is, all users (whether computer naive, literate, or expert) should be able to enter most queries themselves without the intervention of a programmer. (Many DBMSs now have powerful English-like query languages for the use of nonprogrammer users).
- Ease of data manipulation. The system should permit
    - Rapid searching through single and/or multiple charts
    - Sorting information contained in one chart or sorts performed on data aggregated across multiple charts
    - Rapid aggregation of data across patients, units, and departments
    - Data to be abstracted from charts throughout the patients' stay in the system. The user site should be able to determine the schedule and content of abstraction reports. (In hospital systems, data may need to be abstracted at every shift as well as at discharge. In office practices, this may need to be done monthly, semiannually, etc.)
- Separation of data items. The system should separate data usage from data collection and storage. Data needs to be viewed as an organizational resource, and not owned by the programs or department that collect or are the primary users. The system should be designed to ensure that data are available to support patient care, clinical and administrative decision making, and the requirements of third party payers and accrediting agencies. It should support the hospital's ability to meet and document compliance with the requirements of regulatory and oversight bodies, and finally, it must support billing and reimbursement.
- Subset access. The system must support the ability of users to access subsets of the data. That is, retrieval by patient name, admission date, and hospital number is wholly insufficient to modern data aggregation requirements. The system should mimic the ability of a relational DBMS to facilitate a variety of retrieval formats and strategies.

Rationale: New demands for quality assurance and cost analysis from third party payers and other interested official groups have radically changed information processing needs in the patient care area. No paper-based system can support those retrieval and analysis demands. An automated system can provide the type of retrieval and analysis facilities described in this specification if specifically programmed to do so. A paradigm shift is now occurring in information requirements in the health care delivery environment and any automated patient record should enable health care professionals to respond in a timely and successful manner to these new realities.

The system must facilitate migration of data into, within, and outside of the automated patient record.

- The system should be designed to permit raw and aggregated data to be moved to another electronic database for further analysis and storage. That is, a hospital should be able to electronically extract information from its patient care database to send to other internal and external (perhaps national) databases if it so desires. For example, the system should permit the nursing department to extract data from the patient record to enter into its patient classification system, or to a consortium database.
- The system should easily accept data entry from electronic monitoring devices and equipment in the patient care area. For example, physiologic monitors should be able to directly record information into the automated patient record rather than forcing the nurse to copy that information from one computer to another.
- The system should be a part of an integrated patient care system. That is, the automated patient record system should *talk* to the computer systems in the laboratory, the pharmacy, respiratory therapy, and all the other auxiliary services so that nurses do not need to manually transcribe information from one computer system to another.

Rationale: Although some patient care settings may be able to implement their entire operation on a single, monolithic system, most large hospitals and clinics have needed to use a variety of products to meet their computing needs. The automated patient record should permit users maximum flexibility in use of their data from all sources. It must be recognized that technology is changing so fast that it is important that users be able to easily integrate existing systems. The need for manual data extraction and re-entry procedures greatly diminishes the value of the system for nursing.

In addition to internal needs, health care delivery organizations need to compare information from their own operations with that of other similar and dissimilar hospitals. It is essential that the automated patient record system enable hospitals to share critical information for their mutual benefit.

The system must reside on a computer system powerful enough to handle the expected workload for the full life of the system. However, it should also be expected that eventually, actual workload may well far exceed anticipated workload. Therefore:

- The system should be designed to isolate the software from the hardware such that when migration to more powerful processing becomes necessary, this can be accomplished easily and quickly.
- The system response time at peak usage should not exceed 2 seconds for entry

and retrieval of direct patient care. (That is, no bedside nurse should have to wait longer for the system to retrieve a patient's chart or for the system to accept charting entries.)

- System response time for activities other than documentation of direct patient care should be reasonable for the particular application. The term *reasonable* will need to be defined separately for different types of activities and cannot be more generally specified here. For example, a simple query from the director of nursing asking about current census, number of Class IV patients by unit or department, and the like should not incur a response time of greater than 1 or 2 minutes. It is understood that other types of more complex queries may need to be entered in batches for longer processing and retrieval time.

Rationale: Slow response time will damage nursing productivity and decrease the value of the system—perhaps so severely that the system becomes unusable. Therefore, response time should be virtually instantaneous (often referred to as eyeblink speed). At its worst, it should never force nurses to wait more than 2 seconds to enter or retrieve their direct care data.

One of the few constants in the patient care environment is the exponential growth in information demands, far exceeding even the worst case scenarios of system planners. Therefore, system designers should plan for significantly larger than expected system workloads.

The system must provide adequate data storage.

- Active patients or cases should be maintained in an online storage facility.
- Inactive cases may be maintained in an online storage facility. If this is not practical because of the large size of the full database, offline storage facilities should be available to meet the needs of the particular cases to be stored. For example, discharged patients should be maintained online for a sufficient period of time to allow for chart completion, discharge charges to be posted, and chart abstraction activities to be completed. Additionally, discharged cases ought to be readily available on rapid access offline storage for retrospective studies for at least a year. Longer term storage may be accomplished through save tapes, write-once-read-many (WORMs) storage equipment, or other types of storage that may not be readily available online.

Data entry ports must be sufficient in number and placement to ensure that no waiting lines form at the terminal.

- Bedside terminals with additional terminals at the nurses' station and in the physicians' charting room should be offered. Some users may not wish to install bedside terminals in all units. Therefore, bedside terminal placement should be an option, not a system requirement.
- Multiple users should be able to access the same chart at the same time (although some restrictions on simultaneous use may be necessary for portions of the chart during data entry procedures so that two people are not trying to chart in the same place on the same chart at the same time).

Rationale: Access to charts and data is a problem with existing manual and automated charting systems. The system of the future should be designed to overcome these problems.

Considerations of User Convenience and System Functionality

The system's user interface must be designed to fit the individual needs of different types of hospitals, home health agencies, and the like, rather than forcing users to create massive changes in their operations to fit the system.

- The system must permit users to tailor data entry and reporting screens to fit their individual needs.
- The system must permit users to customize their printed output formats (hard copy output) to fit their own personal reporting needs.
- The system should permit users some flexibility in customizing language within the system. That is, terms used for clinical phenomena may vary from unit to unit and region to region of the country. The system should permit some flexibility in permitting users to use their preferred terminology. (E.g., one user site may wish to call ventricular tachycardia *VT* while another may wish to see it printed *V-Tach*. Minor variations such as this should be permitted).
- The system must be able to be customized to fit the particular nursing theory and conceptual framework selected by each user.

Rationale: There is no one generally accepted format for nursing. No acceptable system will try to force users to accept screen formats, output formats, language, and frameworks that fail to meet their needs. Also, no such system will be successful in the marketplace.

The system must permit more efficient data entry and retrieval than those of existing manual systems.

- A variety of input devices now exist that can greatly enhance the ease of entering patient care data. For good typists, the QWERTY keyboard is an efficient input device in some circumstances. For poor typists, alternate data entry devices are especially critical. Among these devices are the lightpen, barcode readers, mouse, trackball, optical character reader, digitizers, voice recognition systems, and so forth. These and other labor-saving data entry devices should be included as appropriate.
- Narrative data entry should be discouraged in favor of multiple choice format, checklists, graphics, and the like.
- Narrative data entry must be permitted because some types of nursing information does not readily fit into structured formats. Also, clinical advances regularly require the creation of new variables. However, it should be slightly more difficult to enter narrative data. (For example, the system might require two additional keystrokes to access the narrative entry facility.) This strategy will

discourage people's natural tendency to cling to the more familiar narrative format.

- Chart retrieval should be easily accomplished by patient name, nurse assigned, room number, case number, or whatever identifiers are normally used to retrieve charts.

Rationale: Data entry and retrieval are cumbersome in paper-based charting systems. They can be equally cumbersome in a poorly designed computer system. A major goal of automation is increasing nursing productivity through reduction in the time required to handle information. The desired productivity improvements are most likely to be achieved with well-designed data entry and retrieval facilities.

The system must contain or be linked with powerful analysis programs so that information can be derived from the aggregated data.

- A statistical analysis program must be one of the database facilities, or the system should permit data to be efficiently transferred to a statistical analysis program so that the data can be used in clinical research.
- Additional analysis programs (e.g., forecasting, linear programming trend analysis, system simulation languages, etc.) should be available for further analysis of clinical data.

Rationale: Among the most important changes in the health care environment is the escalating need for documentation of the success of treatment and careful management of resources. These missions have been difficult to accomplish because the operations data of the health care delivery system has been buried in a storage device (the paper chart) that made use of this information economically infeasible. The current environment requires that this data become available to those responsible for evaluating, managing, and delivering care and care delivery systems. Ensuring that both the data and the analysis tools are available is the only way for the chart to serve the needs of users now and in the future.

The system must support documentation of the process of nursing care.

- There is a logical process involved in clinical decision making called the *nursing process*. The system must permit the user to document that process by making explicit the track from problem identification to interventions designed to resolve the problem to evaluation of the success of specific interventions.
- The system must permit the plan of care to be updated as often as necessary. Outdated information must be retained, but clearly differentiated from updated information on plans for care.

The system should provide memory supports to the nurse in order to reduce errors of omission in patient care. These might take such forms as

- Alarms when scheduled medications have not been charted within 30 minutes of scheduled administration time.

- Checklists of nursing interventions (extracted from the plan of care) and ordered medical treatments.
- Proposed work schedules could be updated whenever a patient is admitted or discharged.

Rationale: Modern nursing care takes place in an incredibly complex health care environment. Psychology studies have demonstrated that the average person can retain about seven bytes of information in short-term memory. The average nurse must retain far more than this volume of information in short-term memory. Nurses need access to memory support tools. The system that can function as a powerful memory support tool for the nurse will enhance productivity and the quality of nursing care.

System Security and Data Integrity Considerations

The system must provide adequate protection against unauthorized data access.

- At least two levels of password security should be provided. Normally, this will include both departmental and personal ID codes. Both are necessary to gain access to any part of the system. Alternatively, physiologic access strategies (such as palm print, retinal print, fingerprint, voice print, etc.) may be used to give authorized users access and to bar access to all others.
- The system must permit the database manager to limit access within the system, usually by password level. For example, nurses' aides may be permitted access only to those portions of the chart in which they actually record data (e.g., hygiene record, vital signs record, etc.). Nurses need access to the entire chart of patients in their unit, but normally would not be given access to patients in other units. This requirement will necessitate complex level definitions, but may greatly add to the security of the patient record.
- The patient record must be protected against unauthorized access through phone lines by persons who randomly enter passwords in an effort to gain entry. For example, some systems automatically disconnect whenever the password has been entered twice incorrectly. Notification of an attempted unauthorized access (and if possible, the location from which the access was attempted) would be a beneficial facility of the system.

Rationale: Maintaining the confidentiality of a patient's health information is a legal and ethical responsibility. The system should facilitate manual efforts to protect this information.

The system must provide hardware and software strategies to protect the data from accidental or deliberate loss or destruction of the data.

- Backup storage and processors (or other strategies) should be available to permit care documentation to continue despite failure of one or more system components.
- The system should immediately detect and notify users of any breakdown in

data storage or transmission function. For example, nurses entering data should be warned by the system if the data storage or phone line transmission attempt by the system is unsuccessful.

- Adequate precautions should be taken against loss by fire, flood, or other natural disasters. These strategies will need to be customized to the user site.
- No clinician should be able to suppress or delete any information entered in a patient record since the chart is a legal document. However, as with paper records, some system must be in place to permit users to place a notice that a nurse charted on the wrong patient, or that an entry time was incorrect, or other error was made.

The system must provide a procedure to purge records that have been moved to alternative storage.

- Many systems will need to provide long-term offline storage because the volume of information is such that online storage would soon be filled. Once the record is moved to long-term storage, the system must permit authorized personnel to purge the record from online storage.
- The ability to purge a record must be severely restricted within the system. That is, only a few persons (if any) other than the database manager should have a password that gives them access to the purging facility.
- Clinician passwords should be specifically denied access to purging facilities.
- A record (e.g., an audit trail) of any activity related to altering or purging patient care information must be meticulously maintained.

Rationale: In a variety of situations, clinicians and the medical records director must be able to certify that the chart is intact and has not been altered.

Issues in Meeting the Needs of Nurse Users

Two major concerns emerged from the discussions of the subcommittee. The first concern was that a rigid separation between the nursing and medical portions of the record was not optimal from either an information or an interpersonal viewpoint. From this issue emerged a very intense concern on the part of the nurse member that the special vocabulary and coding schemes for nursing care data that have been developed and are in the process of being developed not be lost.

The concern about separation of the record related to the idea that the patient has *health* problems, not strictly nursing problems or medical problems. In fact, it was the consensus of the committee that there be a fully integrated patient problem list rather than separate problem lists for medicine, nursing, social services, pastoral services, etc., because physicians need to know about the entire progress of the patient. There was discussion about the fact that some physicians are quite opposed to integrating physician notes with notes written by nurses and other health care personnel. From both information and patient care points of view, this nurse author has no difficulty with an automated record that facilitates total integration of the notes and records of all health care providers in the agency or institution. However, the acceptance of automated patient records may be impeded if users are not given the choice of whether to integrate or maintain separate sections of the patient record for different providers.

The chief danger to a totally integrated patient record, from a nursing point of view, involves the danger of loss of critical information. The focus of medicine is the diagnosis and treatment of disease. Nursing has a double focus. First, nurses assist the physician with the implementation of the medical plan of care. Second, nurses diagnose and treat patients' nursing care problems. Nursing care problems are discussed in a variety of ways, depending upon the writer's preferred theoretical framework. In general, however, nursing problems usually relate to the patients' ability to take physical care of their bodies (e.g., nutrition, shelter, cleanliness, protection from injury or further injury, etc.) and to cope with the psychologic, social, and spiritual implications and effects of illness.

These two areas of responsibility are sometimes called the dependent and independent functions of nursing. A third area must also be recognized, namely, nursing administration. For the dependent functions, medical terminology will usually suffice. However, for the independent and administrative functions of nursing, existing medical vocabulary and coding schemes are inadequate.

Thus, nursing has developed special vocabularies, taxonomies, and some coding schemes to use in discourse about these areas of practice. For example, the NANDA group has both a vocabulary and coding scheme for nursing diagnoses. Loss of the ability to use these vocabularies and coding schemes will have serious adverse consequences for the ability of nursing to document aspects of patient care and patient outcomes. This in turn will adversely affect the ability of nursing to contribute to quality care, quality assessment, and the development of advancements in nursing practice through nursing research. It is critical that the Institute of Medicine (IOM) avoid even the appearance of discounting the importance of this work.

Strengths and Weaknesses of the Paper Record

As part of its work, the Use and Users Subcommittee members were asked to review the existing paper medical record. From their own professional perspectives, subcommittee members were asked to identify the strengths and weaknesses of the paper-based chart.

Strengths

The paper-based record is familiar to a large number of users. This is an important benefit at this time in history because any change in the documentation system will require a concurrent change in human knowledge, skills, and behavior. Because documentation skills have been learned through considerable effort, and charting is a fairly ingrained behavior, retraining costs will not be insignificant. Furthermore, the range and significance of the changes described in this chapter will require considerable behavior change on the part of the nursing staff. There will be resistance to these changes to one degree or another, disruption of established work patterns, and thus a cost in productivity during implementation. Finally, there are many changes in the health care environment that are forcing a variety of changes in the way nurses function. The need documentation system is largely driven by environmental forces, but it is happening concurrently with a large number of other changes in the way nursing care is organized and delivered. The need to add another large change in an already distressed environment is cause for managerial concern and great care in the planning of the change process.

The paper-based charting system is relatively simple to use for data entry. It merely requires reading and writing skills, and these skills are possessed by existing staff. However, the automated patient record will require different data entry skills. Many people are unfamiliar with computers and have limited typing skills. Other data entry technology exists and will be employed to facilitate data entry, but most automated data entry will continue to require some typing skills.

It is fairly simple to teach use of the paper-based patient record to new employees. Nurses learn to document on paper-based patient records. Learning a new paper-based system does not constitute learning a new skill. It merely involves applying an existing skill in a different format. A small amount of time must be invested in teaching the new employee where the different data items are to be found and documentation details unique to the organization. In contrast, learning to use a fully automated system would require the learning of new skills by some employees.

It is easy for individual agencies and users to customize paper-based systems to their specific needs. For most paper-based systems, users prepare samples of the modified or newly developed forms to be submitted to a printer. Thus, users are able to perform much of the forms design work themselves and, in some cases, to pretest the new form prior to printing. Many automated systems require programmers to reformat screens and to reprogram the computer for new reports. It will be important for automated systems to be designed in such a way as to preserve the users' ability to exert control over their forms.

It usually can accommodate all necessary data elements. (Some data can only be accommodated as reports or summaries of source data, e.g., radiology reports.) Paper-based systems can accept handwritten narrative, data output from computers on sheets of paper, rhythm strips and other small sheet reports, and data that can be glued or taped into the chart. It will be necessary to carefully plan how externally generated information that needs to be included in the chart will be accommodated by automated systems.

To the extent that narrative reports are supported, new data elements can usually be instantly added to the paper form. Even highly structured forms can usually support instant addition of new data elements in sections reserved for comments or other items. Clearly, health care is rapidly advancing in many specialties. As new knowledge is developed, the content of clinical documentation needs to be included in the patient record. To the extent that users can restructure forms on the computer as needed, the ability to respond rapidly to changes in clinical practice will be retained. However, many computer systems today require the services of highly skilled programmers and much time to add, restructure, or delete data items and change screen formats. Such time delays will hinder rather than facilitate users of the system. It will be important for automated systems to permit the requisite flexibility in changing data elements to match clinical practice for the full value of automated records to be realized.

It offers relatively good security against unauthorized access since readers must physically obtain the paper record or a copy in order to read it; and copying activities are controlled fairly easily in a paper-based system. Although security is not perfect with existing paper-based record systems, it is still true that an unauthorized user must gain physical access to the only copy of the record before reading it. With an automated system, consideration must be given to the multiple access through the various computers linked to the system. Essentially, every workstation or bedside monitor can obtain a copy of the record. If remote access is possible through telephone lines, every terminal with a modem and a phone can serve as a *window* through which the patient record can be accessed.

Weaknesses

Manual data entry is extremely expensive and contributes to the nursing shortage by consuming so much nursing time through

- Its requirement for tedious manual note writing
- Redundant data entry requirements
- Inefficiencies in data entry formats
- Restriction of record viewing to one user at a time
- Need for transcribing data from one paper form to other forms
- Few and weak supports for memory and work organization

Nurses are in short supply. Few employers can afford to use them in an inefficient manner. Two studies have documented that nurses spend up to 40 percent of their time handling information (Jydstrup and Gross 1966; Richart 1970). Manual narrative notetaking is tedious, time consuming, and subject to the vagaries of human memory, energy, and knowledge base. The result is an information system that has a high level of variability in legibility, completeness, and detail. Important data may be missing while an excess of trivial, irrelevant, or inappropriate items are found. Much of the information may be redundant.

Some users may document in a narrative, free-floating format while others may use a highly structured format. Much of the content of free format narrative notes could be handled in a highly structured flow sheet. That approach can greatly reduce the amount of time needed to document care. Since some narrative is essential, paper chart systems must provide forms for narrative notes. Unfortunately, no paper system can serve to limit or control the amount of narrative. Blank nurses' notes and progress notes may even duplicate information that has already been entered in a structured format document such as a flow sheet. Another inefficiency of the paper record becomes apparent whenever more than one person needs to perform documentation tasks at the same time. A user either has the chart or not. An automated system can be designed such that every workstation is a window into the chart. Many users can access the same chart at the same time so there is less time wasted by personnel waiting for the chart.

In a paper-based system, data needed in more than one form must be duplicated by hand. This reality generates a large amount of transcribing of data from one document to another. Transcription is both time consuming and error prone. Furthermore, with the increasing complexity of patient care, there are more details that must be remembered. If the system demands that nurses perform at a level beyond the limits of human memory, then there will be quality problems. Care quality can be enhanced by systems designed to reduce clinical errors through warnings, reminders, reference materials, and tentative schedules or checklists of tasks to be completed on the shift. Properly designed, the system could function as much more that an automated patient record. It could function as a powerful tool to increase both the quality of care and clinical nursing productivity.

It is physically bulky, and therefore difficult to transport and expensive to store and maintain. Paper records require considerable space to store. Consequently, medical records departments must invest in large amounts of floor space for storage of old charts. Because papers charts are bulky and heavy, it is also labor intensive to retrieve, carry, and handle them.

It is expensive to design, produce the layout, and to print paper forms. Some computer systems have programs that permit users to easily and rapidly create and update forms. Forms programs can be made available on automated patient record systems. Considerable expense savings for layout and printing of forms may be realized if users themselves can design and update their forms directly on the computer.

Alteration of a paper form incurs fairly high redesign and reprinting costs. Revision of a paper form may require users to choose between wasting stock of previous versions of the form or delaying implementation of the updated form (and simply living with the inadequacies of the old version for variable lengths of time). Most printing companies have a pricing structure that rewards large volume orders. Thus, when forms need to be updated, it may happen that a decision about what to do with thousands of copies of the old form needs to be made. It is also important to realize that storage costs of the preprinted paper forms will no longer be incurred if the forms are automated.

Data retrieval is manual and therefore very expensive. With paper charts, searching for a specific data item in one chart is relatively quick and simple. Finding one data item in a thousand charts is tedious, time consuming, and expensive. Considering the amount of data retrieval demanded by regulatory bodies, third party payers, accrediting agencies, internal auditors, clinicians, and others, the full cost of data retrieval from paper charts may be difficult to calculate. In a well-designed automated patient record system, much of the data retrieval requirements could be preprogrammed and automated. Significant full-time equivalent (FTE) staff reductions could be realized if much of the data now manually retrieved could be automatically retrieved.

Data aggregation is expensive—often prohibitively expensive. Once retrieved, data must often be sorted, combined, summarized, or otherwise organized. At least part of this work must be performed manually when the data are extracted from paper based record systems. These data aggregation activities are very expensive if performed manually. When the original database is paper-based, at least some of these activities must be performed manually before the collected data can be entered into a computer or another paper database. Clearly, these activities cost additional FTEs.

Data retrieval takes a long period of time; thus, the ability to retrieve data in a timely fashion is often nonexistent with manual paper-based systems. Reports generated from data aggregation activities may be seriously delayed, thus hampering operations and management decision making. Today's health care environment is changing rapidly. Managers do not have the luxury of spending many months obtaining data and conducting prolonged studies of trends and options prior to making strategic decisions about their organization's operations. It may be that rapid access to internal data combined with the ability to employ statistical analysis and computerized decision support technology in problem solving may be factors in the organization's survival.

Once data are retrieved from a paper-based system, they must either be reentered into a computer for further analysis and report generation, or the analysis and report preparation must be performed manually. For routine purposes, these analyses and reports can be preprogrammed and run at selected intervals. The reports generated from an automated database can be more timely, contain more information, and be presented in a variety of formats, depending upon the needs of the user. (In fact, this can also be a weakness of automated systems. Routine reports are so easy to generate that they may become a blizzard of material crossing the manager's desk. They may also be poorly designed with incomplete information, sent to people who do not need them, or may bury the important information in a mass of irrelevant facts.)

Overview of Requisite Data Elements

A complete listing of all data items that nurses require in an automated patient record is beyond the scope of this chapter. However, there are some data items that can be identified as essential elements of the clinical record. Many of these can be grouped into categories of data that will be needed in most care settings. These categories include, but are not limited to:

1. Direct and indirect measures and observations of patient condition and body system or psychosocial functioning. This will include vital signs; neurologic checks; cardiac rhythms and sounds and parameters (pulmonary capillary wedge pressure, pulmonary artery pressure, etc.); lung assessments; fluid and electrolyte balance; assessment of skin healing and integrity; cast checks; psychiatric evaluations; factors in the patients' social environments, and the like.
2. Identified patient problems and needs derived from patient assessment data.
3. Goals toward which the plan of care is directed.
4. Specific interventions planned and carried out to address patient problems and needs (e.g., personal hygiene, feeding, dressing inspections and changes, resuscitative measures instituted, patient teaching, comfort measures, referrals, psychologically supportive measures).
5. Activities related to discharge planning.
6. Records of treatments and medications ordered by physicians and administered by nurses.
7. Ordered medications/treatments that were withheld, and the reason(s) for withholding them.
8. Reports of patients' progress toward care goals (i.e., patient care outcomes).
9. Laboratory reports and reports of other testing services (e.g., radiology, nuclear medicine, physical therapy reports, the catheterization lab, psychological tests, etc.).
10. Identification of assigned caregivers. This includes records of attending and consulting physicians, records of individual nurses and the care they provide (e.g., medication nurse, primary nurse, team leader, IV team nurse, etc.), respiratory therapists, occupational therapists, physical therapists, and so forth.
11. Physicians' phone orders.
12. Responses of the patient and family to the patient's condition, progress, care, expectations, needs, etc.
13. Information about adverse reactions to medications or treatments.

References

Jydstrup, R. A., and M. J. Gross. 1966. Cost of information handling in hospitals. *Health Services Research* 1:235–261.

Richart, R. 1970. Evaluation of a medical data system. *Computers in Biomedical Research* 3:415–425.

4
Hospital Administrators' Needs for Computer-based Patient Records

Elaine Ullian

The first part of this chapter outlines the needs of hospital administrators for computer-based patient records (CPRs) in five key areas:

- Administrative responsibility for medical records
- Administrative uses of medical record information
- Administratively significant functional requirements of medical record automation
- Data elements
- Critical aspects of the medical record that account for its current strengths and/or weaknesses

The second part of the chapter represents the perspectives of hospital administrators combined in responding to subcommittee members commenting on the outlined material both during the session and in written remarks submitted subsequently.

Hospital Administrators and the Medical Record

I. Administrative responsibility for medical records
   A. Ownership and services
      1. The medical record is regarded as the property of the hospital and is maintained for the benefit of the patient, medical staff, and the hospital.
      2. The administrator is responsible to the governing board for implementing a system for maintaining medical records on every individual who is evaluated or treated as an inpatient or outpatient.
      3. The administrator is responsible for safeguarding medical records against loss, defacement, tampering, unauthorized use, and fire and water damage.
   B. Organization of medical record department
      The administrator is responsible for providing a medical record depart-

ment with a qualified manager and adequate staffing, equipment, space, and facilities to perform the required functions.

   C. Hospital compliance with medical record department
The administrator is responsible for enforcing hospital and medical staff rules and regulations on the completion, accessibility, and authorized uses of the medical records.

II. Administrative uses of medical record information

   A. For prospective and retrospective evaluation of the quality of patient care through review and analysis of patterns of care as documented in the medical record.

   B. For promotion of effective and efficient use of facilities, equipment, services, personnel, and financial resources through statistical analysis of information abstracted from the medical record.

   C. For the determination of a hospital's case mix in terms of patient diagnosis, age, and other variables required for reimbursement from third party payers.

   D. For identifying legal risks and maintaining financial losses in litigative matters.

   E. For documentation of voluntary compliance with standards for accreditation of the institution.

   F. For documentation that demonstrates conformity to government regulations.

   G. To follow up the care of patients with long-term illnesses and assessment of the efficiency of the care given.

III. Administratively significant functional requirements of medical record automation

   A. Adequate medical record documentation. Regardless of the medical recording system used, the quality of a record is highly dependent on its documentation.

      1. Clinical documentation should be appropriate, accurate, and complete.

      2. The record must contain all the necessary signatures.

      3. Only those abbreviations approved by the medical staff should be used in the documentation of patient care.

      4. Entries regarding patient care should be made in a timely manner. Discharged patient records should be promptly completed.

      5. All documentation should be legible.

   B. Functional requirements of future record systems

      1. User accessibility

      2. Full system integration. The system must be capable of integrating all patient information.

      3. Security and confidentiality. Legal and ethical concerns require a system with limited access.

         a. Regulation of information entry

         b. Protection from information tampering

        4. Economic feasibility
          a. High systems and start-up costs
          b. Eventual reductions in staffing, space, and storage expenses
        5. Interfacing capability with hospital, physician, and outside agency information systems.

   C. Potential administrative benefits of future medical recording systems
        1. Electronic attestations and other signatures
        2. Record completion tracking
        3. Digital and voice recognition dictation
        4. Improved coding systems for reimbursement maximization
        5. More rapid information flow and record completion
        6. The development of a more accessible database of patient information for use in quality assurance, utilization review, planning, and statistical analyses

   D. Feasibility of a paperless medical record
        1. Importance of paper record
          a. Paper is currently needed for litigation, continuing care, insurance, and the like. A computerized system would have to be capable of generating hard copies.
          b. Paper often is used as a backup for computerized systems.
          c. Paper records are generated by ancillary services.
        2. Likelihood of paperless record
          a. Nearly impossible in foreseeable future. A completely paperless record would necessarily require every user to be online.
          b. A movement towards a paperless record would have to be phased in over the course of many years.
        3. Legality
          a. Only the Department of Mental Health requires that a paper medical record be kept. It is legal, therefore, for hospital records to be paperless.
          b. Access to a computerized record system would have to be regulated.
        4. Prevalence of computerized systems
        Although many hospitals are partially automated, few, if any, are completely paperless.
        5. Necessity of a sophisticated hospital information system
        It is possible and preferable for an entire hospital to use one computer system. Such a system would operate on one large database. Functions within the system would be separated into modules accessing the one database. Use of the modules would be regulated, and interfacing would occur easily. Such a system would facilitate the incorporation of bedside terminals, as well as physician and ancillary service terminals.

IV. Data elements

The administrator requires the data elements found in the Uniform Hospital Discharge Data Set (UHDDS). This data set consists of the following items:

- Personal hospitalization number
- Date of birth
- Sex
- Race
- Social characteristics
- Residence
- Admission data
- Discharge data
- Admitting physician
- Attending physician
- Consulting physician
- Principal diagnosis
- Other diagnoses
- Procedures and dates
- Disposition of patient
- Source of reimbursement
- Charges

V. Critical aspects of the medical record that account for its current strengths and/or weaknesses
  A. Completion of record upon discharge
    1. Complete identification, financial, social, and clinical patient information
    2. Discharge summary
    3. Physician attestation and other signatures
  B. Quality of documentation
    1. Appropriateness
    2. Legibility
  C. Systems integration within the hospital for use in record compilation
  D. Physician compliance
  E. Effective coding to maximize reimbursement
  F. Space and staffing demands

Major Points

The following questions and responses reflect the hospital administrator's perspective in combination with the issues/concerns raised by the subcommittee members.

Which hospitals are interested in substantial changes/improvements/automation of medical records? The academic medical centers in the United States, with a deep commitment to academic medicine and strong health services research interest represent the principal audience for the Institute of Medicine (IOM) analysis and recommendations.

There are roughly 5,500 nongovernmental acute care institutions in the United States, with a majority represented by community and rural hospitals with fewer than 250 beds, operating at an average occupancy rate of 60 percent. These hospitals do not pursue academic research, nor are they particularly concerned with extraordinary measures or data that will facilitate even more in-depth review of clinical practice.

Conventional wisdom is that the federal peer review organization structure coupled with the stringent quality assurance/utilization review orientation of Joint Commission on Accreditation of Healthcare Organizations (JCAHO) and state insuror policies provide more than sufficient data for review of clinical practice.

Can a revised, twenty-first century medical record be used as a tool for paring costs, monitoring physicians, and length of stay analysis? Why shouldn't a hospital be interested in such tools? Current medical records systems coupled with existing utilization review systems provide sufficient data for all hospital administrators and physicians to identify which physicians consume patient days and order procedures that are beyond *normal* practice patterns. Although some systems are far more sophisticated than others, the basic information that enables discover of those clinicians and quantification of the *excesses* exists presently.

The challenge is not to have more data or an automated system to generate the data. The challenge is how to confront a physician practicing beyond the norms when the *offense* may not affect quality of care (which is much easier, albeit delicate to raise) but resource use. From a practitioner's perspective, the last thing a hospital chief executive officer wants to do is to alienate physicians in any way that would promote their use of another proximate hospital which appears more *physician friendly* and eager for the physician's patient volume.

In addition, many of the comments raised during the subcommittee discussion referred to the importance of a medical record appearing *amoral*. This issue also appeared in the written comments forwarded to me. Whether *amoral* means that the data cannot be used as a tool to restrain resource use is subject to debate.

Hospital administrators should strongly support automation of the medical record for efficiency and cost savings purposes—why should there be any resistance? This statement, also raised in verbal and written comments, is true to a point. The cost of a new system, an automated system, cannot be measured in terms of software and hardware expenses which in and of themselves will be substantial. The greater cost will be the education and retraining of myriad hospital workers who presently interact with the medical record. This includes unit secretaries on the patient floor, laboratory technicians, utilization review staff, nurses, physicians, therapists, interns and residents.

Management engineers should compute this cost, which arguably exceeds the capital expenditure component by a factor of three. The question then becomes, Is it worth it? For whom? Can we quantify the benefit of this investment? What is the payback period?

Priorities and the issue of tradeoffs are paramount to hospital administrators and governing boards, particularly in light of consecutive cutbacks in federal and state support of acute care. Wouldn't the funds be better used through recruitment of several new physician specialists needed on a medical staff? Couldn't the incremental operating costs associated with automation of medical records be better spent on increasing salaries and wages for nurses and technicians in short supply? In terms of capital expenditures, would automation yield more for the patients, for the institution than a new MRI or lithotripter? These are the questions that will be raised by hospital administrators whether they oversee small, rural facilities or major academic medical centers.

In light of these concerns, is there any hope for an automated record? Yes, there is interest for a major revision to the manner in which the data are collected, maintained, and used. The approach for most institutions must be to phase in the process so that the education and training of hospital staff can occur in a manageable fashion. Phasing in also enables an institution to procure the hardware and software without forfeiting the purchase of clinical equipment or new technologies which are highly visible and valued to an institution.

There was general support for a phased in approach among the subcommittee members.

Additional Comments

Many subcommittee members commented that automated medical records will be an important tool for *outcome* measurements. One member suggested that publicizing differences in outcomes would channel more patients to a particular facility. This may be correct. Presume, however, that the outcomes and quality of care—to the best of anyone's knowledge—are already satisfactory and consistent with general medical practice. The difference then becomes, What are the outcome differences *at the margin*? And who oversees these issues? Those topics fall under the aegis of the physician responsible for that service or the medical director of an institution.

5
Patients' Needs for Computer-based Patient Records

William H. Buckley

Introduction

If the question being asked of this subcommittee had been asked 20 or 30 years ago, I suspect that the patient would not have been seen as one of the primary users of the medical record. Indeed, most patients who were a part of preceding generations probably never gave much thought to their medical record, its content, or its potential usefulness outside of the inner sanctum of the physician's office or hospital.

The patient record of the present is certainly a document more patients are aware of, many patients seek access to, and most would agree does not meet all of their current needs for one reason or another. The patient record of the future will surely be a more important document to the average patient than it is today and will be used for more diverse purposes.

In this chapter, I present the following outline: (1) What patients use the record for now and in the future; (2) the current strengths and weaknesses of the medical record from a patient's point of view; (3) some examples of the sort of data patients are interested in now and will likely be interested in the future; (4) the important functional elements significant to patients; (5) observations and cautions.

   I. What patients use the record for
      A. Now
          1. Obtain history for care providers
             a. Second opinion
             b. New physician
             c. Specialty consultation
             d. Home care
          2. Information for other third party
             a. Insurer
             b. Employer
             c. Attorney or other personal advisor

      3. Personal use
        a. Curiosity
        b. Participation in health planning
        c. Instructions for follow-up care, medical regimen
   B. In the future
      1. Participation in care
        a. Full understanding of medical situation from caregiver perspective
        b. Decision making
        c. Follow-up instructions
        d. Accuracy of information
        e. Plan for future vis a vis any limitations imposed by conditions or treatments
        f. Caretaker participation
        g. Record results, observations, questions in record outside of formal healthcare setting
      2. Obtain history for care providers
        a. Second opinion
        b. New physician
        c. Specialty consultation
        d. Home care
      3. Information for other third party
        a. Insurer
        b. Employer
        c. Attorney or other personal advisor
      4. Other uses
        a. Family
           i. Genetic information
          ii. Accurate family history
        b. Billing and other business issues
II. Strengths and weaknesses of the current medical record from the patient's viewpoint
   A. Strengths
      1. Existence of the record
      2. Legal access to the record
        a. Review/copy of hospital record (State of Massachusetts)
        b. Summary of care from private physician
      3. Typed discharge summaries (when they exist)
      4. Problem lists (when they exist)
      5. Care plans (when they exist)
   B. Weaknesses
      1. Availability
      2. Understandability
      3. Legibility
      4. Chronology

      5. Cost of copying

      6. Correction of errors

III. Data elements required by patients now and in the future

Examples of the data elements that patients would find useful might include:

- History
- Findings, including meaning in importance to the specific patient
- Options with some benefit analysis or recommendations, with reasons
- Discharge plan with instructions, medication doses, and a list of possible problems or complications to watch out for
- Goals

Further discussion could include many additional data elements that might prove useful to patients.

IV. Functional requirements of the medical record significant to patients

In thinking about the various features the medical record of the future must have to satisfy the functional needs of the patient, one could review the current strengths and weaknesses and state that there is a need to ensure that the current strengths are maintained and improved upon and that the current weaknesses are corrected. To add emphasis to those points that seem central, the following list is provided with the understanding that others could be included as well:

1. The record must be readily available to the patient.
2. The record must be understandable to the patient.
3. The record should be in chronologic order and preferably indexed.
4. There must be a provision for absolute confidentiality together with an ability to sequester certain sensitive information the patient may not want revealed to those with sanctioned access.
5. There should be integration of the ambulatory and inpatient records for patient convenience.
6. There needs to be a designated area for the patient or family to record their findings and observations.

In addition to these items:

1. There needs to be a clear designation of the notator in every instance, including name and title.
2. Patients should be able to find easily all records of informed consent given by them.
3. There should be a common format (perhaps national) for the record so that the same information appears in the same way from one care provider to the next.

V. Observations and cautions

Until recently, patients did not expect nor were they expected to be full participants in their health care. Like the rider on a Greyhound bus, they were expected to sit back and "leave the driving to us." While one could debate the advantages and disadvantages of this phenomenon, it is clear that the times are changing and that the old fashioned delivery and acceptance of medical care are disappearing.

We appear to be on the cusp, with the future providers of medical care giving more responsibility to the patient and his family members as full partners or collaborators, especially in chronic conditions. Patients and their families will be asked to participate more in the care giving and the decision making. Patients will be asked to be more responsible for their health.

For these and other reasons, the patient record will need to evolve into a document that is user friendly to the person whose name appears on its jacket. People often ask patient representatives, "What is the most common problem at your hospital?" I usually answer the question by stating that the most common underlying factor in almost every problem in the hospital relates to a failure in communication. Traditionally, the patient record has been a communication vehicle for caregivers and caregivers only. Now and in the future, this communication must also be with and for the patient.

Present and envisioned technology should allow for many of the requirements that will make the record useful for the patient to become at least partially automatic. Technology that now exists for sharing information between emergency medical technicians caring for patients in the field and emergency centers could have applications for patients in the home setting and their doctor's office or hospital.

With the proliferation of this technology, however, we must make absolutely certain that the patient's primary right of privacy is fully and vigilantly protected. While the potential for privacy abuse of the electronic and computer-based record certainly exists, this technology can also provide for access by parties other than the patient on a need to know basis *only*.

6
The Computer-based Patient Record: The Third Party Payer's Perspective*

Cary Sennett

Functional Activities of Third Party Payers

The needs of third party payers are most comprehensible in the context of the various functional activities that payers currently are asked to assume. The business of health insurance comprises three separable core activities, each of which requires information that might derive from the medical record. These are claims processing, health care management, and risk pooling.

Claims Processing

The claims processing function is meant to describe those activities that are directed toward the reimbursement of providers or patients for health care services delivered to beneficiaries of an indemnified group. Efficient claims processing depends upon access to an accurate description of the nature of the services that were provided to a patient; the agent to be reimbursed for those services; the amount charged for those services; and sufficient information about the patient to permit linkage to a file that identifies the nature of the health insurance policy that is relevant to coverage decision making. The medical record (at least as it is conventionally regarded) has not been the primary source for information for purposes of claims processing; its use is relevant to this discussion because:

- There is no reason that the medical record could not be used as a primary source for information about any of these.
- In any event, access to the medical record is desirable to support the claims processing activity, insofar as such access provides a means by which to verify the accuracy of the description of services recorded elsewhere (e.g., the submitted bill).

* Disclaimer: The views expressed in this paper are those of the author, and do not necessarily represent the position of Aetna Life Insurance Company.

The functional requirements for the record will depend upon whether the record is to be used directly as a claim document or whether it will be used secondarily to support another transaction record. In either case, information in the medical record would need to be

- Accurate
- Accessible at low cost and in timely fashion
- Extractable (that is, accessible according to selective criteria)
- Sufficiently detailed (see data elements)

As rapid claims turnaround is desired by all parties to the transaction, the functional requirement for timeliness is that *turnaround time should be no slower than that in the current claims processing system*. This implies a routine turnaround time measured in days.

The necessary data elements will depend on whether the record is to be a transaction document or a verification document. In either case, data must include a description of the service (CPT4 identifier), the provider of the service, and the recipient of the service (in a form that can be linked to beneficiary data files). In the former case, charge information must be included.

The major weakness of the record with respect to the claims processing function has been its relative inaccessibility. Although access to the medical record may be legally permissible, the costs of and legal constraints on access to it have prohibited its routine use as a claims processing document. If the record is to be important to the claims processor, access to it must not only be guaranteed; it must be facilitated. As access is increased, the major weakness will be the amount of data in the record that is extraneous to the claims processing function.

The major strength of the record in this regard relates to the integrity with which medical services must be described in a document which serves primarily as a source to inform those charged with the care of the patient. As such a document, it is least subject to errors of misrepresentation; that is, it is likely to be a document that has reference authority with respect to the services involved in any health care transaction.

Health Care Management

The health care management function is meant to describe those activities which attempt to facilitate the delivery of medical care that is appropriate and to discourage the delivery of medical care that is not. Increasingly, payers are being asked to assist the employers to whom we are responsible to construct programs which increase the *value* of purchased health care. These programs attempt to identify care which is inappropriate (in order to prevent it) or to identify the option for care which is lowest cost among equally effective alternatives (in order to encourage it). Such programs derive from what is described as the health care management function.

Health care management of this sort clearly requires the ability to evaluate the logic of planned care. Consequently, access to that logic is critical; the medical record is a document which is invaluable as a source of information on the medical logic relevant to decision making that pertains to the services delivered to an indemnified patient.

The functional requirements for such use depend upon the exact use that would be made. To evaluate planned care *before* it is delivered requires access to the medical record at the (time) point-of-service. If necessary care is never to be delayed because of the review process, then there is a functional requirement for information flow which is, more or less, that the interval between planning care and its review always be less than the interval between planning care and its appropriate delivery. Evaluations of planned care, *after the fact*, will require much less timely evaluation of the medical record. Such evaluations support a variety of current health care management programs, and the capacity for retrospective review will continue to be important to the health care manager. However, retrospective review offers less opportunity to rationally manage care; constraining the payer to retrospective review mechanisms is to be discouraged as the medical record is reconfigured.

Access to the clinical information necessary to evaluate care implies the need for a comprehensive medical record. So long as data necessary to validate care is distributed across many unlinked records (or present in none: e.g., in the attending physician's recollection), the logic necessary to validate that care often will not be transparent from review of any one.

Identification of patterns of care, and providers of care, which (who) are to be encouraged or discouraged implies the need to evaluate care over time and in relation to outcomes. The capacity to use the medical record to assess care longitudinally; to aggregate clinically related events into units of analysis (episodes); to aggregate care for persons served by a common provider; and to summarize these data into comprehensible reports are all especially important to the health care manager.

The data elements required for such evaluations are predictable and comprise those that are relevant to the clinical decision maker. In general, the nature of the planned service must be described; the patient must be described in sufficient clinical detail to support the application of clinical logic; and the provider of that service must be described to permit consideration of possible alternatives. Given that routine transmission of all such data is not desirable, there would be advantage to the development of a mechanism that will permit payers to identify the data elements relevant to their review of a case, and a mechanism to select from the larger medical record only that information which is required.

The major weaknesses of the medical record with respect to the health care management function relate to the difficulties with respect to access considered above; the inability to isolate relevant data from the larger data set; and the absence of a single document describing care provided to a beneficiary in the variety of settings in which care can be delivered.

The medical record, perhaps by definition, is the reference source for information relevant to the care of a patient. As such, it is clearly the preferred source for information relevant to the logic of care planned or provided.

Risk Pooling

The risk pooling function is meant to describe those activities which relate to the management of the financial resources necessary to guarantee adequate reserves to cover the anticipated costs of care for a group. The third party payer, as indemnity insurer, always has had the need to estimate the costs of care for individuals or groups of individuals; such estimation depends upon the ability to evaluate risk and is necessary to price insurance services properly. As large employers increasingly assume the financial risk that is the insurance function, third party payers are assisting them to estimate that risk and to plan financially for it.

Risk pooling depends upon the ability to estimate aggregate expected health care costs in populations. This can be accomplished either by estimating individual risk and aggregating across individuals, or by estimating group risk.

The medical record may provide an instrument to assist in the risk pooling by facilitating evaluations of individual or group risk. The former is clear; access to clinical information should permit much finer estimation of an individual's future health care needs. Group estimates can derive either from summation across individuals or from pooling individuals to describe a population in clinical detail. Detailed clinical information about a subject population will permit more accurate assessment of its anticipated health care expenses.

The use of the medical record for these purposes implies the ability to access clinical data, and the ability to aggregate across persons who are related by virtue of a common insurance mechanism. The former requirement has been discussed already; the latter requires the capacity to aggregate across populations that are related and almost certainly would be enhanced by the ability to aggregate along a number of dimensions (e.g., age, sex, race, clinical condition). Further, the ability to aggregate (e.g., health care use) over time (for an individual or a population) would be value added.

The data needed for risk selection are routinely available in the medical record; they comprise those demographic and clinical indicators known to be predictive of morbidity and mortality. The medical record is an inefficient source for this purpose, in that it contains much information that is superfluous. It is, however, the most current and accurate source for much of the information that would be required for risk evaluation.

Recommendations

The needs of third party payers should be considered when recommendations for revision of the patient record are presented. Third party payers have need for the information contained in the patient record and can use that information responsibly in ways that will benefit both the patient and society at large. Benefit accrues directly to the patient when the record is used to facilitate payment or to permit more efficient evaluation of planned health care. Because society clearly values the functions that third party payers perform, benefit accrues to society in general when payer operations are made more efficient through better information.

Third party payers may also play a strategically important role in motivating the adoption of revisions to the patient record. To the extent that reimbursement for care is a lever that can be used to change the behavior of those in the health care industry, support from the third party payers for revision of the patient record may permit a variety of strategic options to facilitate acceptance of those revisions. These options may be foreclosed should the needs of third party payers fail to be considered.

The revised record should include financial and billing information, patient and provider identifiers, current procedural terminology (CPT4) codes or other detailed descriptions of services provided, and charges. Inclusion of this information will facilitate the use of the record as the single instrument for clinical transaction recording and will likely enhance the accuracy of all transaction records. Furthermore, it will facilitate the development of electronic claims payment systems, which will increase the efficiency of the claims payment process.

The revised patient record should include sufficient clinical detail to permit the medical logic of clinical decision making to be evaluated by a third party. At a minimum, the record must include information about the patient's diagnoses (relevant *International Classification of Diseases*, 9th edition [ICD-9] codes) and the signs, symptoms, and laboratory data relevant to planned care.

The revised patient record should permit longitudinal evaluation of medical care; that is, it must be configured to permit care at all sites at which a patient has care to be assessed and the temporal relationships between care at different sites to be defined. Increasingly, payers are being asked to provide services that are well described as *medical management* services—better information about the process and the outcomes of care needed to permit these services to be provided efficiently and effectively. Access to clinical detail in the patient record and to information that describes care provided to the same patient at different sites and at different points in time will enhance the efficiency and effectiveness of these management services.

The electronic system in which the revised patient record exists should permit timely evaluation of clinical decision making by third parties. The electronic record system will fail to support meaningful third party assessment of care if assessment cannot proceed without imposing unacceptable delays to needed care. This implies that the electronic system must permit access to patient information that enables review and response within an acceptable time frame. A reasonable upper boundary on that would be response within 72 hours; in general, the more rapidly information can be made to flow, the better.

The revised record should permit records of persons who are similar in some important respect to be aggregated. Both management information and actuarial risk analysis depend upon the ability to aggregate the experience of some group.

The revised record should be flexible with respect to aggregation along a large number of clinical and demographic dimensions.

The format of the patient record must be standardized, with a finite vocabulary of elements and clear and widely accepted definitions of terms used. The electronic patient record exists to facilitate information exchange. The nature of that information must be considered, as well as the nature of the system that is to facilitate its flow.

Issues

Resistance to providing patient information to payers must be overcome.

- There is confusion (and disagreement) about the proper role of the payer in the health care transaction.
- There is confusion (and disagreement) about the value of efficient payer operations to social welfare.
- There is poor understanding of the insurance contract and of the legal and ethical obligations of those who are party to it.

Confidentiality of information must be assured.

Explicit guidelines for the use that can be made of certain sensitive data elements must be specified, and systems developed to assure compliance with those guidelines.

Payer use of an electronic record will require considerable capital expenditure and may require reconfiguration of systems at a very basic level. There will be resistance among payers to developing systems to take advantage of an electronic record, if sufficient return on those expenditures is not apparent.

The electronic patient record must be sufficiently robust to permit information needs to continue to be met as information needs change. This is particularly evident as new reimbursement systems—such as prospective payment based on diagnostic related groups (DRGs) and physician payment based on resource-based relative value—change the relative importance of various data elements.

The format and language of the medical record are highly variable across institutions and providers. This variation will frustrate remote users' efforts to interpret the record and may significantly reduce the usefulness of the record, if efforts to reduce that variation are not incorporated into plans for its revision.

7
Health Care Researchers' Needs for Computer-based Patient Records

Allyson Ross Davies

The term *health care researcher* refers to a diverse set of professionals, academicians, and policymakers who study topics related to the organization, process, quality, and outcomes of health services delivery. This chapter concentrates on the uses and requirements of those who focus on medical care services, including mental health services but excluding dental care. Among the disciplines who work in health care research are clinicians (physicians, nurses, psychiatrists, clinical psychologists, and clinical social workers), economists, research psychologists, sociologists, political scientists, and epidemiologists, in addition to those trained specifically in public health and health services research.

Uses of the Patient Record

This diverse set of researchers uses the patient record in a seemingly endless variety of ways. A few of these involve abbreviated interaction with the record (or, perhaps more accurately, with record-based files). The most notable example would be use of patient record data for *sample identification* (e.g., by case type, visit type, problem type, or time period).

Most uses appear to involve more detailed examination of many, if not all, data elements in the record. Among the broad categories of research into which these uses can be grouped are the following:

- *Quality of care evaluation.* This category includes studies of *clinical competence* (e.g., decision making, accuracy of diagnosis, recording behavior); *appropriateness* (e.g., of diagnostic and therapeutic interventions and procedures used); and *effectiveness* (e.g., of treatment procedures, drugs, and technology).
- *Patterns or variations in services.* Grouped here are a wide range of descriptive studies of the use of providers, resources, procedures, tests, drugs, treatments, and the like by geographic area, patient type, specialty or provider type, and location of care (e.g., teaching versus community hospitals). While many of the preced-

ing examples represent studies that take a *macro* view, the more *micro* studies of the provider/patient relationship that rely on patient record data also belong here.

- *Utilization studies.* While studies in preceding categories consider use of services in addition to the primary topic, the studies grouped here consider utilization as *the* topic of interest. Among them are those investigations that use patient record data to define episodes of care, to create *dummy claims forms* (e.g., for comparison of utilization in prepaid and fee for service settings), and to calculate *disaggregated utilization rates* (e.g., of preventive versus palliative services) regardless of whether the service was reimbursed.

- *Outcomes analysis.* Studies that obtain information on patient outcomes from the record include investigations that require data on *case mix*, *severity*, and *comorbidity*, *disease-specific morbidity*, *mortality*, and *sentinel or adverse events*. At present, many of these investigations also obtain such data from special purpose databases (e.g., hospital discharge record abstracts; utilization review or risk management files) that are derived from patient records.

The above list should be considered an illustrative rather than an exhaustive inventory.

Desired Data Elements

Not surprisingly, given the variety of users and uses of the patient record in health care research, virtually every available data element appears to have been used at one time or another. In addition. some data elements currently not present in the record would be extremely useful to current investigations in health care research. The following inventory, grouped by major topic, represents an initial attempt to define the intersection of the *used* and *useful* sets. The inventory probably represents a *wish list*; I am not aware of any data that would accurately identify the *most* used and/or useful.

Identifiers
  Patient (medical record number or other unique ID)
  Provider (unique ID)
  Facility/location (unique ID)
Characteristics
  Patient (birthdate, gender, ethnicity, payer, marital status, education, income, family size, zipcode)
  Provider (responsible physician, referring provider, specialty or provider type, location or type of practice, physician signature)
  Facility (type)
  Visit type (e.g., scheduled, elective, emergency; appointment, walk-in; new or established patient, etc.)
Dates
  Service (admission, discharge; visit)

      Procedures
      Prescriptions (ordered; filled)
      Tests (ordered; filled)
      Results
Codes
      Visit type
      Procedure, service
      Diagnosis
Clinical Indicators
      Chief complaint (in patient's words)
      Indicators
      History
      Physical examination findings
      Diagnoses, primary and secondary (admission, discharge; visit)
      Severity (admission, discharge; visit)
      Comorbidities (admission, discharge; visit)
Process of Care
      Diagnostic tests, procedures, and results
      Therapeutic regimen, procedures
      Prescriptions ordered, filled; dosages
      Lab and path tests ordered, filled; results
      Counseling, health education activities, topics
      Sentinel or adverse events
      Duration (of visit, episode, hospitalization)
Disposition
      Referrals, transfers
      Follow-up plan/type of care
Outcomes
      Mortality
      Physiologic measures
      Disease-specific functioning
      General health status (functional status, well being, general health perceptions)

Note that costs of care do not appear specifically on the list since they are usually imputed from service or procedure codes or obtained directly from financial management systems. Nonetheless, patient record data are an important primary source of information for studies of costs of care.

Desired Characteristics

Desired characteristics of both the patient record itself and the data elements it contains are as follows:

* *Accessibility.* Ideally, all the needed records should be *available* rather than misfiled or lost (a common complaint among health care researchers who use

records). Accessibility would be enhanced if the researcher were able to *link* patient record data across files within and across institutions; at a minimum, this means *common identifiers*. Records must also be *obtainable* via institutional or individual permission, a key consideration for most health services researchers who use the patient record.

- *Standardization*. The more standardization, the greater the usefulness of the patient record to health care researchers. This includes not just *formatting* conventions and *coding* schemes (and the application of the rules that underlay them), but extends to the *definition of the variables* themselves. Because most studies require large samples, standardization must apply not only within but *across settings* to maximize the usefulness of the patient record.

- *Simplicity*. Patient records that were simple to access and use would be a boon to health care researchers. Standardization of format as noted above would increase simplicity, as would the availability of *documentation*, particularly for the contents of electronic record files.

- *Accuracy*. For the health care researcher, accuracy refers not only to the *data elements* themselves, but to associated *documentation* (e.g., of access rules; file contents, location; variable definition, values). Data in the records themselves, as well as those in record-based sources (e.g., discharge abstracts, disease registries, mortality records), must be *reliable* in that they reflect reality and agree across sources.

- *Completeness*. Critical here is that the record represent as much of what happened during care as possible, hence the usefulness of a *unit record*. A unit record with partial information may not, however, be more useful than *multiple records that can be linked*. Another critical issue is whether *missing* data can be interpreted as indicating normal values and usual (i.e., not adverse) occurrences or representing errors of omission.

- *Cost effectiveness*. Patient records that fulfill the above requirements would be a cost-effective source of data, another key consideration for health care researchers.

Strengths and Weaknesses of the Current Patient Record

A review of the strengths and weaknesses of the current patient record must necessarily be based largely on anecdotal evidence, because rarely do we study empirically their accessibility, standardization, accuracy, and completeness. More specifically, if such studies are done (e.g., by professional review organizations, medical specialty societies, residency training programs, inhouse quality assurance programs), they do not appear in the widely read health services research literature. All but one of the few I have identified (e.g., Fessel and Van Brunt 1972; Lyons and Payne 1973; Cooney 1973; Osborne 1975; Gerbert et al. 1987) were completed 15 to 20 years ago and, with the exception of HRET's study of community hospitals (Cooney 1973), focused on small samples of physicians and/or institutions.

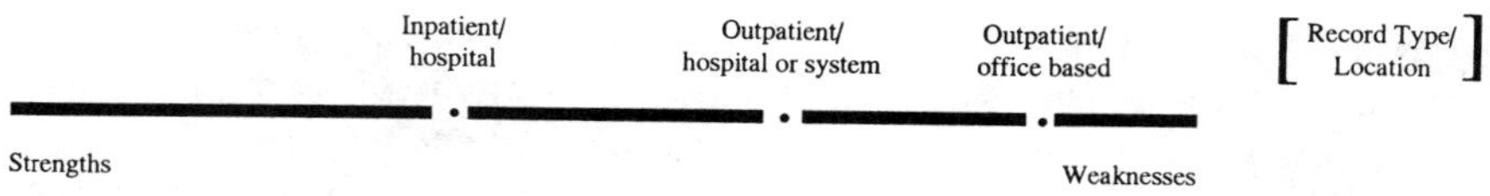

| Inpatient/
hospital | Outpatient/
hospital or system | Outpatient/
office based | [Record Type/
Location] |

Strengths   Weaknesses

Figure 1. The Patient Record: A Continuum

By reputation, the patient record is long on weaknesses and short on strengths. On this continuum, health care researchers would probably rank various records as shown in Figure 1.

While researchers might debate the distance between the entries on this continuum or how far to the left the hospital or health system records might fall, I am confident that the above ordering is correct and the deficits of office based records of ambulatory care are noteworthy.

To be somewhat more specific, still in the absence of empirical data, I believe the following generalizations reflect at least plurality opinion:

Records in General

- Incomplete (with respect to the totality of care and services, as well as the range of desired data elements)
- Unstandardized (on virtually all parameters and particularly for outpatient care records)
- Poorly documented (if electronic database)
- No patient-based data, namely on generic health outcomes

Outpatient care records

- Unstandardized, particularly in office practice
- Generally inaccessible, except in some hospitals and large health plans
- Incomplete
- Inaccurate

Hospital inpatient records

- Standardization spotty (e.g., while coding schemes are generally universal, coding rules often are not)
- Expensive to use
- Incomplete (as a unit record; to describe entire stay, often must link across records or files)

Why Ask for Patient-based Health Status Information?

The listings of data elements considered important by health care researchers included the entry *general health status*. They are not alone in this judgment. Others beginning to request general health status information, or patient-based health outcomes assessments include the policy makers, foundations, and corporations who fund this research, purchasers (e.g., insurance companies and employers) and payers (e.g., HCFA), regulators, clinicians, and administrators. All ostensibly want this information for use in decision making about treatment options, benefits design, purchasing contracts, reimbursement policies, and the like. As Shortell and McNerney (1990) have ably summarized, the desired information falls into three categories: *treatment outcomes* (disease specific physiologic parameters or end-points), *functional health status* (broadly speaking, health status information based on patient report), and *patient satisfaction*.

Focusing, as requested, on the patient-based health status measures, two characteristics of these assessments speak to their usefulness to such decision making:

- Measures of general health status describe *health in the patient's terms*. The disease-specific physiologic indicators of system and organ functioning captured in the current patient record tell us little or nothing about how the patient is doing or how the patient feels.
- Measures of general health status, specifically because they are not disease specific, provide a much needed *common definition of outcome across disease or symptom groups*. Currently, most studies of effectiveness or benefit (cost, treatment, procedure) use dollars alone as the common unit of comparison across different options. Moreover, policy studies that require comparisons across different disease or symptom groups rarely compare more than differential expenditures. Because they would plunge us into the problematic world of apples and oranges, comparisons of the few disease-specific health status measures now in the record are not done.

The current, considerable interest in general health status measures in fact represents renewed recognition of the relevance of such information to the provision of health care and to health care research. Among the earliest recognized requests for outcomes of care in patient's terms (e.g., indicators of recovery, relapse, restoration of function) were those of Nightingale (1983) and Codman (1914). Writing two decades ago (during an earlier peak of interest in using consumers' data in quality assessment), Donabedian (1966) noted that

> outcomes [health status, consumers' attitudes toward care] remain the ultimate validators of the effectiveness and quality of medical care.

Several experts participating in a 1972 conference on a minimum data set for the ambulatory medical care record noted the relevance of patient-based assessments of functional status and general health status to health care and health policy research (Akpom et al. 1973; Cassel 1973; Freeborn and Greenlick 1973). As

Cassel (1973) noted at the time, however, few practical and well-tested measures of such outcomes were available for use, whether in health services research or clinical practice, although a number of developmental efforts were then underway.

Current State of the Art of Patient-based Health Status Assessment

Those efforts to which Cassel referred in 1973 have yielded valuable results. Currently, available measures are extensively used in health care research and they are increasingly used in clinical trials of drug therapies, where *quality of life* (aside from treatment-specific side effects) is a relatively new consideration (e.g., Croog et al. 1986). Several studies (e.g., Brook et al. 1983; Ware et al. 1986; Nelson et al. 1986; Jette et al. 1986; Tarlov et al. 1989) indicate the feasibility of assessing patient-based outcomes in diverse settings and monitoring them over time.

Several available measures meet key criteria for usefulness, which will be familiar to users of any type of data:

- Practical considerations
- Comprehensiveness
- Psychometric standards
- Reliability
- Clinical standards

Practical Considerations

The time required to administer the measures should be *brief,* so they place little burden on the patient and so it interferes as little as possible with the usual flow of patients through the care process. The measures should be *easy to score and to interpret* to minimize the burden to the analyst and increase their relevance to the user. They must often be *available in realtime* to increase their usefulness. In many cases, this may require direct data entry (e.g., by the patient) and rapid scoring and feedback of results.

Comprehensiveness

Extensive work has resulted in the identification of a minimum set of general (i.e., not disease specific) health status concepts. These include:

- Functional status—behavioral indicators of physical, social, and role functioning or performance
- Well-being—feeling states related to mental health, vitality, and pain
- General health perceptions—self-evaluation of health in general, without reference to dimension (as above) or disease state (e.g., the commonly seen rating of one's own health as excellent, very good, good, fair, or poor)

Psychometric Standards

The term *psychometric* is often greeted with expressions that range from the simply curious ("What *does* it mean?") to the downright dismissive ("Sounds like witchcraft!"). By psychometric standards and methods we mean that collection of analytic and statistical procedures that allows us to evaluate and improve the reliability and validity of measures of any object, whether it is a physical measurement (e.g., blood pressure) or an assessment of some state that cannot be observed directly (e.g., mental health, attitudes toward care). One of the major advances in our field during the past two decades has been the application of such methods, heretofore used chiefly for physical measurements and in psychologic research and testing, to assessments of health and health care.

Reliability

Reliability refers to the amount of information (versus random noise) or to its repeatability (e.g., the agreement between two blood pressure readings taken over a short interval). *Validity* refers to what the information in the score means and, specifically, to whether the score reflects variations in the *thing* it purports to measure. In lieu of reviewing the extensive information available about the reliability and validity of the illustrative measures, let me summarize quickly. Indicators of reliability (coefficients) range from zero to 1.0; the higher the better, and coefficients above 0.90 indicate scores that are reliable enough to classify individuals. Reliabilities for the multi-item measures of health status are often in the 0.80s and higher, even in patient populations.

From the plethora of information available about their validity (or appropriate interpretation) that which relates to clinical validity is perhaps most relevant. This judgment reflects my assumption that any consideration of the inclusion of patient-based health status assessments in the patient record must recognize that the primary user of the patient record is the clinician.

Clinical Standards

To be considered valid for clinical users, measures (whether of general health status or other variables) should meet the following criteria (with apologies to Ware):

- Distinguish those with and without disease
- Correspond to known differences among diseases
- Vary according to severity within a diagnostic group
- Demonstrate sensitivity to change

Results from the Medical Outcomes Study, also known as MOS (Tarlov et al. 1989) serve to illustrate the ways in which these short patient-based health assessments are being evaluated in relation to these standards. In one such study (Stewart et al. 1989), published data were used to plot standardized health profiles for patients with one of four conditions (hypertension, myocardial infarction, gastrointestinal problems, and arthritis). To construct these profiles, the mean on each of the general health measures for patients with no chronic diseases was set to zero; the chronic conditions were plotted in terms of their difference in standardized scores from the group with no chronic conditions (controlling for the effects of comorbidity and sociodemographics). These data indicated that the measures distinguished among those with and without disease and corresponded to known differences in the effects of different diseases on functioning and well-being.

Other work, as yet unpublished, evaluates indicators (physical functioning, role functioning, and general health perceptions) in relationship to severity levels for patient subsamples, such as diabetics and hypertensives. The findings of these studies are significant and will be reported elsewhere.

Are We Ready for Patient-based Health Status Assessments in the Record?

The demand and the state of the art of current patient-based health status measures together indicate that current efforts to develop, implement, and test routine ongoing systems for collection and use of general health status measures are timely ones. There appears to be considerable consensus regarding the relevance of these measures to health care and health care research.

Some exemplary uses of patient-based health status assessments feature their inclusion in the patient record. The few experiments with feedback of general health status data to clinicians (Kazis et al. 1987; Rubenstein et al. 1988a,b) reported results in the style of laboratory test results and intended for insertion in the record. Nelson et al.(1986) have recommended that patient-based measures of function and related indicators of health status should be added to the repertoire of vital function assessments used in routine office practice. By their analogy to information on vital signs, they suggest that these measures belong in the patient record. To my knowledge, however, there has been little discussion of these intentions or recommendations regarding the appropriate location of this information.

I believe the Institute of Medicine (IOM) Committee on the Future of the Patient Record could provide a useful catalyst by initiating such a discussion. In considering whether to recommend inclusion of patient-based health status assessments in the patient record, several factors must be examined. Some of these factors clearly support inclusion. These assessment are closely analogous to vital signs, already a key element of the patient record. They are about the patient (in fact, they come directly from the patient) and reflect the process of care; as such, they are analogous to virtually all the history data in the record (which itself often comes directly from the patient). One point on which the evidence is not yet in, however, is their usefulness to the everyday clinical practice of medicine. Theory, debate, discussion, and rhetoric all suggest that these measures can and will be useful to and used by clinicians. I am a strong believer in collecting only data that will be used. I personally believe that whether and how clinicians make use of such measures should be the litmus test. If used regularly by clinicians in diagnosis, treatment, and management of patients, they should be included in the patient record. If used chiefly at a more aggregated level, they might be better stored in free standing databases. As this subcommittee's previous discussions have already noted, the issue of which data elements appear in the patient record folder may well be a moot point as we move toward electronic databases that can be readily linked.

Finally, neither the legal nor political implications of the presence of patient-based health status assessments in the record have, to my knowledge, been explicitly addressed. In Massachusetts, at least, information in the physical record (i.e., that owned by the provider or institution) has a very specific and highly regulated legal status. Many physicians, beleaguered by external (and generally critical) reviewers who read the records over their shoulders, may be loath to have any more information about results in the record than already appears there. The interest of health care researchers in having this information and the current state of the art of obtaining this information with practical, reliable, valid, and comprehensive batteries, are *not* at issue.

References

Brook, R.H., J.E. Ware, W.H. Rogers, et al. 1983. Does free care improve adults' health?: Results from a randomized controlled trial. *New England Journal of Medicine* 309:1426–1434.

Codman, E.A. 1914. The product of a hospital. *Journal of Surgery, Gynecology, and Obstetrics* April:491–494.

Cooney, J.P. 1972. The community hospital: ambulatory services, statistics, medical care record data. *Medical Care* 11(2:supplement):158–169.

Croog, S.H., S. Levine, M.A. Testa, et al. 1986. The effects of antihypertensive therapy on the quality of life. *New England Journal of Medicine* 314:1657–1664.

Donabedian, A. 1966. Evaluating the quality of medical care. *Milbank Memorial Fund Quarterly* 44(pt.2):166–203.

Fessel, W.J., and E.E. Van Brunt. 1972. Assessing quality of care from the medical record. *New England Journal of Medicine* 286:134–138.

Gerbert, B., and W.A. Hargreaves. 1987. Measuring physician behavior. *Medical Care* 24:838–847.

Jette, A.M., A.R. Davies, P.D. Cleary, et al. 1986. The Functional Status Questionnaire: reliability and validity when used in primary care. *Journal of General Internal Medicine* 1:143–149.

Kazis, L., R. Meenan, et al. 1987. The clinical utility of health status information in rheumatoid arthritis patients: a controlled clinical trial. *Arthr Rheum* 30:512.

Lyons, T.F., and B.C. Payne. 1974. The relationship of physicians' medical recording performance to their medical care performance. *Medical Care* 12:463ff.

Nelson, E., J. Wasson, J. Kirk, et al. 1987. Assessment of function in routine clinical practice: Description of the COOP Chart method and preliminary findings. *Journal of Chronic Diseases* 40(supplement 1):55s-63s.

Nightingale, F. 1863. *Proposal for Improved Statistics of Surgical Operations.* London, Savill and Edwards.

Osborne, C.E. 1975. *Criteria for Evaluation of Ambulatory Child Health Care by Chart Audit: Development and Testing of a Methodology.* (Final report on contract no. HSM 110–71–184) Evanston, American Academy of Pediatrics.

Shortell, S.M., and W.J. McNemey. 1990. Criteria and guidelines for reforming the U.S. health care system. *New England Journal of Medicine* 322:463–467.

Stewart, A.L., A. Greenfield, R.D. Hays, et al. 1989. Functional status and well-being of patients with chronic conditions: Results from the medical outcomes study. *Journal of the American Medical Association* 262:907–913.

Tarlov, A.R., J.E. Ware, S. Greenfield, et al. 1989. An application of methods for monitoring the results of care. *Journal of the American Medical Association* 262:925–930.

Ware, J.E., R.H. Brooke, W.H. Rogers, et al. 1986. How do health outcomes at an HMO compare with those of fee-for-service care?: Results from a randomized trial. *Lancet* 1:1017–1022.

8
Record Administrators' Needs for Computer-based Patient Records

Margret K. Amatayakul and Mary Joan Wogan

The goal of the Institute of Medicine (IOM) project is to improve the patient record by addressing the content, format, and potential uses of automated patient records. A project of this magnitude requires concordance of thought regarding the major subject of the study, the patient record. We believe a baseline set of definitions and principles would assist in focusing discussion and provide a clear understanding of the project limits.

In any large health care institution, there is a variety of records maintained throughout the institution containing medical data on patients. These are in addition to the conventional medical record. It seems appropriate to clarify whether or not the IOM study will address the needs of those who originate these various records. Definitions would assist in this clarification and resolve such questions as: Is any medically related data that exists on an individual considered a patient record? If not, where is the line drawn? Will the study be limited to patient records generated in health care facilities? If so, what about home health records? Should the study be concerned with the needs of those who use patient record data but obtain it from a source other than the original patient record (e.g., drug store pharmacists, news media representatives using Medicare files)?

We believe concise definitions are needed which limit the subject of the study, excluding data that do not fit the definitions. In addition, we believe a minimum core data set should be identified and become the focus of this study.

Therefore, this chapter will describe the variety of patient records which exist in a typical, large health care institution. Using this information as a background, we will describe the underlying fundamental considerations which we believe are important to the IOM project. The discussion will incorporate the experiences of the authors in the medical record field. Where appropriate, definitions and principles will be recommended to facilitate understanding.

This chapter will describe and define the following:

- Primary patient records
- Secondary patient records

- "Separate" patient records
- Minimum core data set
- Other considerations
- Ownership of the primary patient record

The Primary Patient Record

Practitioners in the health care field tend to define the patient record based on their experience and exposure to it in various health care institutions. It may be called by one of its many synonyms. In various settings, it is known as a medical record, health record, clinical record, office record, client record, chart, encounter form, and database, to name a few. Not only does the patient record have a variety of names, it exists in different formats—paper, microfilm, monitor strip, optical disk, computer tape—or a combination of the above. Regardless of what it is called or the medium in which it exists, the primary patient record has characteristics by which it can be defined. For purposes of the IOM study, the primary patient record is defined in the paragraphs that follow.

Definition The primary record is defined as: (1) the original, patient-identifiable documentation generated by health care providers as a result of direct interaction with the patient (and/or interaction with individuals who have personal knowledge about the patient); and (2) the documentation under the control of an individual designated by the officers of the institution or the owners of the record as the primary patient record data manager.

It is recommended that this definition be used in the IOM study to define the patient record. The definition is broad and is intended to describe primary patient records in all health care settings.

The first part of the definition refers to the record contents and those who are responsible for creating it. To be considered a primary patient record it should consist of the original documentation of all direct interactions between patient and care givers.

Direct interaction between the patient and care givers includes activities such as discussion with the patient, observation of the patient, the results of studies conducted, the types and results of treatments, and instructions given to the patient. An example of specific record content for a typical hospital record would include sociologic data, consent forms, history, physical examination results, consultations, surgical procedures, progress notes, orders, diagnostic and therapeutic interventions, reports of nursing care, and discharge summary.

In instances where the patient is unable to interact directly with the care giver, information for the record is provided by one who stands in place of the patient (e.g., the parent of an infant). In special instances where input in addition to the patient's is desirable, interaction between the care giver and a significant other may be recorded in the primary record (e.g., the spouse of a drug abuse patient).

The second part of the definition refers to responsibility for the record after it is generated. It should be under the control of a designated data manager to fit the definition of a primary patient record. This requirement means the record is subject to standard practices of record processing and control. It means the record content is subject to quantity and quality controls. It means the record is released in accordance with rules and regulations established by law or, in the absence of applicable law, by direction of the owner of the record, in keeping with patient rights. In short, responsibility for the record is fixed, and controls are in effect which represent acceptable record keeping practice.

Secondary Patient Records

In addition to the primary patient record, there are numerous other types of patient-identifiable records containing medical data that are kept in health care institutions. For purposes of discussion, these will be divided into *secondary* patient records and *separate* patient records, and each type will be discussed.

The patient records commonly called secondary records can be defined as patient identifiable data taken from the primary patient record to satisfy the needs of specific users. Included in this category of secondary records are abstracts of primary record data, logs, indices, registers (e.g., trauma registry), carbon copies of portions of the primary record, photocopies, and computer-generated copies of the original record. The existence of these records should be acknowledged in the IOM study because they meet the special needs of users which are not met by the primary record.

Secondary records are kept by their users for a variety of reasons, including the format of the primary record precludes easy location of the data, the primary record is inaccessible when needed, or summary data only is needed. Secondary records can be divided into three types, differentiated by the level of record control:

Type 1. Record resides in the health care institution where it originated and is under the control of the designated, primary patient record data manager.
    Examples: Joint Commission on Accreditation of Healthcare Organization's required disease index; tumor registry

Type 2. Record resides in the health care institution where it originated and is not under the control of the designated, primary patient record data manager.
    Examples: carbon copies of emergency room reports retained in the ER; log of discharges and diagnoses on neonatal intensive care unit (NICU) patients maintained by department secretary

Type 3. Record is transmitted from the health care institution to an outside third party, becomes part of the third party's file, and is under the control of the third party.
    Example: HCFA's Medicare file

Secondary record types 1 and 2 should be of minor concern in the IOM study. Most of them are nothing more than a summary of specific data items in the primary record or copies of the primary record. They are the kinds of records expected to be integrated into a computerized system and thus the need for their existence as a separate, secondary record is eliminated. An up-to-date report in the desired format can be obtained upon request for legitimate users.

Type 3 secondary records contain data that are usually abstracted from primary records. They also can consist of photocopies or computer-generated copies of all or portions of the primary record. The data in these secondary files has been supplied by the owner of the primary record to be used for a specified purpose. It is supplied with the patient's consent, except when release is required by law. However, once transmitted, it is made a part of the third party's file and is no longer under the control of the primary patient record data manager.

Type 3 secondary records should be considered in the IOM study to the extent the needs of the original user are satisfied. It should be remembered that once this data is submitted, it is no longer subject to the controls exercised over the primary record. For example, it is rarely feasible to update this type of record when the primary record is updated. The IOM study should be concerned only with the needs of the original user for the original use. The needs of others who use the date residing in Type 3 secondary record files should be outside the scope of the IOM project.

Separate Patient Records

A third type of patient record exists in many health care institutions. This type of record is not the same as the primary patient record, but it fits the first part of the definition. It consists of original, patient-identifiable documentation generated by a health care provider (or providers) as a result of direct interaction with the patient. This record, however, is kept separate from the primary record. Its contents are seldom if ever incorporated into the primary record, even though a primary record usually exists in the health care facility. Separate records do not fit the second part of the definition of a primary record, relating to control.

There are many reasons why care givers think it is necessary to keep a separate patient record. Typical examples are

- The sensitive nature of the data
  Example: A psychiatric history containing explicit details of the patient's fantasies and behavior
- The method of patient payment
  Example: A physician with a faculty appointment in a teaching hospital also sees private patients, utilizing the teaching hospital's facilities; the records of these private patients are kept separately in the physician's hospital office rather than made a part of the medical record system of the hospital
- The caregiver's interest in research
  Example: A physician who is both a clinician and researcher in a teaching hospital keeps separate records on research patients which contain detailed data relative to the research project

Although these separate records legitimately can be called patient records, they are not primary patient records because they are not under the control of the primary patient record data manager. The greatest problem in relation to these records is being aware of their existence. It is often only the originator of the record who uses them and is aware of their existence. It is common for the originator to take the records when leaving the employ of the health care institution. In these cases, originators of these separate records mistakenly believes they own the records. Unless there is a written contract to the contrary, such records are, in fact, the property of the institution, not the individual who generates the record.

It is recommended that separate patient records, as described above, be included in the IOM study and thus brought under the control of the primary patient record data manager. However, it would be necessary to make a decision about the disposition of the detailed data in these records. This is discussed in the following section.

Some records can be considered either secondary or separate because they fit parts of both descriptions. A tumor registry, for example, contains data abstracted from the primary record and thus might be considered a secondary record. In addition, however, the registry contains other data obtained from the patient and from health care providers outside the facility regarding the patient's tumor status and thus might be considered a separate record.

It is recommended that records containing this type of additional data, not all of which is available in the primary patient record, should be included in the IOM study, but the additional data should not be part of the minimum core data set. Instead, any data not appropriate for inclusion in the primary record should be incorporated into an expanded (or secondary) data set. Both a core data set and expanded data set are discussed in the next section.

Minimum Core Data Set

Reference has been made several times to a minimum core data set. It is not our intention to define the contents of such a data set in this chapter. However, we propose that a major outcome of the IOM study should be a minimum core set of data that can be electronically processed. This data set would conform to the definition of a primary patient record. It (or a defined subset) would meet the basic needs of all those specified as primary patient record users. To be effective and meet the needs of users, the minimum core data set would have to be a requirement. This means that those responsible for documentation would have to adhere to requirements such as format, content, and timeliness of entry.

A part of the process of determining the core data set would be consideration of the needs of all three types of secondary patient record users. Most of the data elements from these secondary records would be identified as those deserving placement in the core set. A few data items may be considered important but not appropriate in the core set and would be made part of an expanded (or secondary) data set.

Separate patient records should also be considered in determining the core data set. The needs of originators of these records should be carefully explored. The outcome would likely be that some of the data in these separate records would become a part of the core data set, particularly in those instances where the records are kept separate for the convenience of the care giver.

It may not be appropriate for the detailed data in these separate records to reside in the core data set. This would include data that have been kept separate because of their sensitive nature or because they are not germane to the ongoing care of the patient. In these latter cases, a decision may be made to make this detailed data a subset of the core data—that is, a part of the expanded data set.

It is probably beyond the scope of the IOM project to state in any detail the contents of this expanded data set. However, some of the issues which should be addressed are as follows:

- A determination of development priorities, that is, how and when the detail of an expanded data set would be determined
- The responsibility for data acquisition, data entry, and quality control
- The methods of determining the right of access and the methods of controlling access.

The expanded data set probably would not be given priority in development. Once developed, it would be accessed only by authorized individuals via a separate function code. It would not be considered part of the primary record. The expanded data set would not be available for review when the core data is reviewed unless the reviewer has specific authorization and has entered this section of the record. The responsibility for generating the detail and allocating it to this special category would be determined based on the nature of the data.

A minimum core data set coupled with an expanded data set would meet the needs of all users of the primary patient record. The needs of those who want patient or provider-identifiable medical data but use sources other than the primary patient record should be outside the scope of the IOM study.

Other Considerations

Once a minimum patient record core data set has been identified, there are a host of additional considerations. The first of these would be establishing the fundamental requirements regarding data generation, that is, who is responsible for data generation and when.

An electronic record system by its very nature requires a degree of precision that is not a part of patient record generation today. Documentation of patient care must become a new imperative. It will require a mindset that puts the documentation of medical events on an equal basis with other aspects of patient care, rather than being viewed as an afterthought. It will no longer be possible to leave decisions about the format, time, and place of documentation to the patient's care giver. This means that those who have regarded documentation as an activity tangentially related to patient care and who have provided marginal or inadequate documentation long after the events took place will be forced by an electronic record to change this view and these habits. Since poor documentation procedures have been tolerated for so long in health care institutions, the transition period required to master this new imperative may be a difficult one.

Other considerations of importance relate to the technology involved in achieving a truly integrated patient record. The methods of data linkage which make the record available to care givers at multiple sites must be determined. How to update the core data set and the responsibility for doing so also must be determined. Access to the data by the many legitimate users is a major consideration.

Over and above the technologic considerations are the issues of acceptance of an electronic record, training, confidentiality, and ownership. The subject of ownership is briefly addressed in the following section.

Ownership of the Primary Patient Record

Although ownership is a well-established principle with regard to the traditional paper medical record, it could present difficulties in the context of an electronic, integrated record. It may be helpful to briefly review the ownership principles in relation to the traditional record because this is a subject which often is not clearly understood by health care practitioners.

The medical record is a peculiar type of property because a distinction is made between ownership of the record itself and the information contained in the record. The institution responsible for creating the record owns the record itself (that is, the record media, the paper, computer disk, or tape). However, the patient has an ownership right in the *information* contained in the record. It is generally conceded that the patient owns the information in the record, as distinct from the record itself.

This means, for example, a patient cannot come to the medical record department of a hospital and take possession of his/her primary patient record because that document is the property of the hospital. However, a patient can request in writing that information from the record be forwarded to a third party, and this request must be honored. The basis for honoring the request is the principle that the information in the record belongs to the patient. (It should be noted that governmental facilities may have different policies.)

These same principles of ownership apply outside the hospital. For example, a physician in private practice owns the physical record, but not the information in the record. Therefore, the physician cannot refuse the patient's request to forward information to another provider because, for example, the patient has not paid the physician's bill. This refusal would be inappropriate because of the patient's ownership rights to the information.

These principles are relatively easy to apply in the traditional and familiar system of paper records. It is not difficult to transfer these principles to an internal or inhouse computerized system. However, as databases are transmitted and shared between institutions with the ability to add to and update the information from a variety of settings, each of which may be a separate legal entity, the principles of ownership begin to blur. While an integrated patient record is being developed, the principle of who owns the physical record should be considered as part of this development. Ownership, as well as the other considerations mentioned above, may differ from the conventional wisdom when an integrated electronic patient record is implemented. However the problems are solvable with the cooperation of all those involved in this effort.

In summary, in this chapter, the authors have attempted to provide a focus for the IOM patient record project so that it is clear what is included in the study and what is beyond the scope of the study.

Section 2
Technologies for Computer-based Patient Records (CPRs)

1
Current State of Computer-based Patient Record Systems

Allan T. Pryor

Development of medical information systems has an extensive history covering more than 20 years. The early research which was centered in computerized electrocardiographic analysis, laboratory management, administrative record keeping, and the like has become the basis of many commercial medical information systems today. One of the goals of this research and commercialization has been the creation of an electronic computer-based patient care record (CPR). Although a 20-year effort has been made toward this goal, a realizable complete CPR does not exist today. In order to understand the current state of CPR systems, therefore, it is first necessary to define what constitutes a CPR system. Given a reasonable definition of a CPR, one quickly discovers in researching today's systems that there exist only successive approximations of a complete CPR. At what point does the completeness of a system's medical database qualify it to be considered a true CPR system? Is the system's database design sufficiently inclusive and flexible to become a comprehensive CPR system? In order to report on the current state of CPR systems, in this chapter I suggest a possible definition of CPR systems, outlines the general state of CPR systems, and finally reports on several systems that currently qualify as CPR systems.

Definitions of CPR Systems

Since all medically oriented systems contain some portion of the patient's medical record, it is necessary to define the point when a system qualifies as a CPR system. For example, several vendor-supplied automated electrocardiogram (EKG) systems contain patient demographic data, EKG measurements and interpretations, partial medication history, and sometimes patient diagnoses. However, the intent of these systems is not to record a comprehensive patient record, but to serve the needs of a cardiology service and, where possible, transmit this information to a CPR system. Because of the intent of such systems, we can exclude from the definition of CPR systems all departmental systems which are designed primarily to serve the needs of a single department, regardless of the type and amount of information contained in their databases. Departmental systems are not designed as vehicles for access to a complete patient record. While access to their records may be provided remotely, they are not intended to allow review of information not specifically recorded by the system. Using this definition we will also define as departmental systems, financial or administrative systems whose primary emphasis is restricted to admitting functions, order entry/charge capture and patient billing. Also included under the definition of departmental systems are pharmacy systems, laboratory systems, radiology systems, nursing systems designed exclusively for use by nurses, and intensive care unit (ICU) systems that are limited in scope to the ICU.

The definition of a CPR system, therefore, is restricted to systems whose design is management of the entire patient care record. Such a design could involve a physically distributed system with logical central control of the entire record or a centrally located complete CPR in a single database. The key factor is that through some mechanism there is central knowledge, control, and organizational integrity of the entire record. This central control should allow a single terminal to access the entire record regardless of the location of the data. More than just access, there is the need to integrate the data in ways that are not possible in the single departmental system where the data may have originated. The central controlling system should provide integrated and coordinated use of the data, which is impossible as a function of the originating systems. Examples of this extended use include integrated reports, generation of alerts and reminders, and complex data searches across many departmental data elements. A CPR system should ensure consistent terminology across all of the data elements in the patient record regardless of their origin. It should also prevent redundant definition or entry of the same data in the patient record from multiple sources. For example, vital signs entered by the respiratory therapist should be equivalent in the database as vital signs entered by the nurse with the only differentiation being the ID of the person entering the data. Finally, the physical design of the database must ensure that common conventions be followed for the storage of differing data elements. For example, the mode of time tagging the elements must be common, the structure of records should be similar for similar data types, and so forth.

While the distributed design has recently gained great appeal, currently all systems which qualify as CPR systems use a central integrated physical design. Since even those systems that qualify as CPR systems today do not, as part of their systems, provide all of the possible applications for acquisition of patient care data, today's CPR consists of data entered directly into the CPR using applications programmed on the CPR system and data transmitted to the CPR system via interfaces with departmental systems. One of the major differentiating factors between current CPR systems is the extent of their use of networks to departmental systems.

General State of CPR Systems

On reviewing systems that currently qualify as CPR systems, one discovers that the most notable examples are those that have developed at academic institutions.

The commercial world has focused primarily on either departmental or administrative systems. The commercial efforts have been driven by both the expertise of the company and the needs of a market place. The market place to date, however, has been dictated by health care administrators whose computer system needs have not required a total CPR. The administrator has focused on the administrative and financial needs of the hospital, leaving the patient care needs to be solved by the medical staff. Medical department chairpersons have initially been motivated by the desire to increase the effectiveness of their service, not necessarily to improve the overall management of the patient. Unfortunately, this departmental focus has led to the state where many medical information systems exist, but interface standards to connect the departmental systems do not. Fortunately, these standards are being developed by Health Level 7 (HL7) and MEDEX. The work of these groups should overcome the need for individually developed and maintained interface standards between the departmental systems. The database design of the departmental systems is, in most instances, insufficient to meet the flexibility required to extend the system to a true CPR system.

One of the most promising new products being developed by commercial vendors is standard interface software for connecting departmental systems and workstations. This effort is one attempt to create a CPR without having to reprogram all of the existing installed departmental systems. Unfortunately, since most of the work on development of standards addresses only the protocols of transmission and not the content of the information, utilization of the information in a central system remains a major effort of cooperation between the systems being interfaced. Efforts such as those by the American Society of Testing Materials (ASTM) and the National Library of Medicine (NLM) to create a Unified Medical Language System (UMLS) will help to make such linkages possible. Because of the absence of a common medical vocabulary, the efforts to create a CPR system using an interfaced approach still remains an academic effort with each institution required to develop its own solution to the design and use of the CPR.

The academic systems that clearly qualify as CPR systems share several common traits. First, they maintain a large data dictionary to define the contents of their CPR. The design of the data dictionary is sufficiently flexible to incorporate the expanding medical data required for the new applications, as they create new applications or interface to other systems. Unfortunately, there is no common approach to the design of the data dictionary, but the recognition of the importance of a comprehensive data dictionary has been appreciated by all of the system developers. The use of a data dictionary emphasizes the importance given to a coded database by these systems. The coded database not only provides a copy of the CPR in electronic form, but allows usage of the information contained in the CPR for purposes other than data review in only the precise form in which the data was entered. Additional uses of the data include generation of alerts or reminders for health care providers, and creation of reports or flowsheets incorporating data from many sources.

The second common trait among the database designs of these systems is time orientation. All information recorded in the CPR is time tagged, thus making the CPR a continuous history of the patient's medical care.

Third, the systems provide rich research tools for use with the CPR. This feature makes the CPR valuable not only in actual patient care, but also as a repository of research data on which to perform clinical research and outcome evaluation, and to assist in continuous quality improvement studies in the hospital.

A fourth trait of these systems is the flexibility in reporting CPR data. Because of the comprehensiveness of the data, they no longer should be viewed only in the isolated format reported by the departmental system. These data should be reported in many ways and with other data from the CPR.

While these common traits exist among the systems, many differences are also evident. How they have achieved these traits is very system specific. The actual design of the database is unique and the tools for working with the database all appear to be system dependent. What one is able to conclude is that while there may be unanimity about many of the goals of a CPR, there is no clear, common approach to reach those goals.

Review of Some Existing CPR Systems

Three systems will be reviewed in order to illustrate the extent to which CPRs have been created and are currently used. This review is not intended to be an exhaustive one of all CPR systems, but to merely illustrate through examples the progress made in creating CPRs. The review will cover the topics being explored by each of the other working groups. The systems to be reviewed are HELP, TMR, and Regenstrief system.

HELP Patient Care Record System

The Health Evaluation through Logical Processing (HELP) system has been under development for more than 20 years at LDS Hospital and the University of Utah. One basic design goal of the system from the beginning has been to create a central integrated CPR. The second major goal of HELP has been to provide a knowledge base for use with the CPR. In achieving these two goals, HELP has developed an extensive set of applications that serve both as data acquisition modules for the CPR and test sites for the use of decision support logic in clinical environments. The major application modules of HELP currently are admitting, order entry/ charge capture, results review, nursing, intensive care units (ICUs), respiratory therapy, pulmonary/blood gas analysis, surgery, infectious disease, clinical laboratories, microbiology, cardiology, pharmacy, and radiology. Each of these applications uses HELP to acquire patient data, provide management information about the department, and incorporate computerized decision making to support the needs of the department. At LDS Hospital HELP exists on a Tandem 10-cpu computer with an interface to more than 500 terminals, a laboratory system, an automated electrocardiogram (EKG) system, and a financial system.

The HELP CPR database consists of five primary files. Two of the files, the patient demographic file and the patient data file, contain information on patients who are active in the system. The demographic file is a relational file containing key demographic information about the patient. Information in the patient data file is stored as coded items where the codes correspond to a data model created with the HELP database system. The physical structure of this file has been optimized to minimize access to patient data. The data are stored as event strings, where each string contains information about some logical event. For example, vital signs would be stored as a single event string. All of the information is time tagged and stored in reverse chronological order. Two historical files make up part of the HELP database. The first historical file is an abstract of the active file information. When the patient is discharged, all data from the active files are archived to tape and abstracted to the historical file. The historical file contains both demographic and pertinent medical data. This information is automatically entered into the patient's active file for use by HELP when the patient is readmitted. A second historical file which serves as a case mix file is created from the current file when the patient is discharged. This file contains only that portion of the CPR considered important for case mix studies. The fifth patient file of the HELP database is the transaction file. This file records all of the transaction information needed by the system for managing orders and charges on the patient.

Although these five files constitute the major patient files, numerous other files exist on the HELP database, such as an employee file, departmental files, and the like. At the lowest level, management of the database is through the Tandem's Enscribe file management system. Using the Tandem Enscribe file management system a special HELP database management system has been developed. This database system, referred to as PTXT, provides the user level application interface to the HELP database. Currently, research is underway to explore the use of Tandem's SQL software to replace the HELP-developed PTXT database management system.

While the HELP system continues to support dumb terminals, all of the newer software being written requires an IBM-compatible PC with 132-column graphics as the user terminal. The new applications of HELP incorporate the use of windows, thus necessitating the use of PCs and the windowing packages available on them. Special graphics software on the PC is also being developed to interface with HELP. The graphics software will not only support flexible trend graphs, but also utilize icons and animation. There are no terminals on the system that support either voice or images.

No direct input of data from the patients is required. Data acquisition from health care professionals is, however, a key component of HELP. The nurse serves as one of the primary individuals responsible for data acquisition. Essentially, all of the nursing information including care plans, assessment, history, procedures, and documentation is either currently being entered or in final evaluation for entry by the nurses. Respiratory therapists are also required to chart all of their data or procedures into HELP. Physicians at present contribute little to the data acquisition. They are responsible for some ordering, but little else. Dictated x-ray reports, surgical summaries and discharge summaries are entered into the system, but this is accomplished through use of a transcription service and not directly by the physician. Entry of all data into the system is either directly from instruments such as bedside monitors or from the keyboard of the terminals. With exception of barcode readers in the x-ray department, no special data acquisition devices (i.e., light pens, mouses, etc.) are used by the health care professionals. There is currently no facility on HELP for image processing and storage. An image processing system is available at LDS Hospital, but it is not currently interfaced to HELP.

The medical vocabulary of HELP has been developed as a part of the HELP system. While HELP provides a hierarchic data model for creation of a medical vocabulary, using the query language described below, a relational view of the data is also possible and can be used to manipulate the data in the CPR. The codes used in the data model have been locally defined and are not part of any national effort. Even though the internal vocabulary is unique to HELP, several other medical vocabularies have been incorporated in the HELP vocabulary. In particular, *International Classification of Diseases*, 9th edition (ICD-9 codes), Snomed, and current procedural terminology (CPT4) are included in HELP. In all of these cases, a simple algorithm has been used to generate a code in the HELP vocabulary from the codes of the other coding systems.

Three systems are interfaced to HELP. They are a Lab Force laboratory computer system, a Marquette EKG system, and an IBM financial system. Communication among the systems interfaced to HELP is a combination of unique protocols and, where possible, standard protocols. For example, the interface between HELP and the laboratory computer is based on the evolving MEDEX standards. This interface is built around X25 and X409. The interface, however, to the Marquette EKG system is unique to HELP. Since the Marquette system does not provide a standard interface, specific protocols have been written on the HELP system to capture the data from the Marquette system.

System reliability on HELP is primarily achieved through the built-in features of Tandem. Since Tandem provides a redundant hardware path for every component on the system, it is extremely rare that a hardware failure would result in system downtime. Currently the system is running at better that 99.7 percent uptime 24 hours a day, 7 days a week. The CPR is redundantly stored on mirrored disk drives ensuring maximum data integrity. Security on the system is provided by several means. Within the hospital a logon is required for entry into the system. Because of the need for access to all patient data by the physician, the logon is simple and once used allows access to data on any patient in the active patient file. Phone-in access from physician homes/offices to the patient data is provided only through use of special access disks provided to the users. Access must be from a PC containing a special disk that is encoded with the appropriate security checks. A final level of security is terminal control. With the logon, the terminal is activated with a set of privileges peculiar to the logon. Only those allowed logon functions can be performed from the terminal, thus limiting the activity possible at a single site. Once access is made to a function no further levels of security are in effect. With most transactions, the system does record the user ID, making it possible to track use of the terminal when desired. Confidentiality is therefore maintained by access privileges controlled both by the terminal and the logon.

A special query language has been developed for HELP. This language called PAL (PTXT application language) was developed to support the unique HELP database. It provides many of the features seen in fourth generation query languages. A higher level decision language (HELP) is also available. The HELP language provides an interface to medical experts for the creation of decision logic and queries. The HELP decision rules and queries are compiled into PAL syntax for execution. This feature ensures that execution of the decision making logic and queries will be optimized for the HELP database. Text processing is a research project on HELP. As noted above, some of the entry into HELP consists of free text. An initial project in this area has been the processing of x-ray reports. In this example the text in the dictated report is scanned and the appropriate codes of the HELP coded vocabulary are extracted and stored in the patient data file. This experience is being used as a model for text processing of other textual data being acquired on HELP. Once translated into HELP codes, the data can then be processed by the query or decision languages similar to initially entered coded data.

The only linkages currently available on HELP to knowledge, research, and bibliographic databases are to the HELP knowledge base and internally created research databases. The HELP system is primarily a knowledge-driven system and contains a large knowledge base consisting of medical logic modules. The primary applications of HELP all make extensive use of this knowledge base. Results of the knowledge processing go back into the CPR as additional data. HELP-created research databases are also available to HELP. Researchers may, through appropriate queries of the archived CPR, create their own specific research databases. Once created, these databases may be accessed by HELP similar to the current CPR.

TMR Patient Care Record System

The Medical Record (TMR) grew out of efforts that began in 1968 to develop a computer-based medical record system that could be used to enhance patient care. Early efforts focused upon automating the capture and reporting of patient histories and physical examinations. Experience with computer-based medical records was gained by synthesizing the data from these automated data capture tools into a record for patients receiving prenatal care. Attention was next focused upon providing a database that met the needs of an ambulatory care practice together with the clinical needs of a primary care record. Requirements of a growing user community extended development activities into hospital information system functions and meeting the needs of clinical research. TMR, as it exists today, is more the result of an event-driven response to user requirements and to changes to technology than it is the result of an original comprehensive design.

TMR manages all aspects of a patient's encounter, from making an appointment, scheduling an admission, or scheduling a diagnostic test, through the diagnostic workup or treatment course to the closure of the account. Requirements for administrative management, patient care, and clinical research are met for both outpatient and inpatient environments.

The development of TMR has been motivated by a vision of the benefits of a computer-based clinical record including legible records; data availability in multiple locations; focused data display; expert reminders; time savings; and creation of natural history databases. From the beginning, however, we have recognized that a computer-based medical record is not viable as a standalone entity, at least not at the present time. Practices which are not based in academia have neither the time not the financial resources to support a program that provides clinical benefits but that adds on to, rather than replaces, other information management tasks of the practice. Accordingly, the medical record supported by TMR was designed to be the centerpiece of a comprehensive medical information system.

This design criterion influenced decisions about the type and format of data that would be recorded in TMR. Each of the variety of people who use medical data have a unique perspective. At first glance, a medical administrator's questions may appear to require answers based on different data than a physician's questions. On closer examination, both types of questions will be answered with data about patients, their evaluations, and treatments. The focus or the emphasis is the only difference. Therefore, to address the diverse requirements of patient care, education, research, resource and financial management, and outside reporting, a computer-based medical record must store data according to their true meaning rather than storing them in an interpreted form meeting a preconceived reporting requirement. The data can then be structured and interpreted by one of several output programs to meet the focused needs of the user at the moment. Such an approach increases the variety of users who can be supported by the database from changes in medical thinking about the ways in which patients should be classified.

TMR was designed to permit the secretary, nurse, technician, or physician obtaining data about a patient to enter the data directly into the database during the process of patient care. Source data entry was identified as a design goal for three reasons. Data accuracy is enhanced in situations where questions that the system asks about data that exceed limit checks or that are internally inconsistent are answered by an individual who knows the correct answer rather by a data entry clerk reading a form. If the physician is at the terminal entering a prescription at the time the system generates a warning about drug interaction, the problem can be corrected before the patient receives the treatment. Finally, source data capture reduces the personnel costs associated with using the system. Commitment to source data capture increases the size of the hardware configuration required to support a system. Interactive terminals must be available throughout the practice, system response time must be rapid, and the data must be simultaneously recorded on more than one device to prevent data loss. More critically, the professional must view the system as providing enough personal payback to justify stopping and dealing with the system.

We all recognized that realistically all users would not be willing to interact directly with the video terminals. Therefore, the system had to be designed to work equally well in interactive and non-interactive modes. The result was a commitment to several different forms of input that feed into one storage format. Paper worksheets would be used to relay information to the terminal-shy user and to ask for additional data. A *chartless* record, not a *paperless* record, was the design goal.

We recognized that TMR, to achieve widespread use, needed to function in practices that did not have access to computer-literate personnel or programmers. At the same time, we realized that practices would need to be able to tailor the application software to meet different and changing needs in information content and practice style. The need for a system to be modified at the practice level was not perceived to be a one time installation problem. Any information system worth the trouble and expense that go along with its use will change the patterns and will have to evolve with the practice. We therefore committed to developing a single, universal program which could be used in any medical setting in conjunction with a user-defined and user-maintained text table that contains the rules under which that group chooses to operate. This table, called a data dictionary, is tailored at the practice level by using a text editor. Achieving this design goal meant establishing a data dictionary that contained not only traditional items such as medical vocabulary but also information about patient flow and computer hardware configurations.

Finally, in designing TMR, we recognized that an effective computer-based medical record could only be achieved by breaking with the traditional concepts of the medical chart. We assumed that in the near term the traditional record would continue to exist as a legal document, and that the goal of TMR would be to eliminate the necessity to retrieve it from the record room for anything other than legal purposes. TMR was therefore designed with the ability to produce the necessary encounter notes and discharge summaries to keep the paper chart up to date. This approach eliminated restricting system design to meet the requirements of the medical records committees or the Joint Committee on Accreditation of Healthcare Organizations. Information that needed to be recorded for transient use but did not have long-term significance could be left out of the computer-based record. The approach also allowed the system to be installed in one or more specialty areas within a complex institution, while allowing other units to continue to use the patient chart.

TMR uses a proprietary database management language, GEMISCH, which was developed at Duke University and continues to be enhanced to meet new needs. GEMSICH has been used with more than ten operating systems and with most computers sold by Digital Equipment Corporation since 1968. The language is now being ported to the family of IBM personal computers. Controlling the database management system (DBMS) language has been a critical part in the continued development of TMR. With each new operating system, we have only to modify the DBMS and all applications are operational. Upgrading computers has been equally easy. We can easily and quickly adopt to new requirements. Examples include terminal and printer independence where GEMISCH is able to compensate for nonstandard control characters and network interfacing. We were able to solve simultaneous record updating in a cluster configuration through the DBMS. As TMR needs new functions, GEMSICH is modified to provide them. More than half of the current commands in the language have been developed since the original design. Controlling the DBMS has been one of the most important factors in the long lifetime and continued evolution of TMR.

GEMISCH supports several different types of files: the database record; a fixed length, directly accessible file; a hash file; an inverted file; a B-tree file; and a sequential access file.

TMR uses a number of different types of database structures. Factors determining the choice of structure relate to how the data is to be used and to the relationship among the data items. The basic concept is to handle an unlimited amount of data for each patient—a lifetime record. Both retrieval efficiency and storage efficiency influence the design.

The basic patient data is stored in the GEMSICH database record. This record structure supports variable-length text strings and is indexed through a nine-digit key. The patient record is organized in modules: demographic, which includes payment management data such as insurance or HMO data, provider and referring physician data, protocol management data, and a general database section; appointment data; summary problem data; studies (LAB); subjective and physical findings (SAP); therapies (MED); encounter detail; and accounting. The initial retrieval of data brings the latest set of data in all of these categories. The idea is, with a single reading, to bring into memory all data that is likely to be used. Overflow data in certain modules are paged to archive files in logical sections: studies, encounters, SAP, and accounting. A past record is maintained for all therapies. Grouped data entry such as a diagnostic study, history, or nursing assessment is kept in a separate record with a single date and time as appropriate. This file also accommodates long narrative reports such as those for x-ray. Obviously, the amount of data in the root record will vary from setting to setting and from patient to patient. In a general primary care setting, the root record may contain all data for the past 3 years or more. In an intensive care setting, the record may contain data only for the past 2 or 3 days. In any case, the boundary between the root and paged records is transparent to the user. The data structures are the same in each, and functions are available in either case.

TMR uses a second type of database structure for the data dictionary and for certain logging or "tickler" files. This file is a fixed-position, fixed-length, directly accessible file. The data dictionary, first implemented in 1975, is the brains of the TMR system. It contains vocabulary, parameter definitions, menus, algorithms, hardware definitions, user passwords, privilege controls, decision making rules, and controls flow. Examples of logging functions include record management, report generation, insurance filing, and letter writing.

TMR also uses the database record to store summary data. Examples are financial data that are stored with tags for date, place of encounter, provider, patient category, type charge, and transaction code. Other files contain administrative summary relating to procedures performed; patients seen with diagnoses; and students, house staff, attending physicians; and so on.

The appointment system uses a combination of the database record for storing the appointment data for a single day for a clinic, a bit-mapped inverted file for availability of resources, and the direct access file for scheduling details. The inverted file is also employed to support query functions. This file uses bit, numeric and date keys for storage of patient data.

TMR uses a daily record to track daily updates for all records. At the end of the day, as part of the backup procedure, these daily files are used to update the backup total files. TMR also uses a number of integrity programs that run nightly to validate the integrity of the database.

TMR records may be retrieved sequentially, individually, or through a *NEXT INDEX* which can be driven by a number of different indexing parameters. TMR supports a hash file for patient retrieval of an alpha-name or partial name search. The names are kept in a B-tree format. Patients may also be retrieved across a network from another system such as IBM's Patient Care System (PCS).

The patient record files use algorithms based on the patient's primary ID to distribute the records among N files, where N is defined by the user. These files could be on different disk units or even computers.

TMR supports a variety of terminals and printers. Our philosophy is to support the least smart terminal for most basic operations, but to take advantage of the capabilities of smarter terminals including intelligent workstations. For example, most graphics are supported in either a character mode or a line graphics mode. Color is supported for terminals possessing those capabilities.

We are presently developing a download capability for intelligent workstations. A patient record is downloaded from the master database to an intelligent terminal where it can be viewed and updated. At the conclusion of the interaction, the patient record is uploaded to the main system for update. We anticipate that this mode of operation to become the primary mode. However, we do believe that "dumb" terminals have their place and we will continue to support them for TMR.

We support a variety of hard copy printers including matrix, laser, and ion printers. GEMISCH provides the interface and the translations to access graphic capabilities or desired font from a printer set.

TMR supports a number of workstation applications. A workstation in TMR means that all the functions and all of the resources needed are integrated into a single screen that is tailored to the particular set of tasks to be performed. Examples include patient management, claims processing, patient rounding and medical review, and query workstations. These workstations have the capability of networking to access any appropriate data on any appropriate computer, including national databases.

Most data in TMR is acquired directly by keyboard input. In most cases, TMR supports a structured English mode in which parameters may be selected by either text or code. The data dictionary provides the translation from test, including synonyms, to code and defines the characteristics of the response including entry limits where appropriate. Response types supported include numeric; numeric with defined separators such as #/# or #:#; yes/no; positive/negative; integers in pre-defined ranges as 1–6; selection from a predefined set of coded data phrases; selection from a predefined list; phase generated from coded sets; calculated; or free text. Most entry is either free form, within a predefined section, or schema driven.

TMR also supports automatic acquisition of data from a number of instruments such as a patient monitor or through downloading from another database. The surgical intensive care unit (SICU) application at Duke receives laboratory data and admission, discharge, transfer (ADT) data automatically downloaded from the Duke hospital information system (DHIS) running on an IBM PCS. In limited applications, TMR can support barcode input. In the past, TMR supported optical scanning, although no current applications use this form of input.

At the present time, TMR does not support, as part of the patient record, any digital image. TMR does support graphics as part of the patient database. The basic image for the graphic is defined in the data dictionary. Modifications or alterations to the graph are stored in the patient record. Types of graphs being implemented include body outlines showing scars, burn areas, or grafts; eyegrounds; and coronary trees, showing lesions and coronary flow anatomy.

TMR is committed to support data exchange standards. We are currently working to implement the ASTM standard for the exchange of laboratory data and to implement the HL7 standards. TMR currently supports the interchange of data between several systems including IBM's PCS and the Hewlett Packard catheterization system. At present, TMR uses a translation table to translate the codes from one system to the other. Duke has a project underway to define a uniform vocabulary for medical data. Using synonyms with the data dictionary, a uniform medical language can be implemented easily.

TMR currently supports a number of network linkage projects. The primary project is the coupling of Duke Hospital Information System (DHIS) and TMR. Patient identifiers; demographic, ADT, laboratory, and appointment data; referring physicians; and diagnoses are linked between several TMR applications and DHIS. TMR uses DECNET to link applications on several DEC computers and Ethernet with TCP/IP through a MITEK unit to link to the DHIS IBM 3090 computer. GEMISCH has incorporated the needed features to accomplish these linkages, which are provided to the applications programmer as a QUEUE command. These linkages are either realtime, on demand, or polled. Application programs provide the necessary patient identification, record synchronization, and error handling.

TMR also supports linkage to PC-based programs using the LOGICRAFT unit. This approach permits PC-based programs to be accessed from a TMR terminal. One example of this application, discussed below, is the direct access to MEDLINE.

TMR also supports the ability to *hot key* between DHIS and TMR. That is, from any designated DHIS terminal, access can be made to TMR, and from any TMR terminal, if the individual has a DHIS sign-on and is permitted, can access DHIS.

One communications project supported by TMR is the linkage to the referring physician. Selected reports, including cardiology diagnostic studies, operative notes, and discharge summaries are automatically mailed to the referring physician via electronic mail. Several times each day, hospitals around the state dial into a TMR computer and the mail is downloaded through a PC for distribution to the appropriate referring physician.

TMR relies on passwords to provide data security. These passwords must be of predefined length and characteristics, are changed at a maximum of every 6 months, and cannot be repeated. User access to data and function is controlled by the data dictionary. Control specificity includes access, review, update, and validate. In addition, all keystrokes of a user are stored along with a date and time stamp. This journaling file may be used at any time to define what a user did and when.

System reliability may be guaranteed to any level desired by providing adequate hardware. TMR retains at least two copies of all data on different media. In addition offsite backup is supported by multiple tapes. Hardware configurations permit operations with various disk configurations, since these parameters are defined in the data dictionary.

As previously noted, a number of programs are run nightly to ensure system integrity. In addition to ensuring the integrity of a single database, these programs also access multiple databases to insure consistency of data across the multiple databases. Programs also exist to check the logical consistency of data within a database.

In addition to the powerful text-processing capabilities of GEMISCH, TMR supports two levels of report generators. The first, and the easiest to use, supports a script language process in which predefined items are automatically extracted from the database and formatted for insert into the textual document. These scripts tend to be focused for a given application such as writing appointment letters or collection/dunning documents.

The report generator provides an English-like specification language for the generation of reports. The report generator supports decision making clauses and comparison of data over time, and understands how to deal with the data structure of a given module in TMR. For example, the report generator can deal with all components of a therapy including name, strength, signum, number dispensed, who prescribed, and so on. The report generator also supports direct calculation of parameters for insertion into the reports.

TMR supports several query approaches. The DBMS language provides the most efficient, but the most difficult to program query capability for TMR. Three packaged query programs support direct query of the database.

Many queries are based on tabulating events with certain specified details. TMR permits the user to define in the data dictionary what events are to be tabulated. These events might be procedures performed with details of when, where, and who is involved. The events might be encounters, diagnoses, length of stay, and so forth. A program extracts this data at specified intervals from the database and creates a fixed-formatted file with the detail. Report programs permit a time-oriented review of this data, sorted by the various parameters.

A second query program supports access to any data element stored in the TMR data files. This query program permits the user to define the selection characteristic for any variable such as AGE 40 or HCT and then combine these variables in a nested Boolean expression. The output may include any variable and has excellent formatting capabilities, including script. The query program can either be driven by an ID list or can be run across the entire database.

The third query program is the most efficient from a retrieval viewpoint. Any data element may be assigned a key value and name and inverted as a bit, a number, or a date. New parameters may be created from the existing database. The user defines the inversion rules, including the ability to align data to dates or events. Searches may be made across the database. Most queries of this file will take less than 30 seconds when the number of patients exceeds 50,000 and the number of search parameters are as many as 20. Supporting functions include graphs, histograms, scattergrams, contingency tables, and means, maximums, minimums, and standard deviations.

TMR has a number of features directly incorporated into the basic programs. Such features include dictionary-defined problem oriented reviews; drug/drug, drug/test, and drug/problem interactions; problem causal linkages; quality assurance algorithms; test/problem linkages; and various management protocols.

TMR supports a limited number of decision support algorithms. One popular feature of TMR is an online acid-base nomogram which shows a series of points over time representing a patient's acid-base status. Any point can be selected, and a direct linkage is made to MEDLINE for bibliographic retrieval of related articles. The user has a menu of options that can alter the canned search. TMR interfaces with the search engine of Grateful MED to conduct the search. The interaction with Grateful MED and MEDLINE is scripted, and the user is shielded from the wordy dialogue. The user is also immediately freed from the search procedure. When the results from the query are returned, they are placed in the requestor's electronic mail box, and the person is notified immediately if logged on or upon logging on. The user may then review the search results, deleting, printing, or saving selected citations. A citation may be linked directly into a patient's medical record to be reviewed by others. We anticipate expanding this capability in a more general fashion over the next year.

TMR supports a direct linkage between the TMR databases and a number of commercial relational databases and spread sheets. TMR may also directly transfer data into a SAS database. The user flags the data in the data dictionary as a SAS data item along with the SAS name. TMR at some specified interval generates the input to the SAS database.

TMR supports a number of research tools including the inverted query file already discussed. Over the years, the Division of Cardiology has developed over the years a model for predicting survival data based on method of treatment. This model can predict pretest and posttest survival probabilities for medical and surgical modes of treatment over a period of 10 or more years. Variations on this theme predict the outcomes of various tests based on similar patients in the TMR database.

Regenstrief Patient Care Record System

The Regenstrief Medical Record System was first installed in 1972 in a 35-patient diabetes clinic. It was designed as a *summary medical record* containing a few clinical variables, results of laboratory tests, imaging and electrophysiologic studies, along with diagnostic impressions and medication history, and stored as a flowsheet in a computer. The system was intended to complement and shrink, but not necessarily replace, the paper medical record. The purpose was to provide rapid access to organized and legible patient data, and to provide automatic reminders to the physician about problems reflected in the patient's data. In 1975, we published the results of our first randomized controlled clinical trial of the effect of computer reminders on patient care (McDonald 1976a, 1976b). In that and in subsequent studies, reminders improved physicians' response to patient conditions needing attention. For example, physicians given reminders provide preventive care to eligible patients at a rate 150 percent to 400 percent greater than that of physicians not given reminders (McDonald et al. 1984).

Currently, the system captures all diagnostic reports and treatment information about patient visits to the outpatient clinics, emergency room, and inpatient visits at Wishard Memorial Hospital. It stores this information in a coded and computer-understandable form so that it is available for both automatic reminders and for research purposes. Last year, the system captured information on 400,000 Wishard outpatient and emergency room visits and 20,000 Wishard admissions. It now carries 30 million separate observations about 300,000 different patients from Wishard hospital and clinics. This system is now being extended to all three hospitals at Indiana University Medical Center and to twenty clinics and nursing homes within the center city of Indianapolis. Physicians with appropriate access privileges will be able to retrieve patients from any hospital or outpatient site within the network from any other site. We anticipate that the yearly volume of visits will triple with the addition of the above-mentioned environments.

Since 1976, the system and the associated clinical management, laboratory, and pharmacy systems, use a stored data definition, common data access routines for reporting, editing, sorting, purging, cross-tabulating, and otherwise managing these data. Some components of the database are relational and other components are hierarchical.

Data are captured in a variety of fashions. Laboratory information is captured directly from the laboratory system and laboratory instruments. Pharmacy and prescription information is captured from the outpatient and inpatient pharmacy systems. Other information about a hospital stay, duration, and diagnosis comes from the hospital's case abstract tapes. Direct diagnoses and administrative details of clinic visits (e.g., who saw the patients, what clinic they visited, when they were there, how long they were there, what it cost, and what the diagnoses were) are captured by the clinic management system. Outpatient problems are recorded on an encounter form by physicians, transcribed by clerks into the computer, and reviewed by nurses.

Other kinds of clinical information, including the impressions of diagnostic studies, numeric results recorded on visit encounter forms, and special purpose data collection forms (e.g., a brief history form) are encoded and entered by specially trained data entry personnel (it takes roughly one person to encode the impressions from 100,000 x-ray reports per year). Physicians enter little data in this system. In the medicine clinic, physicians enter all orders for diagnostic tests. They are entering all orders on a pilot basis on an inpatient service (e.g., medications, nursing procedures, laboratory tests). We do no image processing at the Regenstrief System.

The Regenstrief system is using the ASTM-HL7 medical message formats to transmit information from a variety of systems within the Veteran's Hospital and

University Hospital to the medical record system. The system also uses a standard unified dictionary of terminology that includes surgical procedures, medications, nursing procedures, clinic tests, diagnoses, and observations recorded from those tests. This dictionary now includes 13,5000 distinct terms and 30,000 synonyms. The local dictionary is cross-linked with ICD9, SNOMED and CPT4 codes, as appropriate.

The system operates on a cluster of VAX VMS computers that are connected to their terminals through Ethernet linkages. The hospitals are linked via fiber optic Ethernet. Microcomputer workstations used for physician order entry and chart review are linked to the central VAX computers also through Ethernet netware using Novell software.

The system reliability is managed by mirroring of disks, frequent backups of some disk files, and redundant systems on a clustered network. On the microcomputer network, the reliability is maintained by redundancy in the workstations and multiple alternative network file servers.

Security and confidentiality is controlled by physical, two-level password security. Users change their passwords at 3-month intervals, but may change them more often when needed. Access to patient data is captured at multiple levels. Patients may be defined as VIP patients, in which case only privileged users may access their data. Certain parameters are also defined as VIP parameters, in which case those results are not displayed, except to special users. The Regenstrief System uses very little text processing, though it accepted data such as the discharge summary and the radiology report from work processing systems.

Two general purpose query systems are available for the medical record content. One, called CARE, has very sophisticated capabilities and permits the generation of tailored reminders based on arbitrary logic. It also permits sophisticated queries across subsets or the entire set of patients in the medical record database. With this system, one can find the average potassium within the first week following the first heart attack. The second query system is called the Fast Retrieval System. This is a much simpler system but provides more rapid access through an inverted file system. It can provide clinical users the option to obtain statistical and distributional information about a class of patients, but no information about individual patients. Researchers can obtain information about individual patients on the Fast Retrieval through special privileges.

The system has no linkages to the Bibliographic Retrieval System (BRS) databases, but a substantial amount of research is performed on the clinical database itself.

References

McDonald, C. 1976a. Protocol-based computer reminders, the quality of care, and the non-perfectability of man. *New England Journal of Medicine* 295:1351–1355.

McDonald, C. 1976b. Use of a computer to detect and respond to clinical events: Its effect on clinical behavior. *Annals of Internal Medicine* 84:162–167.

McDonald, C., S.L. Hui, D.M. Smith, W.M. Tierney, S.J. Cohen, M. Weinberger, and G.P. McCabe. 1984. Reminders to physicians from an introspective computer medical record: A 2 year randomized trial. *Annals of Internal Medicine* 100:130–138.

2
Database Systems for Computer-based Patient Records

William W. Stead, Gio Wiederhold, Reed Gardner,
W. Edward Hammond, and David Margolies

Database management systems have evolved and will continue to evolve. Major problems with existing database management systems include:

- The direct tie between programming language and database structure
- Specialization in design to optimize certain functions at the cost of others
- The difficulty of mapping complex logical structures onto physical media

Each of the existing database structures has identifiable pros and cons and will probably play a role in support of the patient record. We do not recommend selecting a single database structure for support of the patient record. We recommend, instead, careful attention to avoiding obsolescence as the hardware and software platform of the patient record changes.

The patient record database should contain detailed information about each care transaction, synthesize information from all facilities that care for the patient, and cover the patient's lifetime. Multiple values for static and time-oriented data must be supported, and the status of the record at any point in time must be reconstructable. The patient record must provide an integrated source of data about the patient including image and sound. Distribution of application function and data storage must be accommodated, but through a mechanism that guarantees synchrony of data. Access to data in the patient record will need to be limited to individuals with a right to know and who are authorized for release of information, and the database will need to accommodate that information together with a log of who has accessed what data. Response time requirements will vary according to what is being done with single item entries and retrievals at the subsecond level and complex interactions requiring several seconds to one or more hours.

The data structure underlying the patient record will be characterized as an integrated distributed database. Individual records will require multiple data structures for retrieval optimization, and a variety of applications will be responsible for generating and using data. Data synchrony must be guaranteed at both the applications level and at the database management system level. Identification must be standardized, and a dictionary of data item definitions must be developed. Avoiding obsolescence will require a progressive separation of the application from the underlying database.

Technology such as the smart card, optical disk, and natural language processing will play a role in the patient record but will not dramatically change the architecture or approach. Three technologic changes will have impact on the systems architecture during the next five years. Communications technology will permit dissociation of the physical location of the database from its site of use. Compound document technology will permit incorporation of material such as images in the record. Development of new memory and parallel processing will permit a start toward addressing the problem of mapping logical structures onto physical media.

State of the Art 1990

Evolution of Database Structures

Databases have evolved with technologic advances in hardware and software coupled to changing application requirements. Early data structures were provided inherently by the programming language structures. The first databases were sequential because the physical media on which data were stored were sequential devices. With the development of random access storage devices, new database structures were possible. Most of these new structures incorporated indexing schemes, so that individual records could be directly retrieved. Indexed sequential database structures provided advantages in retrieval, update, and storage efficiencies. The need for retrieval by any of several key attributes lead to indexed structures that provided indexing by multiple keys. Software developments provided different techniques for these structures including hashing techniques, binary trees, and B-trees.

Databases may be examined from various perspectives. The above view was largely from an indexing perspective. Another view is from a storage structure perspective. Tradeoffs between fixed length, fixed position files which enhanced retrieval characteristics and variable length fields for completeness and flexibility have been examined in detail. Models resulting from a focus upon storage structure include the hierarchical database, the network model, the associative model, inverted files, and combinations of the above. In the 1960s, a group of interested individuals defined a network database model which provided direction for a number of years. The Conference On Data Systems Language (CODSYL) defined a conceptual file which contains record keys and data fields in the records of files. This approach provided considerable freedom in defining a network of multiple relationships between data items, data fields, and data records. The latest direction in database structures is based on an object-oriented concept. The object-oriented databases provide a behavioral view of the data.

Another perspective of databases is provided through application. Some databases attempt to be declarative in nature and others procedural. The declarative approach defines the contents and structure of the database in a form which is understood by people and programs processing the data. The semantic descriptions are influenced by the frame's representation of knowledge. These structural databases permit easy definition of relationships among data items. Procedural databases use implicit structures that are based upon how the data is to be used and controlled by the programs accessing the data. They have limited power when data is used for multiple purposes.

As data-oriented computer applications became more complex, it became necessary to dissociate the design of the logical structure of the database from the problem of mapping the data physically onto a storage medium. Database management science emerged as the study of ways to support that separation. Applications developers, familiar with the content of a database and the relationships between data elements, focus upon the logical structure of the database. Database managers, familiar with concepts of storage and retrieval efficiency, map those structures onto disks. This physical/logical relationship is accomplished through pointer-based mapping of the logical structure onto the physical structure. A database is a collection of related data, together with the hardware and software necessary to record or retrieve data elements.

In general, there has been a direct tie between a programming language and the database structures that it supports. As noted, the early database structures were provided through the third generation languages such as FORTRAN, PL1, COBOL, BASIC, and so on. This relationship has continued with the fourth generation languages (4GL) of which dBASE III is an example. Many 4GLs were designed specifically to implement a new data structure. IBM's structured query language (SQL) provides a retrieval language for the relational database DB2. The language/database relationship continues to the object-oriented databases of which SMALLTALK is an excellent example. The artificial intelligence (AI) languages LISP and PROLOG provide database structures inherent to the language. The tie between language and database structures limits freedom of choice in that the selection of one determines the other.

The nature of data models becomes increasingly complex and specialized as the models match real world applications. This specialization decreases their utility for general purposes. The goal of a database structure is to be able to represent the underlying meaning of seemingly unstructured data so it can be manipulated in powerful, varied, and useful ways. Development of concepts in database design and implementations is a continuing process. Hundreds of articles are written monthly on this topic. Several journals, from highly technical, professional journals to the popular PC monthlies, are devoted to database topics. That there is clearly no one or *right* database structure is reflected in the many disagreements reflected in those many articles. In selecting the most desirable database for the computer-based patient record (CPR), we need to be careful to not become enamored with the current trends but select the database which most completely satisfies the needs of the CPR. In truth, multiple databases may be necessary since no single database structure is likely to be optimal for each of the various retrieval requirements of the CPR.

Current Database Structures

Hierarchical. Hierarchical databases are viewed by some as an obsolete concept, but the CPR will require hierarchal linkages among other representations. We live in a hierarchical world. We are comfortable with hierarchical concepts, from the contents of books to the management structures of organizations. Browsing as a form of review is well supported by hierarchical structure. The Hypertext concept is totally hierarchical in nature. The medical world is no different. Demographic data lend themselves to hierarchical structures. Hierarchical linkages of medical diagnoses show important cause and effect linkages. Subjective and physical findings may be linked hierarchically to show only the depth of detail required for a particular situation. The CPR will require hierarchical linkages, among other representations.

Problems with the hierarchical structure come to the forefront when the data must be examined from more than one orientation. Then multiple hierarchies have to be superimposed on a single data structure or the data have to be copied into multiple structures. The multiple hierarchy approach is exemplified by IBM's IMS system used now for many hospital applications as PCS. It is complex and requires an expert programming staff for its maintenance. The copying approach is exemplified by the use of MUMPS-based systems for patient care and research at Brigham and Women's Hospital in Boston. Since the access hierarchy is based in the first case on the patients, and in the second case on medications, procedures, and diagnoses, the research databases are created by periodic copying from the primary source.

The tree structure, the most logical implementation of a hierarchical relationship, is an effective database structure only as long as the levels of the hierarchy are limited. Retrieving involves retrieving the root record and following pointers to the record in the next lower levels which in turn contain pointers to the level below it. This process is inefficient when the structures have to be mapped sequentially onto rotating disks and each step requires a disk access with the associated latency related to head placement. New, non-rotating, data storage devices may overcome this limitation, enhancing the desirability of this database structure.

Relational. E. F. Codd, in 1969, developed a relational theory of data which he proposed as the foundation for database systems. This relational model is based on a relational calculus concept and defines structure, integrity, and manipulation aspects of data. Several database systems have been developed from this model, although many of them did not adhere closely to the concepts proposed by Codd.

The popularity of the relational database management system (RDBMS) is attributable in large part to the personal computer and the widespread interest in small databases. To use relational database concepts appropriately, one needs to understand precisely what a relational database represents. The relational model of data has a flat, two-dimensional view of the world with all data expressed in the form of tables. These tables must obey a set of normalization rules. The tables have unique rows and columns, and their cells are single valued. If these conditions are met, the models, mathematical operations, and logic will provide provable correct transformations. Consistency and integrity of database content is supported by having minimal redundancy in the normalized relations.

This tabular structure is simple and familiar, hence the RDBMS popularity. It is general enough to represent many types of data and clearly has its place in many medical applications.

There are a number of commercially available RDBMS. These databases run on mainframes, minicomputers, and microcomputers. In the IBM world, the most popular RDBMS is DB2 along with its SQL which has become a standard for query languages. SQL requires an understanding of syntax and semantics of the data structure to be used effectively, limiting its utility in the hands of the novice or occasional user. IBM has provided an additional tool, the query management facility (QMF), to provide a more user friendly, query by example mode that has a report writer. SQL has been expanded with an interface accessible from general programs. The interface, however, is awkward, since the relational queries are set oriented, and programs can only access single fixed records at a time.

Other popular RDBMS include ORACLE and INGRESS which also run on a variety of machines. One problem RDBMS have is poor retrieval response times when the databases are large and the retrieval requires examination of many data elements. In addition, the 4GL tools which are part of the RDBMS do not provide general programming capability. They provide convenient direct retrieval and limited update, but processing for deep data analysis is not supported. At best, result files can be extracted for subsequent processing. Therefore, although these structures may be utilized in the overall scheme of data storage, none of these RDBMS are capable of being the sole platform upon which a CPR may be built.

Text-oriented structures. Hybrid data structures to optimize text retrieval have been derived from IBM's STAIRS. Forms of optimization include text retrieval with positional operators, with variable links, and with some degree of interposed concept mapping derived from fuzzy set theory. Data structures that are optimized for text retrieval are sometimes combined with other structures and engines in order to support hybrid retrieval strategies. For example, an SQL bridge can permit interaction with a relational database engine for the purpose of document selection or document header field storage and retrieval. Text retrieval systems are useful in constructing clinical research databases, and they will play a role in managing existing text documents such as discharge summaries and operative notes.

Object-oriented databases. The latest approach is built on the concept that the database reflect the meaning or semantics of the objects being described. Clearly, a database is a collection of object descriptions which belong to classes that have certain characteristics. In the object-oriented model, an object is a member of an entity which has its own internal storage of values and a public interface. We use messages to instruct the object to report or alter its private memory and to carry out procedures. The set of characteristics and rules that describe the object is called that object's entity class.

Object-oriented databases have grown out of object-oriented languages with some added characteristics to control, manage, and query the database. The data structure and the programming language are closely related in this model. You can program an object-oriented database directly with an object-oriented programming language and include much of the application execution in the database itself. Examination of programming languages such as SMALLTALK, LISP, and PRO-LOG makes this relationship clear. This model permits additional knowledge to be used to optimize queries and lends itself well to concurrent execution of transactions. Some object-oriented languages, such as MDBS's Object/1, allow the objects to reference existing nonobject-oriented databases.

At the present time, there is no single object-oriented model. A number of computer companies as well as individuals carry out research in object-oriented databases. Tool development is the primary focus of such research and contributes to the power of this approach. It is clear that, while object-oriented databases again will not be the total solution, tools and concepts introduced by this research will be a key ingredient of the database structures used to support the CPR.

Lessons from Existing CPR Systems

Complexity of data items and linkages. Medical databases, which must service complex real world settings, are more complicated than databases for other domains. Certainly airline scheduling, financial, and management databases can be represented by linearly linked data items. Medical information contains a richness of meaning only afforded through complex structures. For example, a physical finding may have to support a variety of modifiers to a base term defining where, when, what, how much, and so on. Some or all of these terms may be present. The result may equally be as complex. One or more responses may be present, including a requirement for narrative to express some unique twist to the finding. Linkages vary among items depending on circumstances. Time specification varies with setting and purpose. Some data are viewed as a group, as a diagnostic test; other data are viewed collectively, as a panel; some data are viewed as single items over time; other views show a collection of data at a given time. Structures must support these variations. Many *standard* database structures do not inherently support these structures. In addition, linkage must be provided between structured data items and digitized voice and image data structures.

Need for redundant data storage. All processes in the health care system either generate or use clinical data. Medical information systems, therefore, logically have a CPR as their core. The CPR should be built as a byproduct of care processes rather than as a dedicated task. If systems are designed under the guiding principle that each datum may only be recorded in a single place in a general purpose database, two problems ensue:

- System developers must constantly trade off between restricting database content to produce a longitudinal record of manageable size and providing the requisite level of functional support to the health care worker whose main concern is providing an immediate service.

- It is difficult to optimize response time for different types of retrieval.

A medical information system, therefore, requires multiple integrated structures. The longitudinal record can be kept to a manageable size by archiving supplemental databases independently.

It is possible to divide those situations in which it has been helpful to record data in data structures that supplement the longitudinal medical record into four categories. The first category is made up of databases of work to be done. Specimen collection lists are an example. Such data can be thought of as an index, and does not need to be retained after the task has been carried out because it may be reconstructed from the longitudinal record if necessary. Tracking information is a second category. Audit trails of who does what to whom, and when, are an example. Such data are of use while a task is being carried out and as a source of summary statistics. Although detailed audit data must be retained for legal purposes, those data do not need to be maintained in a readily accessible form. The third category can be thought of as a data entry prompting buffer. An example is information about suspended outpatient medications. The prior content of the buffer can be replaced whenever new information becomes available. Derived variables constitute a fourth category. Data classifying of patients for research purposes is an example. Such data may be deleted when the researcher loses interest since it can be regenerated if necessary.

Overlapping user requirements. Analysis of the information management requirements of the health care delivery constituencies indicates substantial overlap in need between user groups. The participants in the health care delivery process can be roughly divided into three user groups for the purpose of analyzing their information management needs:

- Individuals with administrative responsibilities including people managing health care facilities, operating reimbursement programs, and making fiscal and clinical care policy
- Individuals working in ancillary service departments such as the laboratory or pharmacy
- Direct care providers such as physicians and nurses

A given individual may function for part of the day as a member of one of these groups and the rest of the time as a member of another group. For example, a respiratory therapist may alternate between the direct care function of providing clinical consultation and a support function of supplying respiratory care apparatus.

Each of the ways in which these three groups of users need to look at data can be assigned to one of five categories of data retrieval:

- Historical recall of data about a particular patient or device
- Access to data about the current encounter
- Retrieval of data, not by patient, but about a subgroup of patients or events based upon one or more common attributes

- Access to data for efficient work flow management
- Access to information in knowledge databases for incorporation into decision making processes

There is virtually complete overlap between the set of functions required by the different user populations. The only difference lies in the frequency with which a function will be used and therefore its perceived priority.

Each of the five types of data retrieval place different requirements on the information system. Historical recall of information about a patient or event can be provided by a system that captures data in a batch after the encounter. Database content may be restricted to items of long-term significance such as the start date, stop date, and dosage of a drug. Data storage must be permanent. An ongoing computer-based record of the current encounter must be interactively accessible for update or display during the course of the encounter. Data of even short-term significance, such as that from the dispensing pharmacist, must be entered. Data may be archived as it loses significance. Subgroup analysis depends upon interpreted data. Linear variables such as age must be converted to step functions such as age range. Data must be time aligned to comparable zero-times, such as the start time of a treatment. Work flow management requires all of the features of data for the current encounter plus a variety of indexes.

The functional domain of an information system is defined by identifying the groups of users that will be served by the system together with their needs. If the needs of a group of users could be met by distinct subsets of the above five types of data retrieval, then design of their information system would be simplified by eliminating the requirements of the remaining types of data retrieval. The complete overlap in types of data retrieval between the major user groups in the health care system suggests that one system should be developed to meet the needs of all groups rather than developing a special purpose system for each group.

Problems That Must Be Overcome

Given the absence of a general purpose database management system adequate to support computer-based medical records, a method must be found to avoid obsolescence as hardware and software technology evolve. The evolution problem not only relates to the physical patient database, but also to application programs which are specific to the database design. Obsolescence can result from the following: (1) hardware dependence, (2) database language dependence, and (3) database/application coupling. Application design must be increasingly divorced from database management if obsolescence is to be avoided.

In the long term, new database servers are changing as technology evolves. A single, general purpose data structure for the CPR would be possible only if an economical physical storage medium were available that could support direct mapping of sophisticated logical structures. Alternatively, inefficiencies required when translating logical structures to physical media may be overcome by a combination of parallel processing and exploiting application knowledge to select the most relevant information.

The CPR may require an architecture which includes redundant data storage to optimize response time and cooperative processing by distributed applications. Techniques must be developed to permit centralized control of synchrony at both the database management and application levels.

A nationwide commitment to the CPR will not be effective without a method of avoiding data obsolescence. A dependence upon the electronic chart will require ongoing conversion of existing data to new definitions and designs. In part, this problem may be overcome by paying attention to recording raw data rather than summary interpretations. For example, for a patient with congestive heart failure, the details of their symptomatology should be recorded rather than their class of heart failure. Such an approach permits application of new classification schemes as they become available. More difficult but equally important will be the development of methods for mapping old data item definitions into new data item definitions as medical knowledge and terminology change.

Requirements for Optimal CPR

Record Transaction Level of Data Detail

The database structure must accommodate recording of transaction-level detail if the CPR is to

- Be generated as a byproduct of the care process
- Be a resource for operations or clinical research or
- Serve as the sole legal record.

In other words, the relatively small set of data that are clinically relevant to subsequent care of the patient must be supplemented by who did what, where, when, and how.

Medication data can be taken as an example. Patient management decisions require a record of the daily dose, start date, stop date, and adverse reactions for any treatment. Support of the care process requires a record for each order containing the medicine, strength, form, signum, prescribing physician, number prescribed, number of refills allowed, and the date the prescription was written. In addition, a dispensing record must be maintained for each filling with the order information plus an Rx number, number dispensed, manufacturer, lot, dispensing pharmacist, and cost. An administration record must include the amount, time, and person responsible for each dose administered. Use as a legal audit trail requires the addition of the name of the individual entering the order, individual validating the order, and date/time stamps of all actions.

The data structure must have the capability of dealing with multiple versions of the same data element. Two situations must be accommodated—change in a result and correction of an erroneous entry. Change in patient name at the time of marriage is an example of the former, and a full history of such changes must be recorded together with index searches for both current and prior values because all versions are peers. Correction of an error is different in that the new value is a replacement for the bad data. An audit trail must be made of corrections which take place after a data element has been validated and made available for electronic access, but applications should access only the replacement.

For time-oriented data, valid intervals of observation and state, as well as data entry and correction times are needed. Redundant data copies must be identifiable so that consistency can be maintained. When derived data is stored, such derivations have to be recomputable as well. Continuous maintenance of derived information (*truth maintenance*) can be very costly. It may be best to set an obsolete flag in the derived data and only recompute derived results when needed or as computing resources are available.

Especially in the distributed and autonomous systems that will be prevalent soon, the effort needed to maintain continuous consistency of related information will be great. By formal modeling of derived data and data distribution, it will be possible to specify permissible delays for this maintenance function. Only when adequate specifications are available will we be able to automate this function.

Provide a Single, Integrated Source to Data

The data structure underlying the CPR must be designed to provide a single integrated source to data about the patient. This requirement has implications both for the way in which care providers interact with the record and for the database architecture.

Each datum must be recorded at the earliest appropriate point in the care process. Subsequent interactions with the record should involve verification or update of existing information, together with addition of new information. Such a process would stand in stark contrast to current practices in which new care providers record their own summaries of facts together with their assessments in their own style. With each cycle of care, the record would become more accurate, consensus would be identified, and points of disagreement would be highlighted.

Regardless of the physical nature of the database, users must operate under the illusion that there is only one database—their own. However, users should only enter that data which they are directly responsible for generating. The architecture must permit other information to be transparently available within the user's working space from the patient database. Provision must be made for passing back additions or modifications and resolving conflicts.

Distribute Function and Storage

The architecture of the CPR must take advantage of distributed processing. Distribution is necessary to permit

- Use of different types of processing resources

- Sharing of common data with local augmentation
- Integrated access of autonomous remote information/knowledge database

Each of the available hardware platforms has a place in the operation of a medical information system. Mainframe facilities may remain appropriate as large data storage servers. Workstations have an advantage in memory-intensive operations such as graphics or spread sheet manipulation. Intermediate processing nodes will be required to transform information from dissimilar nodes and make it accessible. These mediating nodes may also provide the required privacy protection. In a given situation, the system mix may mandate use of a suboptimal technology for a specific task. The correct role for each technology changes with each change in the technology. The data structure underlying the CPR must be designed to function in a distributed system supported by a changing mixture of hardware platforms.

The constituencies of a computer-based medical record vary in the level of detail of information about the patient that is needed. As you transcend the hierarchy of users from care provider to department to institution to region, provision must be made to protect *proprietary* information while passing on information of general import. Each user group needs to record information that is of local interest only. The balance between data sharing and local control can best be met through integrated but distributed databases.

Scope of the Database

Historically, each facility caring for a patient was expected to create and maintain its own record. The architecture for the CPR must support an integrated record consisting of information captured at each of the facilities that cares for a patient. Record retention durations have been dictated by statutes of limitation. The architecture for the computer-based medical record must support a lifetime record for the care of the individual patient, and a perpetual record for research purposes.

Confidentiality

The architecture of the computer-based medical record must permit control of access to data by both category of data and category of user. In some cases, it will be necessary to control access at the individual datum and user level.

The data structure must permit notification regarding patient agreement to release individual data items to individual users. The data structure must permit retention of audit trails of each time a particular datum is accessed.

Response Characteristics

The response time requirements for the CPR will depend upon the type of use.

Data entry must be as efficient as manual methods despite the increase in precision that will be caused by computer-based records. In part, this requirement can be met through electronic data capture and data sharing. Techniques such as the use of templates with exception editing will also be required.

Retrieval response time can vary depending upon the complexity of the task. A provider retrieving a single laboratory result will be frustrated if more than 1 or 2 seconds is required. On the other hand, a request to graph changes in the results of two variables over 5 years of a patient's followup can take 20 to 30 seconds without becoming frustrating.

Distinctions can be made between data that must be available for online retrieval and data that can be recovered more slowly. For example, it will be appropriate to keep the interpretation of all patient x-rays online as long as a patient is alive. On the other hand, it would not be a problem if it took an hour or so to retrieve the images themselves or the full body of the text. Likewise, the detailed audit trails which must be captured as part of the computer-based record do not need to be rapidly accessible.

Architecture for 1991 and Beyond

An Integrated but Distributed Database

The data structures underlying the CPR must permit meeting the seemingly conflicting requirements of

* Recording transaction-level detail while providing a lifetime record and
* Providing a single source to data while distributing function and storage

Neither of the two predominant existing approaches will suffice. A large central database would not provide adequate local flexibility or control of proprietary information. Logical integration of distributed autonomous systems will not provide adequate data sharing, conflict resolution, or integrity.

Given the appeal of the latter approach as an immediate compromise solution to existing systems problems, its rejection requires explanation. The model can be represented by three systems—a laboratory system, a pharmacy system, and an integrating system that gathers data on demand from the other two systems to provide a medical record. Data thought to be of common interest is broadcast to all systems to eliminate redundant data entry. Although information flows between systems, there is no mechanism for conflict resolution or to guarantee that the receiving system acts appropriately on the information. Database quality is a function of the weakest system link, and there is no way to guarantee that the databases will stay synchronized.

The appropriate architecture for a CPR will incorporate aspects of both centralized and distributed database models. The database will consist of multiple structures, all or portions of which may be physically separated. At the applications level, client server concepts must be used to guarantee database synchronization and validity. The server supports data of general interest. An individual user will extract a particular subset of that data of immediate interest. Programs for the manipulation of that data can reside on the user's workstation or be part of a server system. Data of interest only to one user can remain on the workstation, but changes in data originating on the server must be transmitted back to the server, where, subject to update algorithms, the server database is made current. A system that is the client in one situation may be the server in another situation provided only one system is the master or server for a particular datum. That datum may be allowed to reside in multiple places, but updates must be handled through a common server algorithm and then flow to all places where copies of the datum exist under positive control.

At the database management system level, a mechanism must be provided to control concurrency for replicas, overcoming the delays and uncertainty imposed by distribution and network communication. Maintenance of integrity means dealing with the effects of operations addressed to more than one destination. These operations are always performed asynchronously and must be managed without either locking all nodes until the update is complete or requiring strict serialization.

Multiple major structures will be required to record patient- or process-related data. Initial data capture should be into a transaction-oriented file containing both the information about the patient and the information about how that information was or is going to be obtained. A variety of transient indexes into this transaction file should support work flow management. Data should flow, selectively, from the transaction file to a summary record containing information of long-term significance. This latter information will be the subset of data available for interactive historical recall and transfer between facilities. Other process-related data should be archived to bulk offline storage. Research files containing interpreted data should be constructed from the transaction files and maintained for the duration of interest. The archiving mechanism for the transaction file should permit reconstruction of the state of the database at any point in time for legal purposes and reconstruction of the research files on demand.

From an organizational point of view, the database can be considered to be a series of layers, each of which needs to be able to obtain or pass data to the layer immediately above or below it. An example of the layers might be the workstation associated with a laboratory instrument, the laboratory database, and the patient record. As the layers are transcended, less transaction detail is required and there is a parallel increase in requirement for information about the patient as a whole.

Standard Identification and Data Item Definition

Provision of a CPR based upon distributed but integrated databases will require development of standards. In general, we have avoided the question of standards because it is to be dealt with by another working group. However, the issue of patient identification and updatable data item definitions should be covered in this section.

In the long term, we should try to move toward assignment of a unique number to each individual at birth as is the practice in certain European countries. In the interim, the way in which identifying data is captured must be standardized. For example, is the first name separated from the middle name? When establishing a patient record, a workstation must obtain the minimum identification data required by the standard. This information should be transferred electronically from the originating system to the server above it. The server should either return an appropriate number, or pass the request to the server above it. Currently, when there is no further server, after the institutional server has been searched, a group at that level should assign a new number that should be subsequently passed down through the chain. Identification will be so critical that numbers assigned on information obtained through oral exchanges should be verified through some process after the fact.

For data to be exchanged between databases in a way in which it can be interpreted, the minimum elements of a data item definition must be standardized. For example, a laboratory result should not be transmitted without including access to the methodology used in producing the result and the expected values. If the database is to have longevity, database item definition updates must be handled carefully. At a minimum a mapping should be provided to permit translation of old items into new items.

A national effort to make progress toward a CPR will fail if it is focused upon generating a system or even a small set of systems that everyone would use. On the other hand, great progress could be made if attention were focused upon development of databases of common medical terms. With these terms in hand, databases of knowledge or information could be developed with them as indices. Any system capable of matching its database to the common terms would then be able to utilize the information. Medications and drug/drug interactions are a suitable example. There should be a common identifier for every medication. Drug/drug interaction databases should then be built around that identifier, and would become accessible to any system which used that identifier as part of its data definitions.

Increase the Separation Between the Application and the Database

Database management science has succeeded in separation of the specification of the logical database structure from the problem of physically mapping that structure onto a storage medium. However, given the tradeoffs required in supporting computer-based medical records, most existing systems utilize multiple logical and physical structures to get the job done. Application code is integrally linked to existing database structures. Given the absence of a single best database structure and the expected evolution of database technology, our architectural effort should focus upon placing a general data manager between the application code and the various database structures. Such an approach would permit change in the database structures while retaining the investment in the intricate application code.

Role/Impact of Specific Technologies

Smart Cards

The smart card will play a relatively small role in computer-based medical records applications. It will have a role in patient identification and sign on control. Smart card will be impractical as a repository of the computer-based record. For example, if patients brings cards with them to the clinic, how do you update items such as laboratory data, whose results are not known until after the patients have already left?

Optical Disks

Optical disk technology will play a role in computer-based records, but it will not alter the fundamental architecture. Optical disks are ideal for permanently archiving transaction records and audit trails. They have a place in preserving the final version of a timed report. Given their write-once nature, they do not have a role as the repository of the patient database itself.

Natural Language Processing

Natural language processing, in its broadest sense, must be limited. Structured natural language will be an important component of the CPR. Interpretation of unstructured text will never be sufficiently precise to permit maximum benefit from computer-based records. For the same reason, storage of images of text will not be useful except as a transition step from the paper record. In that capacity, it can be thought of as another form of microfiching.

New Memory/Processors

In the long run, memory may be developed that will permit physical realization of the promise of existing logical database structures. Alternatively, techniques may be developed to utilize parallel processing to get around the inefficiencies of these structures. Neither of these events will happen in time to permit development of a system beginning in 1991.

Communication Technology

The rapid spread of communications technology and near term increase in transmission speeds will fundamentally alter past concepts of data management. The data will be commonly located at the site of the responsible individuals. As needed, it can be accessed by remote end users. Transformations to select the stored data, convert it, and bring it to the proper level of abstraction of the end user can be carried out by other processors on the network, maintained by specialists in data understanding. The actual display transformation and direct manipulation of the information will take place at the user's workstation.

Compound Documents

Storage, analysis, restructuring, and retrieval of multimodel (image, voice, full text) data elements into compound documents containing static and live-link components may be feasible by 1991. This technology will be important in permitting unified access to structured data items and images as part of the CPR.

Next Steps

The Institute of Medicine study on computer-based medical records should avoid two fatal pitfalls. It should not recommend collection of a nationwide computer-based record limited to summary information such as demographics and ICD-coded diagnoses. Such a record would be misunderstood by the uninitiated in ways best exemplified by the misuse of mortality data in Medicare reporting. The record must contain adequate clinical information to be a meaningful tool for outcome research. It will be equally important to avoid the pitfall of being overwhelmed by the task and saying that we should limit national efforts to provision of some form of national gateway between systems.

We should begin by identifying a form of common patient identification, together with a record of what systems and databases have information about a patient. Initial transfer of information should then take place in a predominantly textural fashion while the necessary standards and data item definitions are developed to permit utilization of structured data and implementation of the proposed architecture.

3
Terminals and Workstations for Computer-based Patient Records

J. Robert Beck, G. Octo Barnett,
Paul D. Clayton, and Ifay F. Chang

In the context of the computer-based patient record (CPR) system, workstations are terminals or microcomputers that are used by providers in performing the tasks associated with charting and care giving. They may be located at the patient's bedside, at a nursing station or clinical workroom, or at the professional's office.

Conceptual Overview

The CPR workstations within a single health care institution will share a common graphic user interface (GUI). The GUI will be an organizing principle for workstations, inasmuch as nurses and physicians will utilize several of them in the course of caring for their patients. The workstations will be connected to a local area network (LAN), that carries data at the maximum allowable throughput within the institution and delivers data to remote sites. They will be available under $3,000 (1990 dollars). Thus there will be two principal decisions governing the acquisition and installation of CPR workstations:

- What GUI will be adopted?
- How will these workstations deliver and receive data over a LAN?

Hardware

Three general classes of workstation will prevail. The simplest will be handheld or semiportable data entry device (the *bedside terminal*). Used primarily by nurses and other front line caregivers, the small device will facilitate either manual or voice entry to the CPR system. A GUI will probably not be a feature of this system.

At nurses' stations and perhaps at patients' bedsides will be *smart terminals*. These workstations will have a CRT screen, keyboard, data entry device (e.g., mouse, touchscreen, voice), and a modest central processing unit (CPU). The GUI will be the central feature of the smart terminal, which will communicate with central file servers and compute servers that house the CPR itself. The terminal's CPU will package input data for delivery to the CPR system, and will configure structured information retrieved from the CPR so that it can be displayed via the GUI. The X-Windows terminals are current candidates for these systems.

The professional's office workstation will be a full microcomputer, with a CPU capable of displaying images, text, and graphical data on a sophisticated GUI. It will have enough memory and storage capacity to enable local archiving of interesting information, as well as the compute power necessary for moderately complex decision support tasks. Within the health care institution's CPR system, it will function as a large smart terminal, but to the end user it will have additional roles. In the early 1990s, the candidate CPUs for the professional's workstation are the 80386 and the 68030 general purpose microprocessors, as well as proprietary chips based upon reduced instruction set computers (RISC technology).

Special purpose hardware may be developed for health care applications. Examples include voice recognition cards and graphical acceleration cards for the workstations, integrated FAX/voice mail/printer peripherals, barcode readers, and touch screen input devices.

Software

The operating system of the CPR workstation will be one of the contemporary ones that support windowing and a full featured GUI. The X-Windows (MOTIF or Open Windows) system running under UNIX, Presentation Manager or Microsoft Windows running under OS/w, NextStep running under UNIX (Mach), and the Finder or Multifinder running under the Macintosh OS are the four leading candidates. The utility of these various systems will be influenced by connectivity, as detailed below.

The desktop workstation software will include the productivity suite of word processing, spreadsheet programming, file management, graphics, and telecommunications. Not all of these basic tools will reside on the smart terminal implementation, but communications and graphics are likely.

A data management system will reside on the workstation concurrent with the productivity suite, and on the smart terminal as the principal feature. Using principles of hypermedia, the data management system will enable the downloading of information from the main CPR system, user controlled display and manipulation, and archiving at the workstation. This software system will include smooth links to the clinical literature and to scientific databases, as well as to local image libraries. Query engines for these databases might reside on the workstation, but also might be housed at intermediate systems such as departmental or institutional minicomputers. Also included will be rudimentary decision support tools, such as acuity indices, clinical cost analysis modules, expert systems for quality assurance, and perhaps diagnostic or therapeutic expert systems.

Communications

The feel of the clinical CPR workstation will be that of the user's desktop, with an *in basket* of electronic communications from colleagues and ancillary services such as the clinical laboratory, pharmacy, and radiology. Files will contain miniature patient encounter indices, perhaps a database of cases of interest to the provider, and continuing educational activities. High density information, such as radiographic or pathologic images, will be requested and delivered electronically, but perhaps delayed in active clinical information systems.

Basic to this vision of the CPR system is a network of high speed data communications devices, file servers and workstations. Whereas the 1970s and 1980s were characterized by terminal-host interactions between the users and their clinical information systems, the 1990s and the 21st century will see distributed information processing. Display, single use computation, and post processing will be conducted at the workstation level, while data storage and instrumental interfacing will be carried out centrally. A large capacity data network is crucial to this environment, as well as workstation system software that can integrate smoothly into a distributed local area network.

4
The Health Care Professional's Workstation: Its Functional Components and User Impact

John S. Silva and Anthony J. Zawilski

Our purpose in this chapter is to describe selected requirements for a health care professional's workstation (PWS). We focus on the use of a PWS as an intelligent intermediary between a provider and an integrated hospital information system (HIS).

Many current provider/system interfaces are character based, keyboard intensive, traditional mainframe system interfaces. They are typically organized in a series of hierarchical, function-oriented menus that access one process for many patients. Thus, physicians or nurses have to translate from their usual practice pattern of many functions for one patient to the system's pattern. When hospital systems go unused, many fault its clinical users rather than the system (Slack 1989). Results of several studies demonstrate that an HIS will not be used effectively if it is too cumbersome, too complicated, or too time consuming (Safran et al. 1989; Hammond et al. 1984).

Blois suggested that a physician's practice pattern has a definable internal structure, that physicians solve problems in a sequential, reasonably predictable fashion. A *personal* workstation should not only help the provider learn how to use the PWS, but also the PWS should learn how physicians work, then anticipate their information needs (Blois 1985). At a minimum, the workstation should provide fast data entry (Cimino and Barnett 1987; Prokosch and Pryor 1988) and result reporting (Stead and Hammond 1987).

Today's medical environment places increased demands on health care professionals' time. These demands are magnified by the need to document each encounter or provider decision. The need for more documentation is driven by

- Advances in medical science and technology that require more data for complex diagnoses and sophisticated treatments
- Quality assurance and medicolegal concerns that require a complete audit trail for almost all decisions
- Management initiatives to control costs and indicate directions for increasing productivity

Most patient care records are created manually by the provider during the clinical encounter. As the time required for documentation increases, the net time available for true patient/provider interaction decreases. If the provider is to use the PWS to record clinical data, the PWS must be as fast and as flexible as current manual methods. Graphic user interfaces (GUIs) with intelligent visual input (Bergeron and Greenes 1987), controlled vocabularies (Cimino and Barnett 1987), or menus and natural language processing (Cristea and Mihaescu 1988) are emerging techniques for rapid entry of clinical data. Light pens, touch screens, and voice entry are among the many technologies under evaluation. Meeting this critical design objective is the most important challenge in the design of a PWS.

The complexity and richness of functions within an HIS require extensive user training. High rates of turnover and continued development of the HIS ensures that training must be repeated at frequent intervals. The cost of the initial and ongoing training programs and the time lost from patient care during training are substantial. Built-in training expertise is also a requirement for the PWS. As the PWS and its attached systems evolve, changes to the provider interface would be accompanied by online help scripts that document those changes. Thus, providers should be able to train on their own workstations, at their own pace, and emphasize their own specific interests.

These and other compelling reasons argue strongly for an intelligent intermediary between the provider, the HIS, and external systems. The PWS *encapsulates* the provider within a simple, consistent, and intuitive object-oriented interface. The commands needed to navigate and operate the functions of the HIS would be imbedded (hidden) in the software of this intelligent terminal. Initially, physicians should be able to configure their PWS to their own practice pattern. Later, after the workstation has collected usage data, anticipatory computing should provide information to the physician *at your service* (Blois 1985). The same object-oriented interface and online training concepts present a consistent user interface to providers who use the PWS as their interface to other medical systems. Again, details of external system commands and navigation are imbedded in the PWS.

The PWS is intended to be the platform for connections and networking among an extensive family of health care information systems (Blois and Shortliffe 1990), what has been called the *Physician's Office Without Walls*. The immediate goal of the PWS described herein is the design and implementation of an intelligent workstation for providers in an HIS environment. An underlying design assumption is that the enhancement of the data capture and documentation processes which occur during the patient/provider encounter is the single most important issue. The objectives of the PWS include

- Increasing provider productivity beyond the present levels by reducing data entry time and eliminating redundant data entry
- Standardizing the provider/system interface by decoupling command and response structures from the detailed command specifications of the HIS while accommodating individual provider practice patterns

- Completing the bulk of the patient care documentation during the patient/provider encounter
- Increasing quality of care through treatment/diagnosis guidelines
- Increasing provider awareness of abnormal or exceptional conditions, information, or data through innovative displays
- Facilitating the management of free text data
- Expanding the providers' interaction with the PWS by utilizing new technologies such as voice input/output, handwriting recognition, and imaging
- Facilitating collection of administrative and clinical data for patient outcome and resource management studies
- Increasing accessibility to medical information through the use of clinical decision support logic, and the provision of easy-to-use links to existing medical reference databases (e.g., MEDLINE)
- Providing easy access to output processes that integrate various result data to display medical information
- Lessening the risk of data loss and mitigating the effects of a system failure through the local collection and storage of patient data (that can be stored for transmission to the HIS after recovery).

Concept of Operations Scenario

This section provides a scenario, with accompanying drawings of proposed screens, that follows a physician through part of a routine day using the PWS. The reader is reminded that this is only a scenario and that technical details have been simplified and PWS capabilities summarized for the sake of brevity. The figures showing PWS screens are visual aids for the scenario and are not to be construed as detailed requirements or final screen designs. In fact, the information density of these illustrations exceeds the display resolution for most workstations. This limitation does not invalidate the concept, nor does it impact on the work flow shown here. After reviewing this scenario, the reader should have a good idea of the desired PWS user interface's *look and feel*, as well as the level of integration expected between the PWS and an HIS. In this scenario the PWS is shown connected as a tightly coupled workstation to an integrated HIS.

The provider's name is Dr. Hippocratus (Dr. H. to his colleagues). He is a physician and administrator at the Tesla Military Treatment Facility (MTF). Dr. H. has been at a conference this past week, and this is his first morning back at Tesla. Entering his name and password brings Dr. H. to his personalized welcoming screen, shown in Figure 1.

The personalization of the sign-on screen was made possible by the Provider Preference Profile which stores provider specified parameters concerning operation of the PWS. It also stores information about Dr. H.'s needs and authorizations. This latter information is used to make the logon and access to the HIS effectively

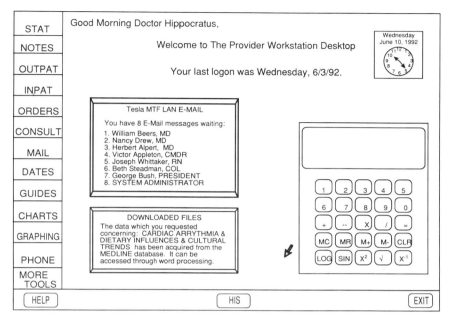

Figure 1. The PWS Welcome Screen

transparent to the provider. The message on the screen concerning research data indicates that Dr. H. has used an advanced PWS facility to query an external database (in this case, MEDLINE) and to download information to the PWS in an unattended mode. Thus, while he was at the conference, the PWS access and download occurred. The calculator shown in the figure appears as part of Dr. H.'s personal profile. It is typical of all PWS tools since it can be operated either by mouse or keyboard, and its results can be selected and transferred as data to any other PWS window.

Activating the CHCS icon initiates a connection with the Tesla MTF HIS and logs Dr. H. onto the HIS. The Provider Preference Profile in the PWS starts a communication script to retrieve messages and information stored on the HIS data repositories and brings up the next screen:

The PWS and the HIS have cooperated to inform the provider that an update of his relevant HIS files has occurred since his last logon, and he is offered the opportunity to wait for the automated update, disconnect from HIS and go into local mode, or use the PWS in a terminal emulation mode with HIS. The Automated Software Update referred to in Figure 2 is a function of the PWS that ensures that the user has the most current release of PWS and HIS applications software. After the download, the PWS formats the data and the screen shown in Figure 3 appears.

Note that this screen has drawn information from different areas of the HIS, as well as some special PWS sources, and has integrated and summarized the information into a single display. Part of the value of the PWS will be its ability to

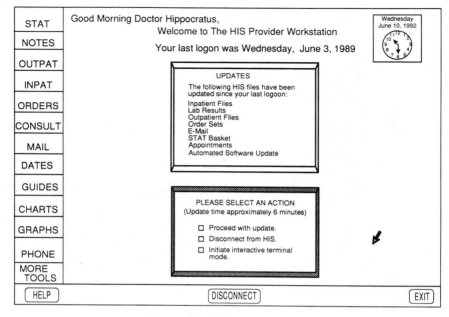

Figure 2. The PWS Sign-On Screen

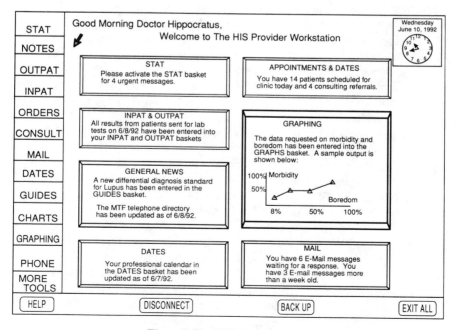

Figure 3. The PWS Detail Screen

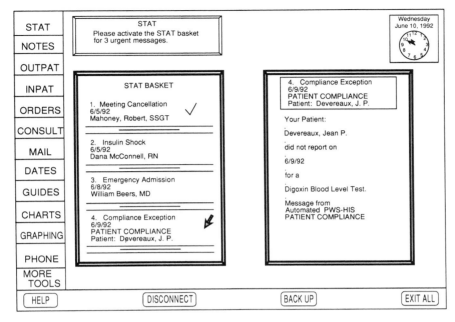

Figure 4. The PWS STAT Screen

convert raw HIS data into information. At a lower level this might mean plotting graphs from tables, and at a higher level it would include the summary and user interface functionalities which would be needed to produce screens such as that in Figure 3.

Clicking with the mouse on either the STAT basket (at the upper left of the screen) or the window that refers to the STAT basket (in the working area of the screen) causes the STAT message screen to appear. Selecting message 4, by either entering a 4 at the keyboard or by clicking with the mouse, causes the screen shown in Figure 4 to appear.

Dr. H. wonders why his patient, Devereaux, has not reported for the required test. He activates the phone tool to call Mr. Devereaux at work and selects a *dial until connected* mode of operation. The telephone function recedes into a background task of dialing until a connection is made.

Reading his next STAT message, Dr H finds the reason for Devereaux's absences and he cancels the telephone function.

Dr. H. selects the OUTPAT icon followed by the CHART icon. This function of the PWS extracts data from multiple areas of the HIS and presents a brief summary of the history, medications, diagnoses, and orders for each outpatient patient as shown in Figure 6.

Since Devereaux is an inpatient, the PWS will present a message to the user asking if the provider wishes to view the inpatient chart. Dr. H. accepts the *anticipated* information and views Devereaux's inpatient chart (Figure 7). He could

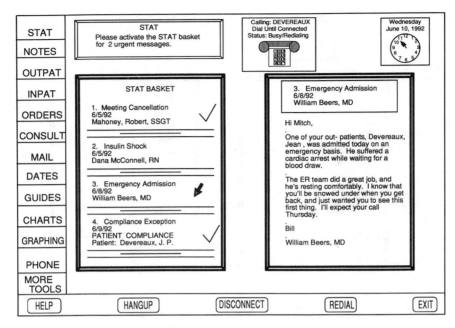

Figure 5. STAT Message with Background Phone Icon

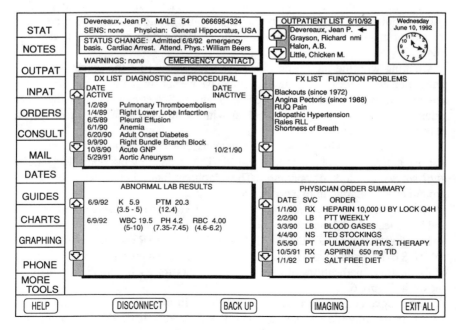

Figure 6. The PWS Patient Review Screen

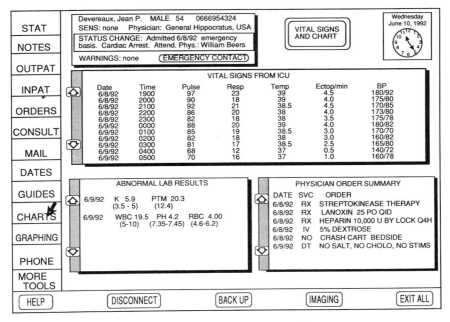

Figure 7. A Patient Vital Signs Chart Screen

obtain the same view of patient information by selecting INPATS and CHARTS icons.

Dr. H. opens the GRAPHING basket and then selects the blood pressure, heart rate, and number of ectopic beats as parameters to be plotted against time. The final graph is displayed on the screen for Dr. H.'s evaluation. Dr. H. opens the NOTES basket and enters a note to Devereaux's chart summary concerning his observations. In this case, the note is entered in free form. The NOTES basket also provides the user with templates to create formatted notes such as that using the familiar Subjective, Objective, Assessment, Plan (SOAP) sections. Figure 8 shows the graph and vitals statistics data partially obscured by the notes being entered into HIS.

Finished with Devereaux's chart, Dr. H. closes it then selects the OUTPAT basket containing the list of patients waiting to see him in the clinic. Figure9 illustrates the outpatient clinic list.

The first patient is Corporal Anne Halon, a 26-year-old woman. She has injured her back in a fall and is experiencing muscle pain. Dr. H. examines her and brings up her summary screen. She is healthy, with no record of chronic conditions. Figure 10 illustrates the use of a text management system that permits a direct, intuitive access to patient data. When Dr. H. uses the mouse to select the *Blisters on Left Foot* entry on the DX list, the text shown in the lower half of the figure appears. This is a synopsis entered by the attending provider during the original

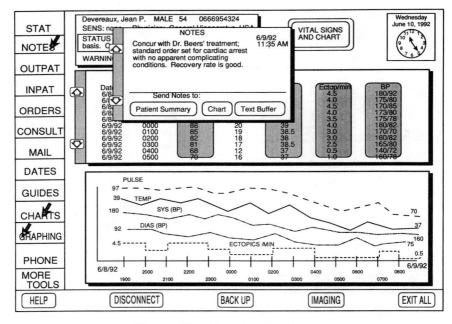

Figure 8. Vital Signs, Graphs and Notes

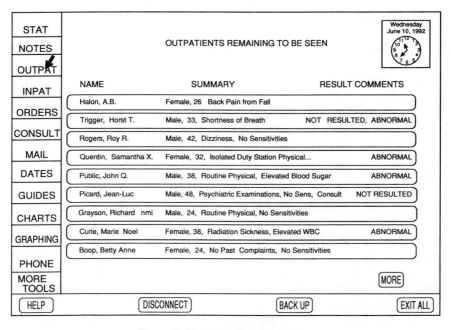

Figure 9. The Outpatient Clinic List

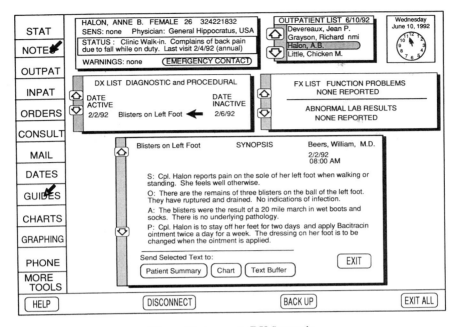

Figure 10. Access to DX Synopsis

encounter. It is in SOAP format which is the standard for DX synopses at the Tesla MTF. By selecting EXIT with the mouse, Dr. H. closes this window when he is through reading it.

Dr. H. has the option of using the mouse to select all or part of the synopsis text for inclusion in his present encounter documentation. By viewing and selecting several synopses for a single patient, Dr. H. can quickly create a chronologic patient history. This same technique can be used to merge information concerning several patients into a single document.

Dr. H. selects the GUIDES icon and selects the BACK PAIN guideline (Figure 11). He compares his examination with the quality of care guidelines stored on the PWS (imported from the HIS) and enters *YES* or *NO* only to those questions listed in the workup guideline that are different from his default values. Note the *International Classification of Diseases* (ICD9-CM) code which is assigned to the guideline. The particular code is for any trunk injury. Dr. H. has the option to accept or reject this code. Any codes entered into the system are later retrieved and used by centralized data analysis routines to create profiles of disease incidence and treatments for the patient population. This figure also shows the NOTES basket open for the entry of some preliminary statements. Dr. H. has opted to enter his notes in a SOAP format (the MTF standard).

When a *NO* is entered as the answer to the question concerning reflexes and the pin prick test, the workup algorithm recognizes a condition that could indicate

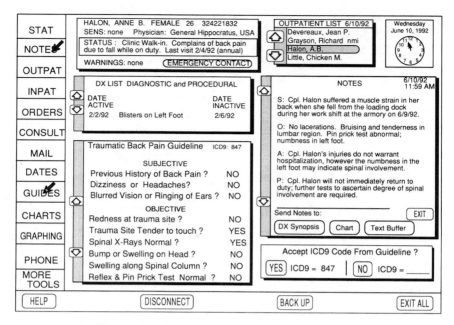

Figure 11. Guideline Screen with Notes and Summary

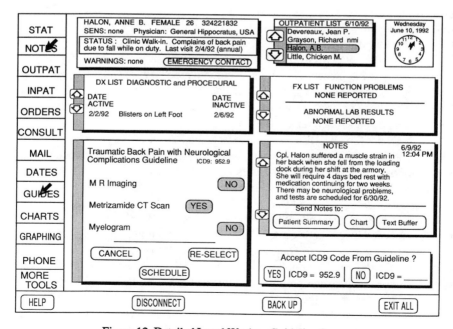

Figure 12. Detailed Level Workup Guideline Screen

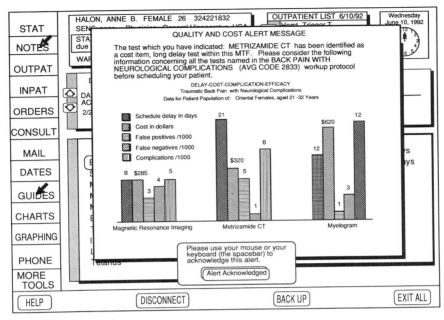

Figure 13. A Workup Guideline Quality and Cost Alert

neurologic complications. The algorithm then switches to a more detailed level of diagnostic guideline and specific tests are suggested (Figure 12).

The more detailed workup guideline appears in the same window, but a new title and diagnosis/problem code are displayed. The window lists the recommended tests that are available at Telsa, and Dr. H. is given the opportunity to schedule his patient for any, all, or none of them. The ICD9-CM code suggested by the system has also changed to indicate possible neural damage.

Dr. H. believes that if there has been disk damage (a possible herniated disk could be indicated by the numbness in the feet found during the pin prick test), then it is subtle and apt to be revealed only by the metrizamide computerized tomography (CT) test. He selects this test by entering *YES* in the proper column. When this scenario refers to Dr. H. as *entering YES*, it does not mean that there was a required keyboard activity. The provider can use the mouse to *click* on the appropriate response. No keyboard interaction is required.

As soon as Dr. H. has entered a *YES* in the column, a Quality and Cost Alert Message appears on the screen. This is shown in Figure 13. The purpose of this message is to present the provider with information about the ordered tests to aid in the decision process. It does not compel the provider to change an order or in any way interfere with any provider action; it is a purely informational device. As a sidelight, the master file containing the quality and cost data used to provide this screen will reside on the central HIS computer. It is envisioned that the central HIS

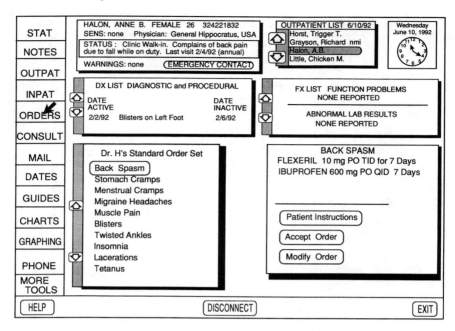

Figure 14. Order Entry on the PWS

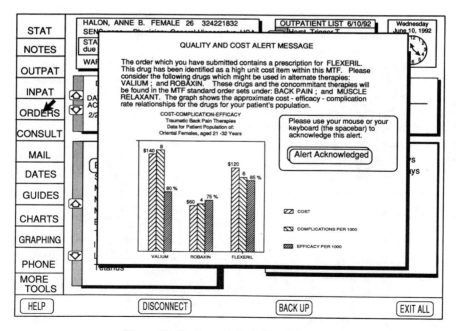

Figure 15. Quality and Cost Alert Message

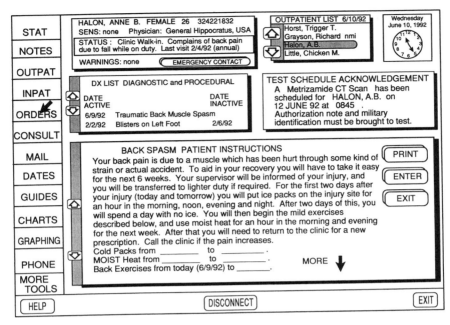

Figure 16. Printing Patient Instructions

file will be periodically updated based on data accumulated at Telsa MTF and the literature, then downloaded to the PWS.

Dr. H. evaluates the information in the alert screen and decides that the metrizamide CT is appropriate, acknowledges the alert, and orders the test. Satisfied that his examination has been sufficiently thorough, Dr. H. amends the text in the *NOTES* window concerning the diagnosis. A copy of the note is also placed into the Text Buffer (a temporary memory storage area) for later use in completing a full report or to attach to the test order. Dr. H. then selects the *ORDERS* basket, and from his personal set of standard orders, selects Back Spasm (his name for the order set) (Figure 14). Dr. H selects the prescriptions with a single mouse click. Simultaneously, the PWS interacts with the HIS order entry module to include this prescription in the patient's records and on the Patient Monitor's list of events. The Patient Monitor is a PWS-HIS hybrid function that monitors the patient's compliance with the provider's instructions. The aspects of compliance that can be monitored include any event that is captured by the HIS including missed appointments, medicines that have not been picked up, and tests that have not been performed. Levels of criticality, which will affect the threshold at which a compliance alert is triggered, can be assigned to different compliance events. As an example, the failure of a patient to report for a blood test may be assigned high criticality if the patient is taking blood thinners and low criticality if the test is part of an annual health examination.

As soon as Dr. H. selects the *Accept Order* command, the quality assurance and cost control guidelines are activated. As part of the management of health care delivery, all drug orders are compared with the MTF database (in the PWS) of high cost or high risk medications. For the purposes of this scenario, the drug cyclobenzaprine hydrochloride (Flexeril) is deemed to be a high cost medication at the Tesla MTF. The Flexeril order has triggered the Quality and Cost Alert Message shown in Figure 15. Dr. H. acknowledges the message, but chooses to use his Flexeril order.

Dr. H. selects Patient Instructions from the ORDERS window (Figure 14) and fills in specific *from date* and *to date* information for cold and moist heat treatments (Figure 16).

Another mouse click enters this information into the HIS. Once the encounter is complete, Dr. H. selects the Print icon, and the printer at the clinic reception desk generates a hard copy of patient instructions for medication and therapy. Dr. H. verbally explains what his diagnosis is and what the patient's responsibilities for her own recovery will be. At the clinic reception desk, the patient picks up the hard copy record of the prescribed medications, recommended back exercises, heat/cold treatment regimen, and the back spasm patient instruction sheet.

While he is working on the patient instructions, the HIS returns an acknowledgement that the CT order has been scheduled (Figure 16). This automatic acknowledgment of orders during the encounter is important since it is a check against a PWS-HIS communications malfunction. If there were some problem in scheduling the test or filling the prescription, the provider and patient can arrive at a solution without going through another *miniencounter*. The PWS is meant to augment the interface between the provider and external medical systems, like HIS, without losing the benefits of such realtime, interactive medical information systems.

The final step in documenting the provider/patient encounter is the completion of the Chronological Record of Medical Care, Standard Form 600 (SF600). Filling out this form requires information that the provider has already entered during the encounter. Instead of retyping the data, the Text Management System provides an intelligent *Copy and Paste* capability. With an electronic version of the SF600 displayed on part of the screen and his template displayed, Dr. H. uses the mouse to select text from the patient summary screen, his SOAP notes, the patient instructions, and the Traumatic Back Pain Guideline for direct insertion in to the electronic SF600. The basic SOAP notes are attached to the patient's problem list. When another provider opens Halon's file, Dr. H.'s SOAP formatted synopsis can be viewed by *clicking* on the muscle spasm entry, as previously described. His completed clinic note, including recommendations, plans, and orders, is automatically sent to the patient's HIS file, to her supervisor's office (in hard copy), and to the Back Pain Registry (a local MTF registry being used for a study of absenteeism).

As the day goes on, Dr. H. sees his patients and uses the PWS to document each encounter. When writing reports, he highlights selected portions of text and saves the text in an electronic notepad (called the text buffer). The contents of the notepad can be copied to order summaries, consultant, or referral letters or other records without retyping. The relevant diagnosis and problem codes are recorded by the system for later use. When placing orders during an encounter, Dr. H. uses the mouse to select complete, predefined order sets from onscreen menus. Thus, without typing, Dr. H. can enter complex order sets directly into the HIS and get the appropriate printed and onscreen documentation.

His day's work continues in this interactive mode. After the clinical work is complete, Dr. H. activates the administrative software found on his system and proceeds to calculate statistics on diagnostic related group (DRG) and ambulatory visit group (AVG) codes, length of stay, and other productivity data. The output of his calculations are processed into a graphic output using a template predefined by his superiors. Dr. H. displays the graph on the screen and then includes a copy of it in an electronic report sent via E-mail. Throughout the day he monitors results on his inpatients, reviews current orders and alters treatment plans from his clinic office. Before leaving for the day, he initiates his semiannual review of the tumor registry. The PWS will perform an unattended query of tumor registry data selected by a set of clinical indicators. After sending a set of electronic messages to his colleagues, he logs off the system and leaves the office. The PWS continues the background task of downloading tumor registry data, and when complete, it severs its network connections. The PWS processes the data using statistical and graphing techniques selected by Dr. H. and outputs a report using a predefined template. It will be ready for review, printing, or inclusion in an E-mail message when Dr. H. next logs on to the PWS.

Functional Components

In this section, each of the functional blocks shown in Figure 17 is described.

Discourse Manager

The discourse manager, as illustrated in Figure 17, is the first line of interface between the provider and the workstation. It is the software that controls all the interface peripherals and takes part in the provider/workstation *conversation*. This

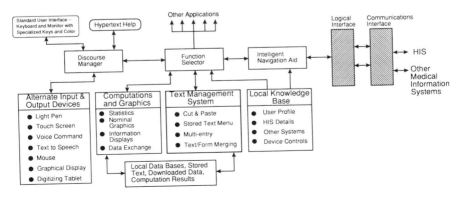

Figure 17. Functional Diagram

replaces the menu system or command interpreter of the traditional provider/system interface. Although the nature of this interface is not specified, the rapid emergence of graphic user interface (GUI) standards using some form of the windows, icons, menu, and pointing device interface style makes the GUI a logical choice for the discourse manager. The dialogue design is key to success of the interface, even if it is GUI based. Traditional usability heuristics for good dialogue design are well established (Molich and Nielsen 1990; Smith and Mosier 1986; Nielsen 1990). Guidelines for human/computer interfaces have also been described (Goodwin 1988; Heilander 1988). New use paradigms based on agents, drama, anticipatory computing (Blois 1985; Laurel 1990; Mountford 1989) and video games offer great potential to improve the provider/system interface. The Department of Defenses prototype of a PWS based on the X-Windows GUI was reported recently (Silva, Zawilski et al. 1990).

The discourse manager taps data in the PWS for the exact description of the peripherals attached to the PWS and then provides the required low-level commands (drivers) for their use. This is an example of the PWS expandability since peripherals can be added to one workstation without affecting the HIS (or other systems) and without requiring changes in software remote to the PWS.

The discourse manager also acts as the gatekeeper for the various levels of help (available in an online mode) that assist the provider in the operation of the PWS. As with the peripheral drivers, custom help information can be added to the local PWS standard help messages without affecting changes at the central processor level. The discourse manager will be the software that will handle natural language interaction between the provider and the intelligent navigation aid (Cristea and Mihaescu 1988).

Function Selector

Once the provider's input has been interpreted by the discourse manager, the proper internal command is passed to the function selector to access a specific PWS function. The function selector relies on the local knowledge base to select the appropriate function. It blends information about the provider with schedule, patient, and other relevant system data to select the proper internal application software for activation. In some cases, this software will recognize that the requested action will require an interface with an external system and will pass an internal request for services to the intelligent navigation aid. In other cases, it will provided coded responses to the discourse manager software which will provide a meaningful response to the provider through the screen, printer, or other peripheral. As the PWS builds usage data, anticipatory processing will enable the PWS to present context-sensitive information and choices to the provider.

The text management system (TMS) is activated by the function selector. A complex subsystem in its own right, the TMS integrates simple text management functions (such as copying text or merging data into forms) into a single, high level functionality, which transcends individual data sources. In this way, for example, the TMS gives the user the capability to enter text information once at the keyboard and to have it automatically posted into different parts of the patient's record and onto different required forms. Another example is the menu selection of stored, standard text (boilerplate) for inclusion in reports or notes. The TMS improves provider productivity and data accuracy by decreasing redundant data entry.

Intelligent Navigation Aid

The intelligent navigation aid (INA) interfaces directly to external systems. The INA uses locally stored data about the external system command and menu structures to activate the appropriate external system module in the most efficient and direct way possible. The burden of knowing all the *shortcuts* and details of the external system is removed from the provider and embedded in special INA knowledge bases resident on the PWS. When changes are made to an external system, the appropriate knowledge base is updated in the PWS. The provider is electronically notified of the changes. In most cases, the INA knowledge base will absorb the impact of the changes and, procedurally, the provider will not notice any difference in the PWS interface. Thus, the provider can continue to use the external system without formal retraining. If any training is required, this training is conducted on a self-teaching basis using the PWS. Training data, exercises, and help screens are downloaded to the PWS along with updated software. The implementation of an INA and the subsequent updating of its knowledge bases will require cooperative programming on the external systems. This is especially true if the updates are to be performed without operator intervention, relying on a startup dialogue between the PWS and the external system software.

Logical Interface

Although the INA will request and deal with functions and actions from external systems, the logical interface actually formats commands and menu calls into the required forms. This is a second layer of isolation between the PWS and the external system. It follows the object-oriented paradigm of encapsulation (information hiding) and promotes the use of low complexity, easy-to-maintain software modules. The logical interface need not be adaptive software; unlike the INA, it can be a specific piece of dedicated code that is replaced or updated as required.

Communications Interface

The communications interface is the final functional block. It represents the software which controls communications peripherals and passes the commands of the logical interface to the installed communication network(s). In a similar fashion, it returns the outputs of the external system to the logical interface for processing at the PWS. For the HIS, the communications interface and the logical interface will be the software modules most dependent upon the central processor hardware and software architectures.

Summary of Impacts

It is expected and intended that introduction of the PWS into the medical environment will change the way medicine is practiced and managed. The PWS must be an enabling technology which permits the collection of complete clinical information at the time of provider/patient interaction. This will provide the data needed for quality of care and management initiatives. Similarly, by having the PWS adapt to the practice patterns found at different hospitals, clinics or private offices, the PWS will present providers with specific, relevant and useful information in much the same way that assistants provide clerical and information gathering support to physicians. While no claims are being made that the PWS can replace a human assistant, it can be claimed that the PWS will impact the users by reducing the number and extent of the routine data tasks that providers must now perform manually.

Training

Present HIS training is often intensive and detailed or excludes providers. Proficient use of these systems requires that the provider receive explicit instruction with each function, menu selection, and option of the system. Training requires a formal classroom environment in full-day sessions that are usually held outside of the work environment. The time requirement is effectively doubled since additional personnel must be assigned to service patients while the providers are in class.

In the traditional systems approach classroom training must be repeated when new or enhanced functions are added to the HIS. When a user moves to a different area, clinic, or hospital, retraining is again required because of differences among systems, the number and type of functions implemented, and/or operational differences among organizations. The PWS philosophy is to provide a single, umbrella interface that deals with all external system details without involving the user. A knowledge base of external system interface details is used by the INA and logical interface modules to manage the dialogue between the PWS and the external systems. As such, changes made to those external systems accessed through the PWS will require changes to the PWS knowledge base and, in some cases, the logical interface and INA software.

The PWS absorbs the shock of external change through the INA and logical interface. The presentation of information to the provider through the discourse manager may remain unaffected. Thus, the PWS promises to alleviate the training burden by focusing on a common, object-oriented interface with the provider and a separate, internal set of modules which deal with the details of interfacing to external systems.

The discourse manager is the PWS module which standardizes the provider interface. All PWS and system functions are presented to the user as *objects* (in the form of onscreen textual and graphical icons) and their associated messages and actions (interactions among the objects). Formal training gives the provider a basic orientation to PWS screen objects and their usage. These fundamental elements of the interface, with their expected behavior and dialogue, enable the user to perform more complex functions. It is envisioned that the short formal training will give providers orientation on how to navigate within the PWS interface and to set up their personal provider profile of special functions. The online help and self-paced training is intended to obviate the need for additional formal training.

As new systems or new versions of established ones are implemented, the PWS modules are updated. This may require additional windows, new objects, and/or actions. Since the behavior of all objects is defined in a consistent manner by the discourse manager, the provider will see the same interface and dialogue design in the new or updated functions. Online training scenarios will acquaint providers with the new capabilities without their having to learn a new system interface.

Training organization will need to be reoriented to provide courses for all providers on the use of the PWS and its interface philosophy as opposed to courses on the details of external systems. The training programs for trainers, technical, and maintenance personnel will require change accordingly.

Decision Support

The PWS decision support software is intended to support health care decisions during provider/patient encounters. With decision algorithms available and integrated by the PWS, providers may base their clinical decisions on local, hospital-wide, or national guidelines or standards of care. Authority and responsibility for health care delivery decisions has always rested with providers. Access to decision support software and associated information bases of therapeutic effectiveness and cost and policy impacts may guide the provider in the selection of more cost-effective or outcome-oriented courses of action. This function of the PWS will more than likely require the formation of review groups to examine the decision algorithms and to synthesize the information used to support the algorithms, like the model of Advisory Boards for the Physician's Data Query of the National Cancer Institute.

Since the PWS software will encourage the acquisition of complete patient information, patient care data can be tracked at any level ranging from the national, to regional, to a single hospital, to an individual provider. Resource allocation decisions that have previously been *guesstimates* will be derived from models using quantitative data from the PWS. The managerial community will become users of the information collected by the PWS. It may be that hospital administrators will create one or more groups to handle the decision support activities needed for administrative and managerial support. Similarly, the amount of information collected may justify a separate administrative information system with decision support functions. Such an executive information system (EIS), which presents summarized data to higher level administrators, could lead to a separate EIS group within the hospital organization.

Maintenance and Support

With centralized systems, the user's involvement in maintenance consists of calling a telephone number when the system is not working. With the PWS, the user will be using a computer, and must know something about the use and abuse of such devices. Further, since the providers will be encouraged to customize the interface of the PWS for maximum comfort and efficiency, users unfamiliar with computers will need additional support.

Among the solutions to the support problem used in industry, the formation of user support groups from ranks of knowledgeable and experienced users has proved to be consistently successful. Providers with previous microcomputer experience or those who have been using the PWS for a period of time can provide valuable insight to other providers in their own jargon. Specialized training in more technical aspects of the PWS can be made available to these providers, and they in turn can pass on this information on an informal, as-needed basis to other users. The formation of user support groups is to be encouraged and will require technical and logistical support.

User Operational Impacts

The PWS should be the catalyst for a gradual evolution from today's manual operation with isolated automated aids to a true, integrated hybrid practice. It is in progressing towards these goals that the PWS will have noticeable operational impacts. The effects will be most pronounced in those areas where there is direct patient contact and an information exchange between a provider and a patient. Providers involved in such services as pharmacy will see less operational change in the short term since their major work is in an offline mode and not part of the primary provider/patient encounter. As the PWS becomes more widely used, the providers will have more information available during an encounter. The provider will spend some part of the initial encounter with a patient in data entry, but all subsequent encounters will be faster. Redundant data collection, common in manual systems, will eventually be eliminated.

On the other end of the information pipeline, retrieval and review of patient information will also be facilitated by the PWS. Instead of waiting for the delivery of paper records for review, the PWS will give the provider detailed patient information quickly and at the provider's convenience. Further, the highlighting of exceptional conditions (e.g., abnormal laboratory results) on the screen of the PWS will direct the provider's attention to appropriate parts of the patient record. Such highlighting might even occur in realtime when the laboratory reports its results during an encounter. Thus, there will be a cumulative effect that will increase the amount of information collected during an encounter, resulting in more information being available which will allow more specific information to be collected.

The inclusion of order sets which have been customized by a provider will increase the uniformity and quality of treatment. The use of predefined decision-support algorithms at the PWS will let each provider draw on the knowledge of expert providers who created the algorithms. This can be thought of as an *instant* consultation, and will let the providers check their own actions without interrupting other providers. As a beneficial byproduct of this capability, the instant consultation will provide an opportunity for continuing, realtime medical education. Providers can compare their conclusions and plans with the stored information recorded by recognized experts. In the same vein, the capability of the PWS to interface with other external medical reference systems (like MEDLINE) during an encounter will permit providers to explore current medical literature in the context of actual patient problems. If continuing medical education credit hours were assigned to such exploratory sessions, then the providers would find themselves devoting time to learning in the context of a patient problem as a valuable adjunct to formal continuing medical education.

Summary

The provider workstation is to be an intelligent, easy-to-use personal workstation for health care professionals. The integrated suite of application and communications software will connect providers to their integrated hospital information system and the myriad of other medical information systems. Anticipatory computing within an adaptive, object-oriented user interface will enable the user to move at will among these diverse systems. This chapter provides a conceptual framework for the functional components of this workstation, a scenario of how a PWS might be used by a health care provider, and an assessment of some of the user and organizational impacts of the PWS.

References

Bergeron, B.P., and R.A. Greenes. 1987. Intelligent visual input: A graphical method for rapid entry of patient-specific data. In *Proceedings of the Eleventh Annual Symposium on Computer Applications in Medical Care*, 281–286.

Blois, M.S., and E.H. Shortliffe. 1990. The computer meets medicine: emergence of a discipline. In *Medical informatics: Computer applications in health care*, ed. E.H. Shortliffe, L.E. Perreault, G. Wiederhold, and L.M. Fagan. Reading, Mass.: Addison-Wesley.

Blois, M.S. 1985. The physician's personal workstation. *MD Computing* 2:22–26.

Cimino, J.J., and G.O. Barnett. 1987. The physician's workstation: recording a physical examination using a controlled vocabulary. In *Proceedings of the Eleventh Annual Symposium on Computer Applications in Medical Care*, 287–291.

Cristea, D., and T. Mihaescu. 1988. Combining menus with natural language processing in recording medical data. *Journal of Clinical Computing* 16:156–166.

Hammond, W.E., W.W. Stead, S.J. Feagin, B.A. Brantley, and M.J. Straube. 1984. Data base management system for ambulatory care. In *Information systems for patient care*, ed. B.I. Blum et al. New York: Springer-Verlag.

Molich, R., and J. Nielsen. 1990. Improving a human-computer dialogue. *Commun ACM* 33:338–348.

Prokosch, H.U., and T.A. Pryor. 1988. Intelligent data acquisition in order entry programs. In *Proceedings of the Twelfth Annual Symposium on Computer Applications in Medical Care*, 454–458.

Safran, C., W.V. Slack, and H.L. Bleich. 1989. Role of computing in patient care in two hospitals. *MD Computing* 6:141–148.

Slack, W.V. 1989. Editorial. *MD Computing* 6:183–185.

Smith, S.L., and J. Mosier. 1986. *Design guidelines for user-system interface software*. Report ESD-TR-86-278, MTR-10096. Bedford, Mass.: MITRE Corp.

Stead, W.W., and W.E. Hammond. 1987. Demand-oriented medical records: toward a physician workstation. In *Proceedings of the Eleventh Annual Symposium on Computer Applications in Medical Care*, 275–280.

Nielsen, J. 1990. Traditional dialogue design applied to modern user interfaces. *Commun ACM* 33:109–118.

Goodwin, N.C. 1988. *User system interface: Designing for usability, M88–54*. Bedford, Mass.: MITRE Corp.

Heilander, M., ed. 1988. *The handbook of human-computer interaction*. New York: North-Holland/Elsevier.

Laurel, B., ed. 1990. *The art of human-computer interface design*. Reading, Mass.: Addison-Wesley.

Mountford. S.J. 1989. Drama and personality in user interface design. In *Proceedings of the ACM CHI' 89 Conference on Human Factors in Computing Systems*. New York: ACM, 105–108.

Silva, J.S., A.J. Zawilski, J. O'Brian, et al. 1990. The physician workstation: An intelligent "front end" to a hospital information system. In *Proceedings of the Fourteenth Annual Symposium on Computer Applications in Medical Care*, 764–768.

5
Data Acquisition and the Computer-based Patient Record

Allan H. Levy and David P. Lawrance

Data Acquisition

Consideration of data acquisition for the computer-based patient record (CPR) should be accompanied by general understanding of the scope, intended contents and function of the patient record. The medical record serves as an active component of the ongoing care process. It contains information on the origins, progress and outcome of a patient's disease(s) so that optimal care can be provided for the patient over an extended period of time. It contains documentation from all relevant sources. Coupled with medical knowledge bases and appropriate programs for medical inference, the data in the patient record serves as a decision support aid and as a pointer to medical literature (McDonald and Tierney 1986).

In addition to its contemporaneous uses during an episode of illness, the record has many other purposes. As a *permanent record*, it is the prime instrument by which an individual's health status can be assessed, the progress of disease noted, and the effects of intervention assessed. As Weed (1969) has pointed out, the medical record is the tool by which the nature and quality of care is audited, and as such it must serve the needs of health care planners, researchers, lawyers, and third party payers.

An accurate and complete record of care events and their costs must be captured and recorded in the medical record. Table 1, although not comprehensive, indicates the wide variety of information sources which must be considered as a part of a comprehensive medical record. The large variety of sources and uses of medical data poses an enormous problem for the development of the CPR. Consolidating information from many sources remains a substantial CPR research issue. Although major problems have been solved, significant barriers remain. It is a mistake, however, for the CPR planner to abandon serious system design efforts to effectively capture medical data. Progress in improving data acquisition for the CPR can be accomplished simply by using some excellent existing acquisition tools.

This chapter concentrates upon those aspects of data acquisition where either the individual health care provider (doctor, nurse, auxiliary professional) or the

Table 1. Sources of patient data.

	Direct source	Primary recording mode	First recipient of information	Means of subsequent processing	Form in present patient record
1	Patient (or family's) verbal history	Aural	Physician or assistant	Notes by listener	Free text, phrases
2	Patient physical findings, progress	Observational	Physician, nurse, or assistant	Notes	Check sheets, free text
3	Patient physical findings via instrument	Machine (monitor)	Physician or assistant at the nursing lab	Interpretation, clippings	Transcribed extracts, clippings of tracings
4	Patient body fluids (blood, urine, etc.)	Chemical laboratory examination	Laboratory instrument	Electrical signal	Numeric value or categorization
5	Patient's tissue	Gross and microscopic examination	Anatomic pathologist	Observation, notes, dictation	Free text, phrases, diagnostic codes
6	Patient	X-ray imaging	Machine to radiologist	Observation, notes, dictation	Free text, phrases, diagnostic codes, visualized image
7	Patient	Other imaging modalities	Machine to physician-interpreter	Complex signal visualized by mathematical transforms	Free text, phrases, diagnostic codes, actual transformed image
8	Old paper medical records (conventional)	Paper, microfiche	Health care personnel	Copied or collated	Copies, abstracts, diagnostic codes, free text
9	Past medical records (computer)	Computer	Computer	Electronic transfer	Original form of computer record
10	Financial and other linking information	Old paper records, computer data banks	Either clerical or computer	Manual or electronic transfer	Written entries, codes 2° indices

patient is the primary instrument of data capture. Data capture from physiologic monitors will also be discussed, and there will an overview of laboratory data acquisition. This report is *interpretive* of current problems and *prescriptive* of future solutions, rather than purely descriptive.

Acquiring Data from Professionals: Some Propositions and Associated Problems

Specific needs demand customized forms of data entry. A single hardware/software/terminal system does not suffice for the capture of all types of medical data. Two general propositions relating to medical data acquisition are set forth. These are presented not as maxims universally accepted or proven; rather they point to areas needing further consideration and evaluation:

• Proposition 1: Insofar as possible, each event should be recorded once and only once as proximate as possible to its occurrence.
• Proposition 2: Data should generally be recorded by the individual first acquiring it.

Recording information once reduces both error and cost. In practice, it has usually not been possible to design systems that implement this principle to any substantial degree. The second proposition is a matter of debate; it relates especially to data input by professionals.

Regarding Proposition 1: Recording Data Once—Problems and Pitfalls

Although a datum should be entered only once, it often needs to be available at multiple locations. Although summary laboratory reports reach the patient record, detailed records like batch numbers, specimen location, and the like will be kept by the laboratory as part of its quality control system. Information common among knowledge bases and reports may be acquired once but widely shared. The proposition of single entry implies automatic and appropriate forwarding.

Unfortunately, data entry responsibilities are usually relegated to clerical personnel rather than to the primary caregiver (nurse, physician). The reasons are related to terminal hardware, physical factors, software and system design, and to factors associated with professional attitudes and training.

Terminals and Hardware Limitations

Because of their size, large terminals have been restricted to areas with adequate space, even if it was not very convenient for users. In contrast, many recorded observations by nurses and physicians take place *at the bedside*.

Once installed, terminals are not been easily relocated. Not just size, but power consumption, weight, heat generation, and noise are limiting factors. Cabling, inadequate displays, poorly designed keyboards, and awkward ergonomics are often present.

Terminals are often (or appeared to be) difficult to operate. They often have an abundance of switches, buttons, and knobs whose functions are either unknown or unnecessary. All buttons are an invitation to be pushed; extra buttons are an opportunity for malfunction.

Terminal display output affects data acquisition accuracy. Terminals must prompt, show intermediate results, and act as intelligent guides to facilitate primary data capture. Clarity of display, adequate screen size, and the ability to provide displays combining text (with differing font sizes and styles) combined with graphics are all necessary.

Software

Programs for data entry are too complex: complicated logins, command structures with no obvious mnemonic content, reference to obscure abbreviations, and unfamiliar coding schemes for data entry, restrictive field sizes, and data types. Data editing is usually cumbersome.

Personnel Attitudes and Training Factors

Many senior health care personnel have adopted the attitude that data entry is a "clerical" function, unworthy of their time or consideration. The time-consuming, repetitious, and tedious nature of data recording in manual systems was only *intensified* by early automated data entry systems. Data entry, no pleasure at best, was converted into exercises of advanced frustration by the inadequacies of early hardware/software/system design combinations.

Many, but not all, of these problems can be avoided using contemporary design engineering principles. Attitudinal issues can be addressed during undergraduate professional school training. Continued emphasis must be placed on the importance of data acquisition and record keeping by both continued inservice training and by the example of supervisory personnel.

Regarding Proposition 2: Recording Data by the Original Observer

The goal of the proposition is to preserve the quality and the timeliness of the data. These two subgoals sometimes compete.

A principal question is, can physicians be induced to type? Many in the field of medical informatics feel that it is imperative that the primary observer record patient data to ensure its accuracy, validity, and timeliness. Conversely, others observe that systems that relied upon physicians to use a keyboard failed. Most attempts to induce physicians to enter data via keyboards have met with only very low degrees of physician cooperation, and data entry is usually turned over to other personnel.

The reasons are many. Most physicians cannot speed type and therefore avoid such clerical tasks. The greater economic value of physicians' time supports a division of labor where only physicians see patients and only clerks produce legible documents. The ability of the physician to delegate is a factor. A quest for simplicity and speed is another factor. We have not yet approached the convenience of paper and pencil as a data entry device (with the possible exception of voice entry. However, the *subsequent limitations of manual entry* in terms of legibility and analysis are cogent reasons for seeking machine-readable primary input.

Can it be different in the planned CPR? Should direct physician entry of data even be attempted or should we seek alternate methods? In lieu of physician-typed reports, digital voice recordings could be accessible until transcribed. Written notes could be digitally imaged (by whom?) and recalled in that form until typed. Automatic or computer-assisted transcription from continuous speech is an advancing science that will ultimately and dramatically change the role of the transcriptionist. Optical character recognition and automatic handwriting analysis will also modify the transcriptionist's role, reducing the need for typewriter style keyboarding. We can also expect the development of predictive user interfaces anticipating options, presenting at all times an appropriate selection of icons. These could altogether replace free-text editors.

Direct Acquisition of Information from Patients

Branching questionnaires have been successfully employed for years as an effective means of acquiring a thorough history from the patient. The efforts of Slack (1984) in this area have been exceptionally noteworthy. He and others have demonstrated the utility of computer administered histories. A number of studies have confirmed that patients will accept computers as vehicles for providing medical information. There have even been indications that some patients may be more willing to impart sensitive medical information to an impersonal computer than they would be to unfamiliar physicians. Some patients appreciate the unhurried pace of interacting with a computer terminal that is not queued up. Accordingly, this mode of acquiring patient information should be more thoroughly explored and evaluated.

Acquisition of History and Physical by Physicians

No data entry problem is more challenging than that of acquiring data obtained from conversation with and examination of the patient. The importance of the history and the physical examination has been apparent since at least the nineteenth century. The computer provided the impetus for better methods of capturing this information. However, computer implementations have pointed out the unresolved issues of how best to *organize basic medical information*. The form of the medical record is now fixed primarily by habit and custom. Attempts to rationalize and change the basic organization of the medical record have been poorly accepted in practice, although often met with enthusiasm in principle. Because proper data acquisition methods are related to the organization of the medical record, it is useful to note some of the common formats used today.

Traditional Form of the Primary Patient Workup

The prevalent form of the conventional medical record is that of a structured narrative, employing free text with an abundance of key words and phrases. The record is arranged, at least in theory, to provide a broad and complete profile of the patient's background relevant to the presenting illness. Emphasis is placed upon the history of the present illness, nearly always as unconstrained free text. Sections, akin to chapters in a book, form other portions—history, review of symptoms, and the like. This general organization is the conventional mode, although specialties have modified it for particular needs. Increasingly, check sheets with conditions common in a particular field of medicine supplement the narrative history, enabling a briefer, faster recording. Check sheets are also commonly employed for the physical examination, with specialized check sheets and data recording forms being common for specialties.

Problem-Oriented Form of the Primary Patient Workup

There are a number of valuable lessons to be learned from the difficulties of integrating the problem-oriented medical record (POMR) devised by Weed (1969), into a total computer-based patient management system. Weed's suggestion that the single narrative of present illness be clearly divided into separate problem-oriented segments had a substantial influence on medical history taking. The concept was that physician-recorded information became a component of a larger system, allowing expert-derived systems of rules and procedures to guide the physician in the patient workup. Although a substantial portion of the rules and decision support for his PROMIS system was written, the integrated information system did not gain wide acceptance and has not survived in its original or intended form (Fischer 1980). However, the POMR remains a popular patient record format.

The obstacles to acceptance of the PROMIS system should be noted. The use of the system required the concurrent input of data as it was gathered in order for it to be useful for immediate medical management. This conflicted with the conventional practice of physician data entry: note taking during examination and narrative writing later. Furthermore, PROMIS provided detailed advice concerning the workup of patients not necessarily reflecting the practice modes of individual users. Some saw the system as excessively authoritarian. It follows that any system of recording data that suggests subsequent management should, at the very least, represent a consensus or provide gentle advice (McDonald 1984). More than that, it should offer alternates and be modifiable within broad limits by the individual physician or clinic.

The Physician as a Participant in Data Capture for the CPR

Health care providers are a challenge for designers of data acquisition systems. They require the flexibility to permit the gathering a wide variety of information over very broad domains of knowledge. Their practice modes and vocabulary are relatively unconstrained. Time is at a premium. Under these circumstances, what can be done to enhance their active participation of recording data into the CPR? Three factors should be considered:

- Incentives and benefits for establishing a CPR
- The organization of the record
- A changing attitude toward the role of the record

Incentives and benefits. Health professionals should see tangible benefits from direct data entry into a computer-based record. It is unlikely that the cost or the time of data entry will be reduced. However, it is important that the cost:benefit not be increased. If economic return is not a direct result, then what are some secondary benefits? A CPR system can provide the health care provider with better practice management, integrated accounting systems for the office/clinic, and automatic claims filing. The ability to link inpatient to outpatient records will save time and expense. A CPR system allowing dynamic restructuring of the record can demonstrate problem-oriented information displays rather than temporally ordered postings. If information in the CPR system is cumulative, crossing individual patient record boundaries, then institutional level experience is extractable, for example, the HELP system at the Hospital of Latter Day Saints (Pryor et al. 1983).

There are other less tangible benefits. The physician may gain increased job satisfaction relating to the practice of medicine if there is a high quality medical record available for each patient in the practice. The ability to link records with bibliographic and consultative knowledge bases will raise the standards of care and provide the physician with a real shield against unjustified claims of malpractice.

Organization of the record. The form of the medical record has a considerable influence upon the design of the data capture tools. There is no single style of medical record keeping that is currently practiced in the United States. At one extreme, the traditional narrative medical record is commonly employed. Elsewhere, the discipline of the problem-oriented medical record is obeyed. The norm lies in the middle, including a brief narrative for the present illness and a combination of specialized forms for special data recording. For a hospital to impose a single form of record keeping upon all physicians would appear to be an approach destined to end in failure. However, alternate approaches are possible without sacrificing a record with comparable meaning and standards of quality, irrespective of the place or mode of collection. Three such approaches are considered:

- Standardized definitions for medical terminology, with linkages between regional and local vocabularies and coding schemas via comprehensive thesauruses, such as those being developed by the Unified Medical Language System project (Humphreys and Lindberg 1989).
- Defined minimum subsets of record content for various environments and specialties. Thus, the requirement for a CPR from an ophthalmology outpatient clinic would be different from that of a general medical nursing unit.
- Defined protocols for the aggregation of these record subsets into a master patient record.

The Patient Computer Record: Interaction with Hospital and Other Medical Information Systems

CPR data acquisition is only one factor, but perhaps the critical one, affecting the function of any health information system (HIS). (The abbreviation HIS has usually been applied to mean Hospital Information System, but this terminology ignores the fact that care is carried out in many different settings: free-standing doctors' offices, hospital-based clinics, well-baby clinics, and rehabilitation centers, among others.) Examination reports performed in the clinic setting may also become part of the hospital record when a patient is admitted.

Portions of the patient medical record that must be duplicated in both of these settings are already electronically communicable to payers, indicating again the poser of financial incentive. Although the ability to merge provider and provider/institution information sets may yield long-range efficiencies, to whose advantage is this? Independent and small group practices may be unwilling to invest in automating their offices to the primary benefit of their hospitals. Although it is often stated that hospitals might provide this service to small practices as a marketing tool, should we depend upon this?

The extent of and the mechanisms for linkages among medical records kept at different sites is an important issue. Which components of information collected at specialized treatment centers should become part of a centralized patient record is a matter worthy of further consideration.

The institution of an adequate patient computer record must impose few new demands on the basic processes of care given in the nursing unit. It may well require changes in the manner by which other practices are currently carried out. When one considers the time required for primary machine recording of patient care-related information, focus is frequently centered upon the additional time required for data entry into computer terminals. Historically, the formidable nature of some software and the bulky and inconvenient operating modes of older hardware imposed significant additional burdens. *This is no longer a necessary consequence, given the present state of the art.* Smaller terminals, handheld devices, barcode readers, optical scanners, and voice recognition capabilities are easing the mechanics of data entry to a degree where machine entry is only as difficult or less so than present manual methods. Manual recording ("Write once–read maybe") currently exacts a considerable burden upon the medical staff. Even now, the paper and ink notation of an event or an order may be quicker than a terminal entry, but the additional time required throughout the rest of the system in terms of subsequent deciphering, retranscription, and retrieval diminishes this advantage. However, in planning for the specifics of terminal use, defined time and motion studies *using a variety of new terminals and data acquisition systems* should be carried out.

Acquisition of Data from Laboratory Instruments

Over the last 25 years, few areas have seen such growth both in importance to the practice of medicine and in the volume of transactions as has the clinical laboratory. Laboratory testing is now of central importance in the diagnostic workup. Furthermore, in an increasing number of disease/treatment combinations, laboratory monitoring of changes is an important component of management. The number of laboratory tests commonly performed has increased rapidly. If there is a success story to be found in the application of computer-based information systems to the medical care process, it is the laboratory information system. All but the smallest laboratories have at the least automated their analysis instruments. Many laboratories have also automated the acquisition, storage, and reporting of laboratory data through the installation of dedicated laboratory information systems. Laboratory analyzers are sold with built-in interfaces to computer-based information systems.

Numerous laboratory information systems are commercially available; many carry out functions that go beyond the simple recording and retrieval of test results. A comprehensive laboratory information system will accept orders from the nursing unit, generate blood drawing worksheets, log specimens into the lab, accept analyzer results and report them back to the nursing unit. The method of order input varies, including paper requisitions, transmittal via the hospital information system, and separate laboratory system terminals at the nursing unit or laboratory office. These direct clinical functions are usually complemented by a number of laboratory management services. Many laboratory information systems provide facilities for quality control of instruments and analyses, and management information in the form of running statistics on the volume and types of laboratory test used.

The clinical laboratory has become substantially (virtually absolutely) dependent on computer-based information systems. Convincing the pathologist to install a laboratory computer system will not be a problem for those involved with establishing a CPR. Rather, the focus of attention will be the integration into the record of laboratory information *already present in electronic form.*

Problems

Several problems relating to the laboratory require serious study:

* *Nomenclature for tests often differs from system to system.* Standards are being developed but are not yet universally required or used in various systems. The nomenclature for test designation does not unambiguously designate the method by which the analysis is performed, and hence units of measurement and ranges of normal values may not be apparent from a test report.
* *The nature of the data needs to be standardized.* A laboratory information system purchased today is not likely to easily integrate with a hospital's medical record system or an imaging department's picture archival and retrieval system. Not only may separate hospital departments have too narrow an institutional focus to facilitate information sharing, but the same is often regrettably true of different product lines offered by a single vendor. Standards groups composed of vendors and customer representatives are successfully attacking these problems; such groups include the American Society of Testing Materials (ASTM), Health Level Seven (HL7), and the American College of Radiology and the National Electronic Manufacturers' Association (ACR-NEMA).
* *Signal-level and cabling transmission protocols for test results differ from system to system.* It will continue to be desirable for laboratory and other highly specialized units to maintain individual information systems tailored to the particular needs of the clinical unit. However, it is critical that data from each

of these special systems can be received and understood by other components of the system. Network protocols accepted by vendors of both general and special systems are needed. This will permit the design of gateways which can pass information from one network to another.

Acquisition of Data from Patients via Monitoring Devices

Currently, large amounts of data are acquired from electronic monitoring of patients. Coronary care units, medical, surgical, and neonatal intensive care units, and operating rooms are among the units with special instrumentation. Currently, there are no universally accepted standards for either the nomenclature or units of measurement of the patient variables measured, nor do different manufacturers' machines employ common file format, code representation, or physical recording parameters. Many of these devices do allow for ASCII interchange of data via RS-232 interface. However, ready *direct* incorporation of data from monitors into a central information system and thereby into the CPR is uncommon. Frequently, segments of recorded data are manually transcribed into the patient record. In other cases, portions of hard copy obtained from the special monitoring equipment is clipped out and inserted into the paper record. In nearly all cases, only manually selected information is permanently inserted into the CPR.

More effective integration of data derived from monitoring is required as a step in the development of the CPR.

Financial Data and the Patient Computer Record

Capturing financial data is currently the major focus of most hospital information systems (HIS). We assert that instead of this being the primary design goal, financial data acquisition should be treated as an important but *natural derivative* of an adequate patient computer record. The need for hospitals to have adequate information about costs, services provided, and moneys received is undeniable. Furthermore, there is a clear need for billing information to be accurate and available contemporaneously during the patient's hospital admission. This need can be met, however, through a medically oriented information system with the patient record as its nidus—the center of growth for the entire system.

The emphasis on fiscal data has resulted in the development of online systems for data capture of charges and for the development of many independent subsystems for their analysis and subsequent reporting. If the level of effort expended in this direction had been accompanied by equal attention to capturing the content of the medical events that caused the generation of the charges, then the CPR would already be well advanced.

There were sound reasons for avoiding a medically oriented hospital information system in the past. Now, many of the difficulties of data acquisition, human interfaces, and access to stored information have been obviated by progress in technology. There is a renewed imperative for accurate medical data with detailed third party and governmental scrutiny of the details of care.

The ability to better capture both process and outcome information may revolutionize payers' abilities to control both the quality and the cost of care. Incentives to develop CPRs could originate primarily from the payers as complete systems and regulations. However, the uncritical demand for capturable information could result in much more, not less, documentation overhead if the desires for apparently useful indices of quality outpace abilities to automate their capture.

Preliminary Recommendations

These recommendations primarily cover data acquisition in which medical professionals (physicians, nurses, other medical auxiliaries) acquire information through observation or direct physical examination. Recommendations about nomenclature standardization, transmission protocols, imaging, and detailed recommendations relating to terminals and workstations are dealt elsewhere. These are touched upon in this report only as necessary to adequately support and justify the recommendations relating to data acquisition.

Modifying Institutional Behavior: Incentives and Expectations in Health Care Settings

The use of electronic data capture must be encouraged throughout each health care setting. Senior management at each operational level (nursing supervisors, physician chiefs of staff, ancillary department managers) must themselves be convinced that primary electronic data capture of medical events is important to their function and is an imperative for their subordinates and coworkers. The use of terminals and electronic data acquisition systems must be internalized into the corporate/institutional culture of health care settings. This can be accomplished through training, incentives, and individual example.

Training. Use of new systems for data acquisition requires carefully planned training programs. These do have a cost in time of personnel away from normal duties and in the cost of the teachers, trainers, and materials. Although good training is indispensable, it is frequently inadequately accommodated.

Incentives. Personnel should be rewarded in some appropriate manner for use of and acceptance of the CPR. The nature of these incentives is extremely complex. One should not expect employees at any level to perform well if they are ordered to do a job without any understanding of the reasons for the new tasks and the benefits to them. Positive reinforcements should be provided. Personnel should receive some tangible evidence of how other components of their responsibilities are made either easier or more effective.

Care providers must receive benefits from more useful information output if they are to be expected to participate directly and personally in automated data acquisition. The timely availability of accurate, legible information relating to a patient's status is usually considered as the one prime benefit. The value of this should be further tested by formal evaluation. Linking the medical input information to other information and decision making resources (bibliographic databases, automated consultation programs, protocols for treatment planning) is another such incentive; this has a high probability of beneficially affecting direct physician participation in an automated data acquisition process. The need and value of this should also be tested.

Some existing job positions may require reclassification to higher skills levels having increased salaries. This will tend to be unpalatable to hospital and other health care institutional administrators; it may be desirable in the intermediate term because of improvement in institutional efficiency and care quality.

By Individual Example. Senior personnel must be sufficiently motivated so that they themselves use the system for their own job responsibilities. New physicians must not be made to feel odd if they admit to entering data into the computer.

Modifying Institutional Behavior: Patterns of Information Flow

The adoption of substantial levels of automated data processing requires a concomitant rethinking of the general information flow throughout a health care institution. Time lags, redundancy, and duplication that are prevalent in existing manual systems protect data integrity. As automated systems improve efficiency, they may cause increased possibility of errors. The introduction of automated medical data capture should be accompanied by management consideration of the need for changed levels of responsibility and organization. The impact upon employees who may feel they have become subordinate in the process has to be considered. Without explanation and justification, such feelings can turn into resentment against change and covert sabotage of the endeavor. However, even with this caution, management must not lose sight of the advantages that will be realized through more extensive automated data capture and more easily available medical information at a managerial level.

Factors Related to the Data Acquisition System

Software

Software must be easy to use and must facilitate data entry. Command structure of different programs should be *related* and have a *consistent* thread of logical design from program to program. Although data fields in an intensive care unit will be different from those in a general surgical unit, a common mode of information acquisition should be recognizable. Insofar as possible, skills in data entry learned in one unit should carry over to other areas of care administration.

Programs designed to accept data from professional personnel should have machine/human interfaces that reflect the level of training of the personnel using them. In some cases, relatively untrained individuals may be recording items of information (i.e., aides may record pulse, blood pressure, height and weight). These individuals should have access to interfaces that allow very simple data entry techniques. Nurses need to enter detailed observations relating to mental status, general physical condition, and other specialized data. Physicians need to record detailed data but will be less frequent users of a hospital information system than nurses or aides. The set of tools they will require will of necessity be more complete, yet they should not be more complex.

The interface provided all personnel should offer them a relatively broad choice among various modes of operation. *Icon-based* control structures have achieved wide popularity in recent years and various pointers (mouse, trackball, touch panel, joystick) have been used as devices to assist data input. Many users enjoy and are comfortable with these. However, others welcome the opportunity to give *direct* and explicit *commands* through the keyboard without traversing hierarchies of menus or multiple pulldown and pop-up windows. Good interfaces can accommodate both modes, allowing users to shift from verbose to expert modes of data entry as their familiarity with programs increases.

Hardware

Terminals appropriate to the activities within a work area or unit should be used. New construction of health care facilities should include provisions for physical location and *easy relocation of terminals* and other electronic information-processing equipment. Bedside outlets for terminals are now in place at some hospitals. Hospital renovation should include provisions for this.

Adequate numbers of terminals and data recording devices must be placed at convenient locations. Delays or waiting lines should not be an impeding factor for recording data.

The physical attributes of data terminals must be considered. Size, weight, power requirements, and heat production are all important. Preferably, a terminal should be easily portable; failing that, it should be easily relocatable. Studies should be carried out regarding the desirability of *wireless handheld terminals* broadcasting to a nearby receiving multiplexor.

Acquisition of Data Directly from Patients

Patients should be more involved in terms of direct data entry into the CPR. Questionnaires can be administered via computer terminal. In this mode, advantage can be taken of branching logic. As is the case with use by medical personnel, terminal and software design will have to be carefully suited to the general sophistication of the patient population served. If the CPR is coupled to the patient questionnaire, the formulation of questions can be made more specific to the nature of the patient's problems and highly detailed information relating to the specific patient problem can be collected. In this way, the value of computer-based patient records can be further enhanced.

Acquisition of Data from Patients via Monitoring Devices

Provision should be made for the *selective incorporation of data obtained from instruments into the patient record.* Appropriate automation of data reduction, analysis, and interpretation will be necessary in order to make this step practical. It is not simply impractical but disadvantageous to include all the information from all monitors in the patient record in an undigested form. However, the present means of manual selection and transcription can be substantially improved by using automated selection of data. Programs embodying knowledge-based systems can analyze data in trends and flag abnormalities. This will represent an *advanced stage* of development of the CPR. Before this can be realized, standardization of nomenclature, units of measurement, machine output format, and codes will be necessary to avoid the inevitable confusion that will result if there is need for special translation tables to accommodate each monitoring instrument.

Factors Related to Data Transfer and Sharing

Standardized nomenclature for many elements of the medical record should be adopted. Such standards are especially critical for the appropriate incorporation into the CPR of data originating from the clinical laboratory. Much work has already been accomplished in this area through national standards organizations.

It is imperative that this effort receive a *high priority* and that strong incentives be provided to both vendors and users to adhere to such standards.

Standards that are produced should be *amenable to extension* as new tests and methods are developed. Furthermore, a permanent national group with either official or quasi-official status should be clearly charged with the maintenance of such standards.

Medical terminology in general requires better definition. The efforts underway through the Unified Medical Language System (UMLS) project of the National Library of Medicine is a key to accomplishing this. This effort should be considered as a critical component of efforts to produce a useful CPR that will have more than local acceptance.

The proper balance must be found between the ongoing need for free text for the richness of meaning that exists in natural language and the advantages with regard to uniformity and clarity of definition that result the use of standardized vocabularies. Further field trial studies are necessary. In the interim, the computer-based medical record should allow for the incorporation of free text as a component of the record, or make adequate provisions for linkage with free text stored separately from the CPR.

A Master Index for Each Patient Record

Renewed attention should be given to establishing a single master patient record for each individual. In contrast to earlier suggestions for the single patient record, this could now take the form of an index to individual patient records held at various institutions and linked as necessary via network. Suggestions for a master *birth-to-death* record have been made in the past. Citywide efforts to establish this have been attempted without evident success. The proposition to restudy this is made with full knowledge of the attendant difficulties in a country whose system operates at so many different levels as does health care in the United States. However, an alternate approach can be tried, involving not the physical collection of all medical information for a patient at one site, but rather a central index to a patient's subset medical records (clinics, hospitals, subacute care facilities, etc.). The patient's index itself could be transferred to the custody of the care provider with primary charge of the patient at any particular time. Careful attention must be given to patient's rights to privacy and confidentiality. (The particular suggestion is very tentative, made with the realization that many other methods must be studied.)

References

Fischer, P.J., W.C. Stratmann, H.P. Lundsgaarde, and D.J. Steele. 1980. User reaction to PROMIS: Issues related to acceptability of medical innovations. *Proceedings of the Fourth Annual Symposium on Computer Applications in Medical Care*, J. O'Neil, ed. Washington, D.C.: IEEE Computer Society Press.

Humphreys, B., and D. Lindberg. 1989. Building the unified medical language system. *Proceedings of the Thirteenth Annual Symposium on Computer Applications in Medical Care*, L. Kingsland II, ed. Washington, D.C.: IEEE Computer Society Press.

McDonald, C.J., S.L. Hui, D.M. Smith, W.M. Tierney, S.J. Cohen, M. Weinberger, and G.P. McCabe. 1984. Reminders to physicians from an introspective medical record: A two year randomized trial. *Annals of Internal Medicine* 199:330.

McDonald, C.J., and W.M. Tierney. 1986. The medical gopher: A microcomputer system to help find, organize and decide about patient data. *Western Journal of Medicine* 145:823.

Pryor, D., R.M. Gardner, P.D. Clayton, and R.H. Warner. 1983. The HELP system. *Journal of Medical Systems* 7:87–102.

Slack, W. 1984. A history of computerized medical interviews. *MD Computing* 5:52.

Weed, L.L. 1969. *Medical records, medical education and patient care: The problem-oriented record as a basic tool.* Chicago: Year Book Medical Publishers.

6
Data Entry for Computer-based Patient Records

Gregory C. Critchfield

Laboratory Environment

Review of Current State of Technology

In many ways, significant inroads into data entry for the computer-based patient record (CPR) have already been made from the hospital laboratory. This is in part due to the large number of data that originate from laboratory sources (estimates place somewhere near 40 percent of the CPR is derived from these sources), as well as the generally *numerate* nature of the data. Laboratory computers process patient laboratory results and collate them into a computerized laboratory report. Most major laboratory information system (LIS) vendors devise interfaces with hospital information systems so that the machine readable data from the laboratory become available to the CPR.

The workers who generate laboratory information are primarily laboratory medical technologists, cytologists, and pathologists. Currently, there are two major methods of data entry:

- Interaction with a cathode ray tube (CRT), which could be either a terminal or a computer
- Online interfaces to automated laboratory instruments

The terminals support entry of textual information, laboratory results entry and verification, inquiry of the laboratory database, and quality control review. These data input functions are presently well-developed in the clinical laboratory side.

In the case of anatomic pathology (surgical pathology and autopsy, as well as hematology reports), pathologists typically dictate reports that are transcribed and printed. In most situations, the computer is used only for its word processing features. SNOMED encoding (which could have significant utility in the CPR, if accurately and consistently performed) is customarily performed by residents in university settings, while in most community hospital settings this task is carried out either by a secretary or clerk or not at all.

Most laboratories are in the process of assessing the value of integrating various sources of information with local area networks (LANs) for the purpose of speeding the flow of information and decreasing transcription error rates. More recently, the use of image processing systems has received more attention (McEachron 1989; Robb 1987; Weinstein 1987).

Optimal and Practical CPR Systems Achievable by 1995

As far as the laboratory is concerned there are several major areas for growth that can be achieved doable by 1995:

Graphical interfaces to data entry and inquiry. Given the enormous amount of laboratory information, clearer and more intuitive methods will continue to be developed to aid the workers in interpreting the data. One method for doing this will be more extensive use of computer graphics. The graphic user interface (GUI) pioneered at Xerox Park and popularized by the Macintosh will find greater use in helping health care professionals interact with the patient record. Although there is a great deal of interest in developing such systems, significant research into human factors tailored for the medical environment will still need to be performed. The success of such efforts will depend on whether there are advantages (e.g., time, effort, accuracy) over traditional methods for interacting with the patient medical record (Mandell 1987).

Full text retrieval. Anatomic pathology written reports could be stored in their full text format using several commercially available products or adaptations of them. This information retrieval technology is available on PCs, principally of the IBM-compatible variety, but is being ported to other systems.

Full image retrieval. By 1995 images of any anatomic examination could be available as part of the CPR. To store, retrieve, and display such images would require the existence of technology to scan and digitize histologic and cytologic slides, store the data in a compressed format on a high capacity medium (e.g., optical disk drive), and a suitable high resolution display. There are many analogies in image processing of radiologic images as well.

Currently, resolution equal to that of television is attainable on both Macintosh II and IBM PC-compatible computer systems. This quality of display probably would not be adequate for primary review of the material by anatomic diagnosticians, but would be sufficient for cataloging purposes when combined with the textual report of the reviewer's findings.

It is reasonable to expect that advances in technology will permit better performance at more reasonable costs.

High band width communications network links. Irrespective of where information will be stored, full text and full image retrieval presuppose that there will be a means for communicating large quantities of information to the end user. This requires that high band width communications networks be in place, so that graphic and textual information can be transmitted efficiently from the point of creation to the information consumers. Rigorous assessments will need to be made of how much information is to be transmitted for high resolution images, the rapidity of the data transfer, and the time to process the images at the peripheral workstation.

Improvements in SNOMED encoding and knowledge representation. Although free text has traditionally conveyed important information to the end user, it is not in a form that readily supports decision logic in a computer-based system. One means for improving this is to have automatic encoding whereby text is filtered and pertinent diagnostic information is extracted. The extracted data can become the framework for a knowledge representation.

A solution to the high prevalence of inaccurate coding is to improve the algorithms for automatic encoding and allow a higher level diagnostician review of the machine-derived codes. With an appropriate user interface, this review might be a simple (not unpleasant) task that would improve the quality of coding.

Voice recognition systems. At a recent COMDEX (Las Vegas, November 1989), several voice recognition systems (VRS) were demonstrated. (One was demonstrated in which WordPerfect commands were given through a microphone rather than a keyboard.) Currently, VRSs have been shown to have a restricted vocabulary and to perform slowly. However, speed has increased in many of the recent offerings. It is probably safe to project that humans will continue interacting with computers through keyboard, mouse, and lightpen interfaces for the next decade or so (Murchie 1988). Nonetheless, there may be limited areas in the laboratory (and hospital) environment where this technology might improve on the user interface. These systems require a voice recognition board in a computer and the appropriate software drivers. There are still many issues to be settled concerning how such a system would be implemented, including (1) how the system is trained to an individual's voice, (2) issues of security, (3) vocabulary limitations, (4) cost, and (5) compatibility with software. The issue of compatibility with many software packages is addressed by the use of memory-resident software that intercepts the user's voice, translates the verbal commands into scan codes (identical with those of the keyboard), and sends the scan codes to the computer.

Hospital Environment

Current State of Technology

Although there are several systems that can be cited for both pioneering and state of the art development for health care worker-derived information for CPRs, I will discuss a few with which I am most familiar.

The HELP (Health Evaluation through Logical Processes) System at Latter Day Saints (LDS) Hospital has been developed over the last two decades by Dr. Homer Warner and coworkers. The system is an extensive realtime patient care database, with logical frames that are fired as the system becomes aware of new data. These decision frames reflect various levels of concern that a conscientious health care provider would exhibit as information becomes available on a patient. Various levels of caution or warning are provided to the human caregivers based on the decision logic (which is framed by clinical experts and knowledge engineers). The data are derived from multiple sources in the hospital setting, including the clinical laboratory, pharmacy, radiology, cardiac catheterization laboratory, pulmonary function laboratory, nursing, and physicians themselves.

Data acquisition takes place via online interfaces from the clinical laboratory sources. The pharmacy interacts with a pharmacy module in the HELP system. The nursing staff use bedside terminals for each patient into which nursing care plans and information are entered. The radiology department uses terminals into the HELP system, where diagnoses are entered from the radiologists' reports. Physicians use CRTs at nursing stations to look up laboratory information and can enter certain orders via the same interface. In general, the input into the HELP system is performed by menu selection, then data entry (with the exception of online instrument interfaces).

Generally, other medical centers employ the same type of CRT-based technology (Chan 1987; Seiver 1987) but perhaps without the degree of integration seen in the HELP system. Several improvements to user interfaces in many centers have been made with GUI-based systems (Loeb 1989; Quaak 1987).

Optimal and Practical CPR Systems Achievable by 1995

An optimal system for data entry by health care workers would have several characteristics:

It would be based on personal computer/workstation technology. Significant advances in microelectronics in the last decade include the development of 32-bit processors that make it practical and cost effective to build personal computers/workstations that can be useful in the hospital environment. Not all the advances in technology come from hardware, since several important software tools have also become available such as page description languages, hypertext linkages (Timpka 1989), personal computer versions of LISP, C, Modula, object-oriented extensions to languages, and inexpensive database primitives, to name a few.

The system would allow high resolution graphic displays of data (see above). The use of radiologic and pathologic images with textual reports could enhance the CPR (Huang 1987). Although radiology is not discussed above, considerations are similar to the efforts described with pathology.

The workstation would be linked via high band width communications links to other sources of data both in and beyond the hospital environment. Connectivity to many sources of information is critical and will aid the health care worker to improve the quality of the information put into the CPR.

The system would use local (with or without remote), erasable, and read-only optical disk storage. This would allow access to a wide variety of "static" information as well as data that change rapidly in the clinical setting.

The operating system (OS) wold be multi-tasking, so that a variety of tasks could take place simultaneously. The resulting functionality would be transparent to the end user.

This would allow a worker to continue to input data while information from the laboratory or pharmacy was updating the individual patient's record. The system would then operate in realtime.

Versions of multitasking OSs are now available on personal computers (e.g., UNIX, OS2, AUX, etc.).

The system would not be costly. A rough cost estimate (projecting to 1995) of a workstation with the capabilities described above (including realtime image processing) is as follows:

Central processing unit	
30+ MHz process	
4–8 Mbytes memory	
Ethernet IF	$3000
Magnetic hard disk drive, 300 Mbytes	700
Optical disk drive, 1 Gigabyte	500
System software	1000
Voice recognition board and software	800
Scanner and digitizing software	1000
Video camera	500
Applications software	2000
	$9500

Alternatives to the Above Projected Technologies

Several microcomputer interfaced devices could be used by health care professionals to enter patient data into a computer system and by patients themselves. Certainly hybrid approaches may offer the best of many worlds for implementing the varied data entry tasks inherent in the medical setting. Among these could be the marriage of videodisk technologies with the computer for elicited histories from patients, handheld devices (microphones, small keyboards, electronic clipboards, scanners, etc.) that health care workers could use to interact with computers. The communications could take place via radio frequency signals or through LAN or other ports into the computer system. Because of the plethora of possibilities, cost projections are speculative. Nonetheless, there will be a great deal of interest in their development.

References

Chan, D.H., et al. 1987. A microcomputer-based medical record system for a general practice teaching clinic. *J Family Pract* 24:537–541.

Huang, H.K. 1987. Progress in image processing technology relate to radiological sciences: a five year-review. *Comput Methods Programs Biomed* 25:143–156.

Loeb, R.G., et al. 1989. The Utah anesthesia workstation. *Anesthesiology* 70:999–1007.

Mandell, S.F. 1987. Resistance to computerization. An examination of the relationship between resistance and the cognitive style of the clinician. *J Med Sys* 11:311–318.

McEachron, D.L., et al. 1989. Image processing for the rest of us: the potential utility of inexpensive computerized image analysis in clinical pathology and radiology. *Comput Med Imaging Graph* 13:3–30.

Murchie, C.J., et al. 1988. A comparison of keyboard, light pen, and voice recognition as methods of data input. *Int J Clin Monit Comput* 5:243–246.

Quaak, M.J., et al. 1987. Automation of the patient history—evaluation of ergonomic aspects. *Int J Biomed Comput* 21:287–98

Robb, R.A.. et al. 1987. A workstation for multi-dimensional display and analysis of medical images. *Comput Methods Programs Biomed* 25:169–84.

Seiver, A., et al. 1987. Bedside computers in the surgical intensive care unit. *Angiology* 38:248–252.

Timpka, T. 1989. Introducing hypertext in primary health care: a study of the feasibility of decision support for practitioners. *Comput Methods Programs Biomed* 29:1–13.

Weinstein, R.S., et al. 1987. Telepathology and the networking of pathology diagnostic services. *Arch Pathol Lab Med* 111:646–652.

Selected Bibliography

Massey, J.K., et al. 1987. A PC-based free text retrieval system for health care providers: Design and development. *J Med Sys* 11:69–71.

7
Information Retrieval

Allan H. Levy and David P. Lawrance

The purpose of a medical record system is to recall, reorder, and summarize data. Information is its product. If useful information cannot be retrieved, then data need not be acquired. If the product is useful, then the cost of data assimilation may be justifiable, The worthiness of an information system is very much dependent upon the utility of retrievals.

Medical information is retrieved in three principal modes:

- Information from outside the patient record enhances general knowledge useful in the care of a patients.
- Information from the medical record is usually sought in a problem related mode. The record is queried for information specific to a particular patient, often in the context of a clinical situation.
- Information is required to manage urgent situations. Urgency has different meanings and different time frames for different health professionals, ranging from a time scale of seconds for the physician in an intensive care unit to days for an public health director in the midst of an epidemic.

Although overlapping, these modes are a convenient classification for analyzing retrieval purposes. Also, different types of users (patients, physicians, nurses, other health professionals, administrators) will access the same knowledge base with different retrieval goals. These two dimensions are summarized in Table 1.

Each different combination of user class and retrieval mode deserves a distinct analysis in the design of optimal retrieval strategies. Among the factors to be considered are data representation forms, data transformation methods and the systems requirements to achieve them. These include the hardware, size of the data bases, acceptable delay times for retrieval, terminal characteristics, and methods of interactive control of retrieval by the user. Additional considerations include the familiarity of system users and their levels of training must be considered.

Unfortunately, an optimized information system is a compromise of performance among different user classes. For example, it will not be practical—at least, not in the immediate future—to physically store all various patient record and

Table 1. Uses for Retrieved Medical Information.

	Environments in which information is retrieved		
	General	Case oriented	Urgent or emergency
Usual information source for users listed below→	Books & journals; bibliographic databases; collections of records	Medical record; ancillary clinical information	Special monitors; medical record
Patient	Enhanced awareness; Life style modification; Risk avoidance	Choice of Rx Cooperation in Rx	Understanding of risks
Physician	Continuing education; Extending knowledge base	Appropriate medical care	Rapid decision making
Nurse	Continuing education; Extending knowledge base	Enhanced patient care	Participation in decision making
Other health professionals	Education for enhanced capabilities	Appropriate performance	Performance under pressure
Hospital administrator	Continuing education; Longterm planning	Daily management of institution	Coping with rapid changes
Third party payer	Policy planning	Policy execution	Dealing with rapidly changing economic pressures
Employer	Planning of insurance & benefits options	Funding employee health program	Exceptions for special cases

related data bases in different forms, each optimized for a specific use. However, cooperating distributed information systems do permit tailoring. When information is redundantly stored in several distinct geographical locations, the ability of the system to survive and recover from faults increases. When the primary users of a geographical data site have shared retrieval requirements, the local system can be optimized to them and reformatted for less frequent users. For instance, a radiology system can be optimized for its clientele, a laboratory system for that particular department, yet both should be able to retrieve information from the other just as the general hospital information system can request information from them.

Coupling a Retrieval Request with Medical Knowledge

A retrieval system has to know where the information is stored. It should provide reports in the context of who is making the query. It should anticipate additional information, not explicitly requested, that would be useful.

A request by a physician for lab results measured at many intervals for a patient with a chronic illness might generate a time dependent scatter plot but the laboratory report for an acutely ill patient with tests performed only once might be tabular. A consultant may always want to see which laboratory method was used on automated chemistries but a nurse might rather see only the abnormal results and the pending labs. A clinical pathologist may want references to the literature on test methods but the resident prefers references concerning test interpretation.

There are problems associated with providing unsolicited information. Irrelevant information wastes time. A presumption that the system is dictating treatment may cause resentment and rejection. Nevertheless, the goal of "do what I want, not what I say," is worthy.

Many systems factors affect the ability to retrieve information. The appropriateness of the knowledge representation is critical. The querying interface must be adequately expressive and yet humanly comprehensible. The machine/human interface should have an interactive feel and displays should be neat, legible, and easily understood.

General Retrieval External to the Medical Record

A search for information beyond the individual medical record may be an effort to become better informed about a topic or to obtain additional information about a particular clinical case. In other instances, a retrieval request may be aimed at gathering a subset of records from which statistical analyses for research will be conducted. The domain of knowledge embraces a more global area than that of the patient record.

Retrieval Languages, Interfaces, and Boolean Algebra

There is often too close of a coupling of the retrieval language to the database storage system. Since search engines, file systems, and querying terminals may be sold by different vendors, international standards defining the boundaries, functions, and mechanism of communication among operational layers, and specifying the structure of query dialogues is welcome.

Boolean logic or modifications of this technique are the principal frameworks by which retrieval questions are expressed to computer data bases. The familiar boolean operators (AND, OR, NOT) are the mainstays of such systems. In primitive forms, now almost abandoned, reverse Polish notation was required to pose search questions. These and algebraic notational methods have been largely replaced, at least on personal computers, by user friendly techniques that formulate search questions based on boolean algebra, not requiring the user to learn any complicated syntax. Nonboolean methods using statistical characteristics of a text as distance metrics for a search pattern are also used. Search statements can be constructed using graphic icons for concepts, pipes or wires for relationships, and filters for operations, constructed using a pointing device such as a mouse. Such interfaces for constructing dataflow models make it possible for end users to search large databases, without extensive prior training.

Searching via Hypertexts

Hypertext is a new vehicle for transmitting information and making searches. The essence of the hypertext is the ability to allow easy and flexible access of one portion of a text to another without the apparent use of an index. The user is provided with buttons and other hot spot areas on the screen. When activated, they cause the text to branch to the desired segment. In advanced hypertext systems, any part of the text itself can be selected via a pointing device, and the portions selected become the keywords for a search through the remainder of the text.

Free Text versus Index Field Based Searching

The increased computational speed of computers, especially of personal computers, and decreased cost of random access memory now permits searching of free text in order to locate documents containing keywords or phrases. This has led to less reliance upon the traditional indexing fields such as the MeSH controlled vocabulary. The relative merits of free text versus indexed searching is a subject still under active study by library scientists and other information retrieval specialists. Probably, neither technique will suffice. Effective searches will ordinarily require a judicious combination of both approaches. This complicates retrieval system design. The system designer should provide a way to guide the user to an appropriate balance between the constrained vocabulary of an indexing system and the searching of free text. Present day retrieval systems do not usually incorporate tools to do this. Techniques in the domain of artificial intelligence will likely be useful. Free text searching of multiple databases (wide area information servers or WAIS) using massively parallel computers is also very promising.

Retrieval from the Medical Record

The second column of Table 1 illustrates the needs when retrieving information relating to the care of a specific patient. Retrieval from the medical record and ancillary data bases is perhaps the most common context in which physicians and other health professionals access medical data bases. If the retrieval capabilities of the system are inadequate, the prime purpose of the computer based medical record is unfulfilled. Careful attention must be given to the detailed needs of the patient care provider for information in the clinical setting.

The patient's medical record is a single *logical* record with a immense variety of fields, differing in both length and form. The *physical* record may well be distributed on a variety of machines. The user of a distributed system should not need to be aware of the location of the information nor how it is coded. It should be presented a single logical entity. Furthermore, retrieval capabilities must accommodate stored information of vast diversity. Some will be in the form of images, some as digitized sound, and others as electrical signals values. The variety of the information formats requires a wide range of capabilities for making queries and for information display.

General Hardware Requirements for Retrieval

A useful terminal for retrieval shares many characteristics associated with those used for data acquisition. These include the capacity for high resolution graphics, sharp contrast, display stability, low power consumption, low heat production and portability. We refer the reader to our chapter on data acquisition.

Continued Need for Hard Copy

It is particularly important that a system has easy access to hard copy devices. For the indeterminate future, our society will not be paper free. Yet paper copies should be discardable. Indeed, one of the problems of hard copy is that it tends to be retained, both by virtue of tradition, and by a caution born from prior experience of serious loss of data through computer failure. Hard copy, however, *should not be relied on as a security shield* against computer failure. Any system that is designed with paper intended as a backup will be unstable: recovery time after failure will be prolonged and will cause dislocation in normal operations. Rather than relying on paper backup, hardware redundancy and well tested software should be the primary instruments for guaranteeing the security of medical records and health related information.

Handheld Two-Way Terminals—Will They be Useful?

Handheld devices ("palmtops"), particularly those with wireless transceivers, used for the retrieval of and immediate response of medical information should be very useful in the hospital setting. To the authors' knowledge, such devices are not yet in clinical use.

Software for Retrieval from the Medical Record: Providing the User with Tools to Meet Specific Needs

Routine Reports

In the course of normal clinical care, a number of reports are now routinely available to the care provider. Many inpatient and ambulatory systems generate paper reports. These are usually dispatched by messenger from the laboratory to the nursing unit or clinical area where they are manually posted in the medical record. Other hospitals have automated laboratory information systems where laboratory results can be queried by the physician from terminals in the nursing units. Some hospital information systems incorporate laboratory results and other ancillary medical diagnostic information, and can be queried from the nursing unit.

Several enhancements and additions should be considered. Health care workers could be automatically paged when important patient information is available through the HIS. Paging devices could also be used as display terminals. Digital pagers already have the capacity to store messages and to display them on a small screen upon the request of the recipient. Such capabilities should be integrated into hospital systems. Two further points should be considered in connection with this. The recipient should be able to specify for a particular patient what class of information is to be automatically transmitted. Pocket display devices with larger displays than currently available pagers will be desirable.

Displaying Information

On the Importance of Good Form

The ability to assimilate information is governed by its manner of presentation as well as by its intrinsic abstractness and level of detail. The importance of form was forcefully brought to the consciousness of early designers of computer-based medical records in the 1960s. To the surprise of many, and to the disappointment of many more, computer generated laboratory reports were not considered as an adequate substitute for the old style handwritten laboratory report.

At that time, computer printers produced only upper case letters. The concept of fonts and type styles virtually did not exist in the computer world. Reports were difficult to read at a glance. Design devices—shading, boxes, line rules, two color printing and the like—were lacking. Although assuredly more accurately transcribed, and usually received in a more timely fashion, they were almost impossible to comprehend. Computer reports did not become acceptable until upper and lower case print trains became available in the early 1970's and preprinted forms were used.

Retrieval upon Demand

Health care providers should be able to selectively retrieve any portion of the medical record upon demand. The requestor should be able to specify its presentation format. System designers would be well to avoid methods requiring text specification of the output format and investigate mechanisms currently used by data base management packages on personal computers. Interactive graphical design methods allow the requestor to manipulate components of a form on a computer screen. Variants can be devised to provide the same range of capabilities for medical record retrieval components.

Retrieval in Urgent Situations

All of the caveats relating to ease of request and comprehensible displays apply with emphasis during medically urgent situations. The rapidity of information retrieval may be at a premium, but its clear presentation is just as important. In urgent circumstances, the system must especially guard against provoking information overload, which clouds rather than simplifies decision making. The coupling of knowledge based systems with the patient's medical record potentially can provide a useful *knowledge refinery*.* Copious amounts od data in the record are boiled down to a summary combining text and graphics epitomizing the situation and corresponding advice. There may need to be special output devices, combining large screen, overhead mounted displays with sound; but in general the limiting factors will be the quality and relevance of the information retrieved rather than extraordinary methods of presentation.

Security

Provisions must be made to limit the entry and retrieval of sensitive attention to detail. Methods establish user identification, restrict data views and activities to particular individuals and terminals, encrypt files and transmissions, log requisition transactions, and physically secure terminals, computers, and media. Data integrity must also be guaranteed using reliable archival and fault detecting and faulty recovery technologies.

---

* To the best of our knowledge, the term knowledge refinery was first used by Donald Michie and Rory Johnston in *The Knowledge Machine* (New York: William Morrow & Co., 1985).

8

Image Processing and Storage for Computer-based Patient Records

John A. Norris and Jerome R. Cox

Introduction and Background

During the first three decades of work on computer representations of the patient record it has been impractical to incorporate images along with other patient data. It is clear that images have been an important part of the traditional patient record and it is only for technical reasons that they have been absent in electronic versions heretofore.

Electronic displays became economical and widely popular in the decade of the 70s, but were limited in capacity to a few dozen lines of alphanumeric characters. This limit was imposed by the amount of information that could be stored in a handful of memory chips.

By the 1980s, memory densities had increased sufficiently that our handful of memory chips could now store line drawings and graphs. In the 1990s, high resolution images can now be stored in the same handful of chips, removing one of the major barriers to the electronic display of the complete medical record. In what follows, we review definitions to be used, the need for medical imaging, the special requirements of medical imaging, and the future for computer modeling and visualization.

Definitions to be Used

By *medical images*, we mean high resolution (i.e., high contrast and high definition), clinically useful diagnostic images obtained by film scanners, computed radiography (CR), magnetic resonance (MR), computed tomography (CT), ultrasound, and nuclear medicine sources. Data from all of these imaging modalities is being acquired digitally today, and in the near future the images they produce will be available in electronic form routinely in all radiology departments. Other forms of medical imaging that involve computer modeling and new methods of computer visualization will be discussed separately and called advanced medical imaging.

Medical images that appear today in the medical record are two dimensional, still images. When converted to digital form, the intensity resolution (number of measurable levels of gray) of these images varies from eight to twelve bits (from 258 to 4096 levels of gray), yielding the ability to present images with medium to high contrast. Their image definition (spatial resolution) varies from 64 by 64 pixels (4096 total) for nuclear medicine images to 4K by 5K (20M total) for the output of modern film scanners. This image definition can be chosen to suit the image source and can be high enough to capture all the information present in the source.

The information content of medical images can be many orders of magnitude greater than is associated with other aspects of the medical record. For example, a single, high definition chest image contains about 25 megabytes of data. This data content is the equivalent, in terms of information content and, therefore, in terms of storage required, to the data in the 100,000 pages of 300-word typewritten text records (30 million words, or 30,000 times the proverbial 1,000-word worth of a single picture). It is also equivalent to the data in the graphic records of 5,000 12-lead diagnostic electrocardiograms.

Medical images can be contrasted with computer graphics presentations. The latter deals primarily with synthetic images generated algorithmically by the computer and based on parameters supplied by the user. Medical images may be thought of as natural images (or pictures) arising from the detection of energy from ultrasound, x-ray, magnetic, radioactive, or ultraviolet or visible light emitting sources. Both intensity resolution (levels of gray) and image definition (spatial resolution) are much higher for medical image presentations than for all but the most advanced computer graphics presentations. Computer graphics finds its most popular use in business graphics and in engineering design. These fields will contribute to, but not drive, the field of medical imaging.

The Need for Medical Imaging

Modern medical practice makes increasing use of diagnostic medical images. Referring physicians and specialists alike depend upon images in making critical diagnostic and therapeutic decisions. In some cases, the radiologist's written report is adequate for medical decision making by the referring physician, but often, particularly in the case of specialists or subspecialties like surgeons and cardiologists, these images also become an important part of the ongoing medical care process. Furthermore, the radiologist's report may in all cases be required as documentation to justify the actions taken by the health care team.

Thus, images have become an essential part of the patient record, and a medical record without images is incomplete. The physician examining it must turn elsewhere for the part of the record required to make medical decisions. This lack of completeness is a flaw that erodes confidence in any electronic record without images. Completeness of the record is essential, not only to diagnostic and therapeutic decision making, but also to evaluation of the appropriateness and quality of these decisions.

Therefore, as diagnostic images become an increasingly valuable part of medical care, so it must follow that medical images will become an essential part of the electronic medical record. Today these images are limited to ultrasound, MR, CT, x-ray, and nuclear medicine images. In the future they are certain to include advanced and powerful ways to visualize the medical data now presented as two dimensional, still images.

Special Requirements of Medical Images

The popularity of computer graphics in engineering workstations, desktop publishing, simulation, and in computer games has been of relatively little help to high quality medical imaging. The image definition required for diagnostic and therapeutic decision making from an electronic image appears to be at least 2K by 2K pixels, while the intensity resolution required must be between 10 and 12 bits. It is true that less well defined images may be adequate for physicians in non-diagnostic situations, but the radiologist charged with a diagnosis will only feel comfortable if the quality of the image under review is at least as good as film which normally has image definition of 5 to 25 million pixels and intensity resolution of 256 to 4096 levels of gray. The 100 or more gray levels distinguishable on a typical CRT monitor is also inadequate for careful diagnosis unless it is augmented by the ability to control contrast by means of an adjustable intensity window. Such contrast control requires display buffers that store more than 8 bits per pixel and usually 10, 11 or 12 bits per pixel, depending on the imaging modality.

These requirements for high resolution (high contrast and high definition) press the technology beyond the state of the art for computer graphics workstations. Even though raster scan displays have almost completely replaced calligraphic displays, the needs of computer graphics and medical imaging have not yet merged.

The larger information transmission requirements of medical images over that for computer graphics presents an additional problem. Computer backplanes, local area networks, and disk storage do not support the data transmission speeds required for high quality medical images. These supporting or infrastructure developments, however, will be available within the next five years to support the demanding needs for display of medical images.

Picture Archiving and Communication Systems

The picture archiving communications and other special requirements for medical images are of particular concern in radiology where hoped-for new technological developments are expected to lead to a new generation of picture archiving and communication systems (PACS) to be installed in many radiology departments by 1995. A PACS system allows the electronic storage, transmission, and display of medical images throughout the hospital or medical center. A PACS system consists of an archive to store the image, a network to distribute it and multiple display systems to display it. Stored images are retrieved from the archive on a portable medium, usually in the form of an optical disk, are transferred to a central magnetic storage device, and are transmitted over a high speed network to a large number of display stations capable of high definition presentation and interactive contrast control.

The PACS system can deliver many benefits not available with film. Two or more physicians can examine an image at one time by transmission of the same image to multiple locations. No longer will films routinely be lost or misplaced by the reviewing physicians. And now they can, in general, not only be found but retrieved and accessed in a matter of seconds. Also, the amount of storage taken by images stored on optical disk is less than 2 percent of that required by a hard copy film library, and has many advantages over microfilm or microfiche storage. Furthermore, in an electronic archive, all of the images associated with a given patient can be made available at a single location through computer managed image libraries.

The advent of powerful PACS systems in departments of radiology has important implications for the future medical record. Text, graphs, handwritten copy (even handwritten physician or nursing notes), as well as images, can all be made available interactively and in a responsive windowing environment. What this means is that by using tools developed for PACS, for the first time the *complete* medical record can be made available to and be managed by the physician electronically.

The Future for Advanced Medical Imaging

Computer models that help the understanding of patient dysfunction and disease are only in their infancy. These models range from the microscopic to the macroscopic views of everything from molecules to organ systems. All of these models will increase our understanding of health and disease and many will be useful in the care of individual patients.

The technology for generating and visualizing these models is taking shape. Three dimensional rendering of shaded images allows the appreciation of spatial relationships not possible in two dimensional sectional data. The addition of the fourth and fifth dimensions of time and space, as in the case of motion graphics/cartoons, adds even more visual meaning to some images. This and the segmentation of three dimensional, natural images into distinct features (so refined they can be labeled, as in an anatomy textbook) are difficult problems that may take years to solve satisfactorily. Nevertheless, computer generation and visualization of models of the mechanism of action of pharmaceuticals, proteins, DNA sequences, cell physiology, ion channel dynamics, organ behavior, cardiac dynamics, brain metabolism, hip joint mechanics, facial reconstruction and of many more interesting and medically important processes are beginning to be seen. This combination of computer graphics and natural images has a long way to go to be widely applicable clinically. However, the pioneering applications in hip joint replacement and facial reconstruction will likely show the way to many more applications of the visualization of models in medical practice.

9
Data Exchange Standards for Computer-based Patient Records

Clement J. McDonald and George H. Hripcsak

Background

Three facts, though perhaps self-evident, require emphasis:

- Medical records, whether paper or electronic, are composed entirely of data, mostly patient data. Without patient data, there is no medical record.
- Spontaneous generation does not apply to the medical record. All of the data stored in medical records come from elsewhere: from clinical laboratories, pharmacy systems, and radiology systems. Data also come in the form of orders and prescriptions that may be captured from hospital information systems and/or pharmacy systems, respectively.
- For electronic medical record systems to be practical, a medical record must be able to access many of these existing electronic sources of medical information. Such information is already stored in a variety of different formats, so standards for exchanging such information must be established before they can be easily transferred to a medical resource. Hence, the need for data interchange standards (McDonald and Hammond 1989).

The electronic exchange of clinical data requires two different kinds of standards. The first kind defines the message format and structure and specifies such things as whether the fields are fixed or variable length, whether data are ASCII or binary, whether dates are represented as MM/DD/YY or YYYYMMDD. The second defines the codes and vocabularies used to identify tests, diagnoses, findings, and so on.

Present State of the Art

Data interchange standards are well developed. Health Level Seven (HL7) refers to the seventh level of the ISO communication protocol, the application level (Hammond 1991). HL7 consists of a group of hospitals, medical systems vendors and consultants who are defining and standardizing communication among all components of a medical institution (including, but not limited to) admission, discharge and transfer, billing transactions, order entry, result reporting, supply management, and so on.

HL7 is the largest of the standards development efforts. As many as 200 participants attend its meetings. Version 2.1 of the HL7 standards was distributed in June 1990 (Health Level Seven, Inc. 1990). The HL7 network interface has been successfully demonstrated at the last two meetings of the American Hospital Association. The demonstration included registration, admitting, order entry, radiology, and laboratory systems. It is being installed at more than 80 sites, including a number of prominent medical centers.

HL7 efforts are being made in collaboration with the American Society for Testing Materials (ASTM). The ASTM is the oldest and largest of the United States consensus standards groups and a founding member of American National Standards Institute (ANSI) (Megargle 1990). ASTM E31.11 is one of six ASTM subcommittees that are relevant to CPR data interchange (McDonald 1991). (The others will be described below.) ASTM E31.11 published E1238–88 (ASTM 1988), its first standard, in May 1988. This is being implemented now.

ASTM E1238–88 focuses on the transmission of clinical laboratory results, though it has been used for other kinds of clinical data such as spirometries and blood pressure as well. The latest version of the ASTM 1238 (ASTM E1238 draft revision 4.2) will accommodate all clinical data including history and physical admission and discharge notes, electrocardiograms, obstetric ultrasounds, electroencephalographs, consultation notes, and so on. With a few exceptions, the old standard is upward compatible with the revision. The current draft of E1238 has passed subcommittee and committee ballot and now awaits the last level of balloting (Society) before approval.

ASTM E31.11 and HL7 work closely together. They use the same encoding rules, the same data types, and, in the case of the order and result reporting segments, the same data elements and segments. In both standards, the exchange of clinical information is a three-level hierarchy, consisting of patient identifying segments, diagnostic study order segments, and observation segments. In one message, a patient may have more than one order and each order may have more than one observation beneath it. Both standards require that all information be transmitted as printable characters. The number 135, for example, is sent as three separate ASCII characters. Each field within a segment such as a patient's name or a test identifier is variable in length and separated from the next field by a delimiter character. The content of a field may be divided into components (e.g., the first name, middle initial, suffix, and title) of the patient name field, separated by component delimiters. Thus, a patient name might appear as follows: Smith∧John∧D∧Sr∧MD. Some fields may contain multiple values separated by repeat delimiters. The patient name field, for example, may contain multiple names to accommodate aliases and maiden names. The diagnosis field may contain multiple diagnoses.

The HL7 and ASTM data interchange standards use common data types. Date/times are always reported as YYYYMMDDHHMMSS, using the International Standards Organization's standard date format. Accordingly, January 12, 1988, 2:35 p.m. would be recorded as *198812011435*. HL7 and ASTM also use the same specifications for telephone numbers, addresses, personal identifiers, observation identifiers, and diagnoses.

The HL7/ASTM interfaces are now being widely implemented. Academic centers, including Indiana University, Duke University, Cleveland Clinic, Mayo Clinic, and Columbia Presbyterian Medical Center, are implementing ASTM or HL7 interfaces. Fifteen nationally based referral laboratories are using or implementing the ASTM 1238 standard. Mayo Clinic's reference laboratory results has been using the standard since December 1989. Metpath and American Medical Laboratories and Smith Kline Beecham, the largest commercial clinical laboratory vendors, are also using it.

Most intensive care system vendors, including Space Labs, Hewlett Packard, Becton Dickinson, and Marquette Laboratories, are developing ASTM or HL7 linkages so that they can automatically import lab results into their own systems. The same is true of the major laboratory system vendors and the largest HIS vendors such as Shared Medical Systems and HBO. A number of office practice systems are implementing ASTM links to commercial laboratories. With such links, practices will be able to order laboratory results through their office computer and receive them automatically into computer-based medical records.

These standards are being used internationally as well. HPRIM, a consortium of 25 laboratory systems vendors in France, representing more than 95 percent of France's laboratory volume, have committed to ASTM 1238 as their standard interface with office practice and hospital systems.

A sister ASTM subcommittee, E-31.12, has also made considerable progress. They have published a standard for discharge and transfers (ASTM E1239; Murphy 1991) and developed a standard description for the content of a computer-based patient record (ASTM E1384–91). The committee has also worked to define vocabulary and nomenclatures (Gabriele 1991). Forrey and Deto are far along in the development of a standard nomenclature for clinical laboratory tests. A given test name consists of multiple parts including the analyte (e.g., serum potassium or glucose), source (e.g., sputum, urine), the precision of the procedure (e.g., whether it is qualitative or quantitative) and the methodology (e.g., radioimmunoassay, colorimetric). The availability of a standard test name/code will make it much easier for medical systems that receive results from many laboratories to identify equivalent tests from two different sources. ASTM E1238 is collaborating with the Euclides project from Europe (McDonald 1991). Euclides (DeMoor, Euclides Consortium) has defined the most complete and systematic coding system.

ASTM E-31.14, another sister subcommittee, focuses on standards for communication between laboratory instruments and computer systems. This committee has published two standards: E1381, Low-level protocol to transfer messages between clinical laboratory instruments and computer systems (ASTM 1990); and E1394, A standard specification for transferring information between clinical instruments and computer systems (ASTM 1991). Because the message format is the same as ASTM 1238 format, system vendors who use 1238 for communicating with outside systems can use much of the same code for communicating with the instruments within the laboratory. It is likely that both of these draft standards will be formal standards by the time this report is published.

Yet another sister committee, E31.16, is concerned with the standard specification for transferring digital neurophysiological data between independent computer system (Jacobs 1991). In their recent work on standards for the transmission of electrophysiologic signals, they have balloted a draft proposal for the transmission of electroencephalograms (EEGs) and electromyograms (EMGs). This standard uses the same encoding rules, data types, and many of the same segments and fields as ASTM 1238/HL7 but adds the capabilities for sending the tracings themselves as X/Y coordinates. Their specification has the support of most of the EEG and EMG hardware industry and is likely to pass subcommittee and committee balloting by the end of 1991.

The American College of Radiology (ACR) in collaboration with the National Electrical Manufacturers Association (NEMA) published the first standard for medical images in 1985. This was revised in 1988 (ACR-NEMA 1988). It is supported by all of the major manufacturers of PACS equipment and is being adopted for the purpose of transporting images from devices that capture radiologic images to central repositories and from the repositories outward to display systems. It is a flexible standard that can accommodate a wide variety of images and image modalities and includes standards for image compression as well as image representation.

Another important development is the Medical Information Bus (MIB) P1073 (Harrington 1991). This is an IEEE effort to standardize the interconnection between intensive care unit instruments such as IV infusion devices, blood pressure measurement machines, ventilators, urine output measuring devices, cardiac monitoring devices, and so on. The MIB standard is very smart. It permits a device to be attached to a bus, identify itself, and negotiate linkages with the appropriate central system. It has been under development for 9 years and is now in final balloting.

MEDIX P1157 is yet another IEEE effort with goals similar to HL7, with the aim of being fully compliant with ISO network specifications (Harrington 1991). However, no specifics have been published yet. HL7 and ASTM use conventional communication methods that will work in a variety of network environments including electronic mail. The ISO sets forth a more sophisticated method which includes the database definition within the message. It is anticipated that MEDIX will use the HL7 ASTM message contents and convert them into the ISO format.

Another emerging standards effort concerns the format for certain types of logic for making medical decisions. Medical decision support systems have been shown to be useful. Several institutions have already assembled large medical knowledge bases (McDonald 1988, Pryor 1988). There are many conceptual similarities among the knowledge bases, but each knowledge base's syntax is different. In order to facilitate the sharing of knowledge between institutions, a common standard for sharing medical knowledge should be defined.

A Medical Logic Module (MLM) (Clayton 1989, Hripcsak 1991) is an independent entity that can be understood and used without necessarily needing to refer to the rest of the knowledge base. Most real systems do not satisfy the independence constraint perfectly due to nesting and special properties, so this is just an approximation. A single module contains about the amount of information that fits on a single page of text (i.e., anywhere from a paragraph to several pages).

To be useful for sharing knowledge, the MLM standard must have several properties. The first two properties are the most critical:

Readability. The MLMs should be able to be read and interpreted easily by medical experts with little computer training.

Lack of ambiguity. The MLMs should be unambiguous, so that the same module cannot be interpreted in two different ways.

Writability. The MLMs should be able to be written by medical experts with as little training as possible. Note that this is a different property than the first. For example, it is easier to recognize a list of numbers like *1, 2, 3;* than it is to remember that the list is delimited by commas and terminated with a semicolon. No matter what syntax one uses, making the MLMs strictly unambiguous will make them more difficult to write since it rules out the use of natural language. One can produce a specialized editor (e.g., a syntax directed editor) to facilitate writing MLMs but the MLMs should be readable in their native form.

Ease of computer translation. The MLMs should allow easy computer translation. This, however, is less important than the first three requirements. In fact, there is a trade-off between ease for the user and ease for the computer. While a standard that requires the user to write machine code will be a failure, so will a standard that allows the user to write natural language. The standard must be practical to both the user and the computer.

Ease of maintenance. The MLMs should be able to be manipulated and maintained on common software and hardware, especially early on. For example, it should be possible to edit them with common text editors, print them on common printers, display them on common computer displays, and send them on common networks.

ASTM E31.15 has taken on the responsibility of producing consensus standards for representing medical knowledge in an exchangeable form. Its first effort, a standard specification for transferring modular medical knowledge bases, is medical logic modules based on the Arden syntax (Hripcsak 1991, ASTM draft) and is now in initial balloting.

The time is very ripe for all of these standards. Third party payers and governmental agencies are requiring more and more clinical data. Hospitals and clinics cannot afford to continue to add layer upon layer of manual chart encoding. This data should be obtained with the use of standards directly from electronic sources such as clinical laboratories. Physicians and medical institutions are demanding quick access to well-organized and comprehensive clinical information, i.e., an electronic medical record. The utility of computer generated alerts and reminders has been established and the use of such systems is expected to expand substantially.

For those who wish to learn more about these standards or to participate in their development, a list of standards organizations and contact persons is given at the conclusion of this chapter.

Future Proposals

In the 1995 time frame, the ASTM and HL7 standards are likely to be widely implemented and used in the medical care industry. They are compatible with all current technology. They can be used in a sophisticated network environment as well as on simple RS232 data exchanges.

MEDIX, on the other hand, takes advantage of the full ISO capabilities. MEDIX is committed to converging with the HL7 ASTM message structure and provide a means of carrying such messages over full ISO networks. ISO capabilities are likely to be widely available in large institutions in the 1995 time frame, but are less likely to be useful in the office practice environment in this time frame. ASTM and HL7 will be needed by these environments for the next decade.

The American National Standards Institute (ANSI) is now in the process of developing a planning panel to help coordinate various standards groups.

References

ASTM E1238–88. 1988. *A standard specification for transferring clinical laboratory data messages between independent computer systems.* ASTM subcommittee E31.11. Philadelphia: American Society for Testing Materials.

ASTM E1239. 1988. *Standard guide for description of reservation/registration-admission, discharge, transfer (R-ADT) systems for automated patient care information systems.* ASTM subcommittee E31.12. Philadelphia: American Society for Testing Materials.

ASTM E1381.90. 1990. *Low-level protocol to transfer messages between clinical laboratory instruments and computer systems.* ASTM subcommittee E31.14. Philadelphia: American Society for Testing Materials.

ASTM E1384. 1991. *Standard guide for description for content and structure of an automated primary record of care.* ASTM subcommittee E31.12. Philadelphia: American Society for Testing Materials.

ASTM E1394.91. 1991. *A standard specification for transferring information between clinical instruments and computer systems.* ASTM subcommittee E31.14. Philadelphia: American Society for Testing Materials.

Barnett, G.O. 1984. The application of computer-based medical-record systems in ambulatory practice. *New England Journal of Medicine* 310:1643–1650.

Clayton, P.D., T.A. Pryor, O.B. Wigertz, and G. Hripcsak. 1989. Issues and structures for sharing medical knowledge among decision-making systems: the 1989 Arden homestead retreat. In *Proceedings of the Thirteenth Symposium on Computer Applications in Medical Care* 116–121.

DeMoor, G., et al. 1990. Euclides, a European standard for clinical laboratory data exchange. In *Readings in medical informatics*. Ghent, Belgium: Euclides Foundation, State University Hospital.

DeMoor, G. 1991. Euclides coding system. Version 1.40 28.04.91. Ghent, Belgium: Euclides Foundation, State University Hospital.

DeMoor, G. 1991. Euclides syntax manual. Version 1.1. Ghent, Belgium: Euclides Foundation, State University Hospital.

Gabrieli, E.R. 1991. Need for standards in medical communication. *Topics in Health Records Management* 11:27–36.

Hammond, W.E. 1991. Health Level 7: An application standard for electronic medical data exchange. *Topics in Health Record Management* 11:59–66.

Harrington, J.J. 1991. IEEE P1157 medical data interchange (MEDIX): Application of open systems to health care communications. *Topics in Health Records Management* 11:45–58.

Health Level Seven: An application protocol for electronic data exchange in healthcare environments. Version 2.1. 1990. Chicago, Ill.: Health Level Seven, Inc.

Hripcsak, G. 1991. Observations and opinions: Standards revisited; Arden syntax for medical logic modules, data interchange for clinical neurophysiology. *MD Computing* 8:76–78.

Jacobs, E.C. 1991. Observations and opinions: Standards revisited; Arden syntax for medical logic modules, data interchange for clinical neurophysiology. *MD Computing* 8:78–79.

McDonald, C.J., and W.M. Tierney WM. 1988. Computer-stored medical records. *JAMA* 259:3433–3440.

McDonald, C.J., and H.E. Hammond. 1989. Standard formats for electronic transfer of clinical data. *Annals of Internal Medicine* 110:333–335.

McDonald, C.J., D.K. Martin, J.M. Overhage. 1991. Standards for the electronic transfer of clinical data: progress and promises. *Topics in Health Records Management* 11:1–16.

McDonald, C.J., L. Blevins, W.M. Tierney, D.K. Martin. 1988. The Regenstrief medical records. *MD Computing* 5:34–47.

Megargle. R. 1991. Role of ASTM in computer information standards for medicine. *Topics in Health Records Management* 1991. 11:17–26.

Murphy, G. 1991. Standards for automated patient records. *Topics in Health Records Management* 11:37–44.

Appendix: List of Standards Working Groups and Contact Persons

ACR-NEMA: Radiological Imaging Standards
Contact: Steve Horii, M.D., Co-Chairman, Division of Imaging Physics, Department of Radiology, Georgetown University Hospital, 3800 Reservoir Road, N.W., Washington, D.C. 20007-2197 (202-687-5990); or David E. Best, Co-Chairman, Eastman Kodak, Electronic Products and Planning Division, 343 State Street, Rochester, NY 14650–0801 (716-588-2054)

ASTM E31.11: Clinical Data Transmission
Contact: Clem McDonald, M.D., Chairman, Regenstrief Institute, 1001 West 10th Street, Indianapolis, IN 46202 (317-630-7070)

ASTM 31.12: Medical Informatics
Contact: Elmer Gabriele, M.D., Chairman, Gabrieli Medical Information, Statler Towers, Suite 1633, Buffalo, NY 14202 (716-856-2890)

ASTM E31.14: Interfaces for Laboratory Instruments
Contact: Leon B. Wolf, Chairman, E.I. DuPont de Nemours Co., Inc., Medical Products Department, Concord Plaza, Ridgely Building 2A5, Wilmington, DE 219898 (302-695-5685)

ASTM E31.15: Medical Knowledge Representation
Contact: Al Pryor, Ph.D., Chairman, University of Utah, LDS Hospital, 325 8th Avenue, Salt Lake City, UT 84143 (801-321-2123)

ASTM E31.16: Digital Neurophysiological Data
Contact: Ernest C. Jacobs, M.D., Department of Neurology, The Cleveland Clinic Foundation, One Clinic Center, 9500 Euclid Avenue, Cleveland, OH 44195-5221 (216-444-7006)

Euclides
Contact: Georges DeMoor, Ph.D., Chairman, State University Hospital of Gent, Department of Medical Informatics, De Pitalaan 185–5K3, B-9000, Gent, Belgium (32 91 40 3436)

Health Level Seven (HL7): Hospital Network Systems
Contact: William E. Hammond, Ph.D., Chairman, Duke University Medical Center, Box 2914, Marshall Pickens Building, Durham, NC 27710 (919-684-6421)

H.PR.I.M.
Contact: Jean-Yves LeMarchand, Secretariat, 133 Boulevard du Montparnasse, 75006, Paris, France; or Bob Rothstein (32 16 38 07 32)

IEEE Medix P1157: ISO Medical Standards
Contact: Jack Harrington, Hewlett Packard, 175 Wyman Street, Waltham, MA 02254 (617-890-6300)

IEEE P1073: Interface for Patient Monitoring Devices
Contact: Jack Harrington, Hewlett Packard, 175 Wyman Street, Waltham, MA 02254 (617-890-6300)

10
The Unified Medical Language System (UMLS) and Computer-based Patient Records

Donald A.B. Lindberg and Betsy L. Humphreys

General Description of the UMLS

Purpose

The purpose of the Unified Medical Language System (UMLS) (Lindberg and Humphreys 1989; Humphreys and Lindberg 1989) is to make machine-readable information relevant to particular practice and research questions readily available to health care practitioners and investigators. Important biomedical information is distributed among many different machine-information sources. These include databases of scientific literature, patient record, factual databanks, knowledge-based expert systems, and directories of individuals and institutions. Unfortunately, a number of significant barriers separate potential users from the information in such sources. The barriers include the variety of ways the same concepts are expressed in the different information sources and by the users themselves, the difficulty of identifying all the available sources and selecting those most appropriate to particular questions, and the range of access paths and conditions that must be negotiated to retrieve information from multiple sources. Such problems prevent individual users from gaining access to relevant machine readable information and also impede the development of more powerful search interfaces to help these users. The UMLS project is working to overcome these barriers and to facilitate the development of much more powerful and user friendly interfaces to machine-readable biomedical information. The UMLS is not an attempt to impose a single standard vocabulary on the biomedical community. It is an effort to deal effectively with continued diversity in biomedical terminology and information sources.

UMLS Components

There will be two categories of UMLS components: knowledge sources or databases and functional features or components. We expect that at least three new knowledge sources (Lindberg and Humphreys 1990) will be needed for a fully functioning UMLS; a Metathesaurus™ representing concepts and terms present in a variety of biomedical vocabularies and classifications, a Semantic Network identifying the useful and permissible relationships among the broad categories or semantic types (e.g., "Medical Device," "Disease or Syndrome") assigned to all Metathesaurus terms, and an Information Sources Map describing available machine-readable information sources and containing scripts that support successful automated connections to these information sources. Although systems developers will probably have to add information of particular local interest to the UMLS knowledge sources, these centrally maintained and updated databases should substantially reduce the level of effort required to build successful interfaces to multiple machine readable information sources.

A set of UMLS functional features or programs will make use of the information in the UMLS knowledge sources to interact with users and with sources of machine readable information. These functional features will include a query interpreter to determine the meaning of the user's question, a graphical displayer to present information about relationships among concepts to the user, an information sources selector to identify the databases likely to be relevant to the user's question, a query formulator to transform the user's question into a format suitable for searching the appropriate databases, and an output processor to merge, rank, and display the information retrieved in a coherent manner. There are likely to be several different implementations of the UMLS functional features, each tailored to a particular functional environment or hardware/software platform. NLM will develop these capabilities within Grateful MED[R] and its associated expert search assistant called COACH.

Current Status

The current focus of the UMLS project is the development and testing of the initial versions of the UMLS Knowledge Sources. The first versions of the UMLS Metathesaurus and the Semantic Network were issued in October 1990. Meta-1 (Tuttle et al. 1990) as the first version of the Metathesaurus is called, contains about 64,123 concepts and about 208,559 unique terms, including synonyms and slight variations. Meta-1 includes as its base set of terms all of NLM's Medical Subject Headings (MeSH[R]) vocabulary, all terms in the Diagnostic and Statistical Manual of Medical Disorders, 3rd edition, revised (DSM-IIIR) (1987), and terms for clinical problems and a small number of laboratory procedures heavily used at selected COSTAR (Barnett 1984) sites. Terms from the Systematized Nomenclature of Medicine (SNOMED) (Cote 1979), the International Classification of Diseases, 9th edition, Clinical Modification (ICD-9-CM) (1980), and current Procedural Terminology (CPT) (1989) also appear in Meta-1, along with a set of Library of Congress Subject Headings (LCSH) (1989) that were mapped to MeSH by NLM staff. Subject matter experts reviewed all Meta-1 records to add or correct basic information, label the relationships among terms, and edit any incorrect automated matches. The purpose of the editing was to ensure that Meta-1 records accurately reflect the meanings of terms in their vocabulary sources, not to add additional meanings or terms known to the subject experts.

The numbers of terms from each vocabulary included in Meta-1 are as follows:

195,409   MeSH (15,510 preferred terms; 35,307 supplementary chemical
          terms)
   447   DSM-IIIR (267 preferred terms)
   776   COSTAR (776 unique concepts)
 9,489   ICD-9-CM (2,775 preferred terms)
10,301   SNOMED (5,670 preferred terms)
   446   CPT (166 preferred terms)
 5,106   LCSH (7,000 preferred terms)

Although the coverage of clinical concepts will have to be expanded in future versions of the Metathesaurus, Meta-1 already includes terms for the majority of diagnoses frequently encountered in clinical practice. The coverage of patient findings and routine clinical procedures (e.g., laboratory procedures) is not extensive.

Each Meta-1 record contains three types of information:

• Basic facts about the main concept name including the vocabulary sources in which it appears, its semantic type, part of speech, lexical type (e.g., eponym, trade name, acronym), and in many cases a definition.

• Associated terms from the Meta-1 source vocabularies including lexical variants, synonyms, related terms, and hierarchical contexts.

• Usage information including the occurrence of the main concept name, its lexical variants, or synonyms in MEDLINE[R], DXPLAIN, PDQ, QMR, and OMIM (Online Mendelian Inheritance in Man). For MeSH terms, the frequency of usage with specific qualifiers or subheadings and of co-occurrence with other MeSH headings is also represented.

The first version of the UMLS Semantic Network (McCray 1989) contains information about the 131 semantic types or categories to which all concepts in Meta-1 have been assigned. In the Network each semantic type is defined and some of the important and useful relationships among the types are explicitly represented (e.g., *Virus* CAUSES *Disease or Syndrome*).

Meta-1 and the Semantic Network were issued together in multiple formats on two CD-ROMS. For each knowledge source, there is an ASCII relational version, an ASCII unit record version, and a browsable version suitable for loading on a Macintosh computer. One copy of Meta-1 will occupy approximately 200 megabytes. The Semantic Network is very small in comparison. The initial versions of these UMLS knowledge sources are intended for use by system developers. They are *not* be accompanied by applications programs. The first version of the UMLS Information Sources Map will be issued in 1991. We expect to issue the first version of it sometime in 1991.

The strategy for development of the UMLS knowledge sources is to begin modestly and to add coverage and complexity as actual use and experimentation show it to be necessary. The initial versions of the UMLS knowledge sources are therefore available free of charge under an experimental agreement, in exchange for feedback on problems, successes, and promising avenues for enhancement and expansion.

Potential Interactions between the UMLS and Computer-based Patient Records

The UMLS is necessary, but not sufficient, to support effective retrieval of external machine-readable information relevant to specific patient records and to locate and aggregate information from patient record databases. Development of these capabilities will also require more rigorous control over the creation and maintenance of patient data and special user interface programs tailored to patient record environments.

Linking to External Databases

Studies of physicians' information needs (Covell et al. 1985; Osheroff et al. 1991) indicate that most patient encounters generate questions that could be profitably addressed to machine-readable information sources such as MEDLINE, PDQ, QMR, DXPLAIN, etc. These and similar sources can be used to refresh a practitioner's memory about an infrequently encountered problem, to review recent research findings, to suggest other possible diagnoses, to verify the appropriateness of a planned treatment, to locate a relevant practice guideline, to identify an applicable clinical trial, or to find appropriate experts to consult. Physicians who consult MEDLINE regularly report many incidents in which online searching has affected treatment, improved patient outcomes, and reduced hospital risks and costs (Use of the Critical Incident Technique 1989). Unfortunately, most clinicians do not consult machine readable databases regularly. While there are a variety of reasons for such non-use (Shortliffe 1989), the difficulty and inconvenience of accessing multiple machine readable systems are significant deterrents for many health professionals.

An ideal patient record system would allow health professionals to conduct useful searches of external databases at the time they were entering or reviewing information in a specific automated patient record. In such a system a practitioner using a light pen or other highlighting mechanism could select terms from the patient record for use in an automated search of external databases. If the practitioner's question were whether a certain finding could be explained by one of the patient's known clinical problems, all the relevant search terms would probably be present in the patient's record. In many cases, however, the user's question would involve a combination of concepts, some of which would not be present in the patient record. The search interface would therefore allow the user to enter additional concepts at the time of the search. The practitioner could also specify via function key or other easy mechanism certain frequently needed types of searches, e.g., for recent articles, for a practice guideline, for an open clinical trial suitable for the patient represented in the record, for data on patients similar to this one.

The ideal system would accept the terminology selected from the patient record or entered directly by the practitioner. The system would interpret this input sensibly and would interact with the user to verify that the interpretation was correct. The system would then select appropriate information sources based on its understanding of the question, its knowledge of the databases accessible in the user's environment, and stored information about the user's preferences and past information-seeking behavior. With limited interaction with the user at strategic points, the system would convert the original query into search statements appropriate to the information sources selected, make the automated connections to these sources, conduct actual search sessions, assemble, rank, and organize the information retrieved, and present it to the practitioner in a comprehensible display. Data from the patient record might be employed in these output processing steps to identify the retrieved information most relevant to the details of the patient's case. It might also prove necessary to retrieve an interim result from one external information source in order to make a successful connection from a patient record to a second external source. When the information retrieved included citations and abstracts from the published literature, the user would be able to view or order automatically the full-text of articles that seemed most useful.

Given an automated patient record system, the UMLS components, and a concerted development effort, at least an approximation of this ideal system can become a reality. Prototypes of certain pieces of the ideal system are already under development. Yale's Psychotopix (Powsner and Miller 1990) system uses the machine-readable text of a psychiatry consultation as the basis for an automated search of MEDLINE. Massachusetts General Hospital is experimenting with fully automated connections to multiple machine-readable information sources including COSTAR, DXPLAIN, and MEDLINE (Cimino and Barnett 1990). NLM has developed Loansome Doc, an automated connection between Grateful MED and DOCLINE (Dutcher 1989) that allows users to order the full-text of citations retrieved in MEDLINE. Other limited online document ordering capabilities are already available. While the initial versions of the UMLS Knowledge Sources cannot handle all types of queries that might be generated from patient record data, they should support experimental development of systems capable of interpreting and obtaining useful answers to some important questions arising in the course of clinical care. With appropriate experimentation and feedback from patient record environments, the UMLS products should become increasingly useful for interpreting terms present in patient records or entered by users, converting these terms into the vocabularies and classifications used in other information sources, and selecting and connecting automatically to external information sources.

Retrieving Patient Data

Apart from the use of a specific patient's record in the course of providing or billing for care, the purpose of retrieving patient records is often to summarize the data contained within them. A clinician searching for records of cases similar to the ones being treated may be primarily interested in a summary of patient outcomes arranged by the type of treatment provided or a display of the frequency of certain patient findings. Health services researchers wish to aggregate data from many patient records to discern patterns in the efficacy of different therapies, in the level of care provided to different population groups with the same illness, in the outcomes of procedures in different institutions, or in the use of certain therapies in different geographic areas. For such summaries to be meaningful, they must be based on the relevant subset of records, e.g., records for all patients who underwent one of three procedures for a specific clinical problem. Given the existence of patient databases with suitable content, the UMLS should be able to assist in the retrieval of relevant patient records. At least within the next few years, the UMLS project is unlikely to generate products that will help to summarize the data from the records once retrieved.

As they are developed and extended, the UMLS Knowledge Sources will contain an increasing amount of information that can assist in converting the questions posed by practitioners and researchers into search statements capable of retrieving automated patient data. The assumption is that these questions will consist of some combination of terms entered directly by the user, terms selected from patient records, and terms used in searching other sources of information such as MEDLINE. The questions may also include numeric values such as the results of particular tests.

The ideal system for retrieval of patient record data would in essence be the same system described for retrieving information relevant to a particular patient record from external information sources. The clinician or researcher would have an easy method for selecting applicable search terms from a patient record or other machine readable source. Search questions could also be entered de novo by the user, perhaps via a template or other mechanism designed to make the question easier to interpret. The system would accept the terminology entered by the user and then proceed through query interpretation, information source selection, conversion of the user's terms into appropriate search terms, automatic execution of the search, and retrieval and organization of the output. Most of the additional features required for effective retrieval of patient data would probably be in the area of summarization and presentation of results. Again, with appropriate testing and feedback on necessary improvements, the UMLS Knowledge Sources can becomes effective tools for interpreting questions that can be answered by patient records and for converting these questions into search statements suitable for retrieving patient data.

Structuring Patient Records to Facilitate Information Retrieval

There are few existing automated patient record systems that could support the links to external information sources or retrieval of patient data previously described. To allow the development of even preliminary versions of the capabilities desired, automated patient record systems should have the following features:

Standard and explicit designation of at least the key elements in the patient record. Development and use of a standard format for the principal elements of patient records will facilitate information retrieval in patient record systems. Interpretation of even uncontrolled vocabulary is much easier if the specific location of the vocabulary in the patient record is designated unambiguously. The fact that a term appears in the Immunizations Section of the record, rather than the Diagnostic Tests Section, will make its interpretation easier. Even when controlled terminology is used, the context of the terminology must be clearly specified in the patient records *and* be available as a parameter for searching groups of records. For example, a user must be able to retrieve records with *Non-Insulin-Dependent Diabetes* in the Problem List section, without getting records in which *Non-Insulin-Dependent Diabetes* appears only in the Family History section of the record.

A policy of including full terms in addition to codes, acronyms, or abbreviated words in the indices to the patient records and in the displays of patient record data, if not in the physical records themselves. The development of interfaces for searching across patient records and linking data in patient records to other types of databases will be greatly facilitated by the presence in the records of full terms. Acronyms and abbreviations are helpful in data input, but generally inhibit effective information retrieval. Work done in conjunction with the UMLS project has confirmed that acronyms are a primary cause of incorrect automated mapping among different vocabularies and information sources. Patient record systems should therefore convert or map acronyms and abbreviations to the appropriate full terms.

Use of some controlled vocabulary or vocabularies for all new instances of at least selected elements of patient records: i.e., the basic name of each patient problem, the name of each procedure performed by a direct caregiver. These elements of the patient record are given highest priority for vocabulary standardization for several reasons. They are involved in required statistical reporting and billing procedures; they are essential elements for quality control of health care and technology assessment; they are likely to be used as search arguments in a wide variety of inquiries directed to patient record databases; they are the elements that are currently being assigned ICD-9-CM and CPT codes. There are also existing controlled vocabularies that at least in combination cover many of the concepts needed in these parts of patient records. Because these elements of the patient record are already being coded, there will be less incremental cost in controlling the vocabulary in these areas than in using controlled vocabulary in other parts of the record.

To be effective, vocabulary control must involve immediate validation of terms entered in the selected data elements and feedback on any nonstandard terms entered. Caregivers must have the option of approving the incorporation of nonstandard terms when the controlled vocabulary used does not cover the current situation adequately. Even partial vocabulary control of key data elements is much better than none. Managers of patient record systems should begin to implement vocabulary control wherever it is easiest and most convenient (e.g., standard demographic characteristics) and then gradually expand as more efficient data entry and validation methods are developed.

There are no existing controlled vocabularies that can be recommended without reservation for even selected elements of the automated patient record. Therefore for the immediate future individual patient record systems should be free to select the combination of controlled vocabularies they will use. Factors to be considered in selecting appropriate controlled vocabularies include the existence of a machine-readable map between the vocabulary and a corresponding required coding scheme (e.g., ICD-9-CM or CPT) and the likelihood of the vocabulary's inclusion in the UMLS Metathesaurus.

Maintenance of detailed documentation of the various vocabularies used. Because individual patient record systems will make different decisions regarding the selection of controlled vocabularies and the timetable for their implementation, each system must contain documentation of the names and editions of the various vocabularies and classifications in use in records throughout the system. This implies the existence of a central system manager with significant authority and influence. Vocabularies and classifications can undergo substantial changes from edition to edition. Maintenance of basic information about the vocabularies in use during different time periods will assist in updating or linking patient data when vocabularies are modified. Such information will also help to make effective connections among patient records containing terms from different editions of the same source vocabulary.

Minimal use of locally developed classifications and vocabularies. No single existing controlled vocabulary or set of controlled vocabularies is likely to be a perfect match for all local requirements, but this does not justify local development of entirely new controlled vocabularies. However simple the task may appear on the surface, the development of a useful, coherent vocabulary or classification system is difficult and time consuming. If local needs really cannot be served by existing vocabulary systems, the preferred course of action should be to extend an existing system rather than create a new one. If local terms are used, some mechanism for synonym control should be established. Any locally developed codes or terms must be clearly identified as such within the patient record system, and care must be taken not to use any scheme that results in codes already in use in an external controlled vocabulary. Clear labeling of local terminology will facilitate its conversion to an appropriate external vocabulary should one become available.

The greater the reliance on controlled vocabularies in automated patient record systems, the greater the likelihood that these systems can be effectively linked to other information sources via the UMLS. Perhaps the most significant impediment to the use of reasonably specific controlled vocabularies in patient records is the probable increased cost associated with record input and maintenance. In an automated environment, the use of a controlled vocabulary should lead to a tremendous increase in the utility of patient records with little or no increase in the overall cost of the entire patient record process (i.e., input, update, storage, retrieval). Unfortunately, the input and update costs are likely to rise, and these are more visible and readily quantifiable than the cost of retrieval, or nonretrieval, of information from patient records. Use of sophisticated data entry mechanisms can help to control input costs.

Another problem in the lack of regularly maintained vocabularies suitable for some segments of the patient record. Despite excellent efforts by many individuals, professional societies have a much better record of developing such vocabularies than they have of updating them consistently and with reasonable frequency. Some more reliable mechanism for maintaining and updating a core set of clinical vocabularies needs to be found.

Ensuring the Utility of the UMLS in the Patient Record Environment

As previously explained, the initial versions of all UMLS products are experimental. They represent first steps toward facilitating the retrieval of biomedical information from multiple sources. To achieve their full potential, they must be tested in a variety of environments and enhanced based on the insights gained from this testing. If the UMLS is to be effective in the patient record environment, the early versions of the UMLS products must be used in conjunction with automated patient records. Extensions and improvements will necessarily occur in gradual increments. Priorities will be assigned based on the value of the enhancement to the greatest number of those actively seeking to use the UMLS products to solve biomedical information problems.

Because the National Library of Medicine does not collect or use patient date, we are relying on our collaborators and those requesting experimental copies of the initial UMLS products to provide experimental files of patient data for use in UMLS research and to experiment with the UMLS products in conjunction with functioning patient record systems.

Meta-1, the first version of UMLS Metathesaurus does not have extensive coverage of signs, symptoms, and routine clinical procedures. While we assume that expansion in these areas will be needed to support patient record applications, it is not clear which topics have priority for expansion or which existing controlled vocabularies should be incorporated to cover these terms most effectively. NLM is particularly interested in specific feedback on how users expect to use CPT data within the UMLS Metathesaurus. Relatively little CPT data appears in Meta-1 because the complexity of most CPT expressions precluded automated mapping to other UMLS source vocabularies. We need a clearer assessment of the utility of mapping complex CPT expressions to all or some of the more atomic concepts contained within them.

As part of the legislation that created the new Agency for Health Care Policy and Research, NLM was assigned specific responsibilities for the collection and dissemination of information related to health services research, including technology assessment, outcomes research, and the development of practice guidelines. Effective access to information in automated patient records is essential to progress in these areas. With an increased program emphasis on health services research information, NLM is even more concerned that the UMLS products function as effective tools in the patient record environment. The Library expects to provide direct support to a limited number of test projects involving the use of the UMLS products in access to patient record information. The development of a research and development agenda related to the automated patient record would assist NLM in making more effective use of the resources available for this purpose.

References

Barnett, G.O. 1984. The application of computer-based medical record systems in ambulatory practice. *New England Journal of Medicine* 310(25):1645–9.

Cimino, C., and G.O. Barnett. 1990. Standardizing access to computer-based medical resources. In *Proceedings of the fourteenth annual symposium on computer applications in medical care*, ed. R.A. Miller. Washington, D.C.: IEEE Computer Society Press 33–37.

Cote, R.A., ed. 1979. *Systematized nomenclature of medicine*. Skokie, Ill.: College of American Pathologists.

Covell, D.G., G.C. Uman, and P.R. Manning. 1985. Information needs in office practice: Are they being met? *Annals of Internal Medicine* 103:596–599.

CPT. Current Procedural Terminology. 1989. Chicago: American Medical Association.

Diagnostic and Statistical Manual of Mental Disorders, 3rd ed. revised. 1987. Washington, DC: American Psychiatric Association.

Dutcher, G.A. 1989. DOCLINE: a national automated interlibrary loan request routing and referral system. *Information Technology and Libraries* 8:359–370.

Humphreys, B.L., and D.A.B. Lindberg. 1989. Building the unified medical language system. In *Proceedings of the thirteenth annual symposium on computer applications in medical care*, ed. L.C. Kingsland III. Washington, D.C.: IEEE Computer Society Press, 475–80.

Library of Congress Subject Headings, 12th ed. 1989. Washington, D.C.: Library of Congress.

Lindberg, D.A.B., and B.L. Humphreys. 1989. Computer systems that understand medical meaning. In *Computerized natural medical language processing for knowledge representation*, ed. J.R. Scherrer, R.A. Cote, and S.D. Mandil. Amsterdam: Elsevier Science Publishers, 5–17.

Lindberg, D.A.B., and B.L. Humphreys. 1990. The UMLS knowledge sources: tools for building better user interfaces. In *Proceedings of the fourteenth annual symposium on computer applications in medical care*, ed. R.A. Miller. Washington, D.C.: IEEE Computer Society Press, 121–125.

McCray, A.T. 1989. The UMLS semantic network. In: L.C. Kingsland III, ed., Proceedings of the thirteenth annual symposium on computer applications in medical care. Washington, D.C.: IEEE Computer Society Press, 475–80.

Osheroff, J.A., D.E. Forsythe, B.G. Buchanan, R.A. Bankowitz, B.H. Blumenfeld,

R.A. Miller. 1991. Physician's information needs: Analysis of clnical questions posed during patient care activity. *Annals of Internal Medicine* 114:576–581.

Powsner, S.M., and P.L. Miller. 1989. Linking bibliographic retrieval to clinical reports: PsychTopix. In *Proceedings of the thirteenth annual symposium on computer applications in medical care*, ed. L.C. Kingsland III. Washington, D.C.: IEEE Computer Society Press, 431–435.

Sherertz, D.D., N.E. Olson, M.S. Tuttle, M.S. Erlbaum. 1990. Source inversion and matching in the UMLS Metathesaurus. In *Proceedings of the fourteenth annual symposium on computer applications in medical care*, ed. R.A. Miller. Washington, D.C.: IEEE Computer Society Press, 141–145.

Shortliffe, E.H. 1989. Testing reality: the introduction of decision-support technologies for physicians. *Methods of Information in Medicine* 28(1):1–5.

The international classification of diseases: 9th revision, clinical modification: ICD-9-CM, 2nd ed. 1980. Washington, D.C.: U.S. Health Care Financing Administration. [For sale by Superintendent of Documents, U.S. Government Printing Office.]

Tuttle, M.S., D.D. Sherertz, N.E. Olson, M.S. Erlbaum, W.D. Sperzel, L.F. Fuller, S.J. Nelson. 1990. Using Meta-1—the First Version of the UMLS Metathesaurus. In *Proceedings of the fourteenth annual symposium on computer applications in medical care*, ed. R.A. Miller. Washington, D.C.: IEEE Computer Society Press, 131–135.

Use of the Critical Incident Technique to Evaluate the Impact of MEDLINE. Bethesda, MD: National Library of Medicine, 1989 (Available from the National Technical Information Service, PB90–1425 22/GBB).

11

New Communication Technologies for Integrating Hospital Information Systems and Their Computer-based Patient Records

Helmuth F. Orthner

Based on a speculative view of the next generation of hospital information systems (HISs), communications technologies are reviewed and the impact of new technologies is examined. The Integrated Services Digital Network (ISDN) technologies are examined in more detail. ISDN has the potential to become the basis for all user interfaces in hospitals that require several information modalities (voice, text, and/or images) or all those applications that are oriented to transactions. ISDN also enables the HIS to reach out into the community and still maintain a highly secure access through a caller identification feature that ISDN can provide. Current local area network (LAN) technology is affecting the architectures of hospital information systems. As graphic user interfaces (GUIs) and multimedia systems are introduced in these systems, the bandwidth of the current LANs may be insufficient and therefore networks with higher bandwidths are needed. The fiber distributed data interface (FDDI) is a good candidate for linking LANs that are located within close proximity (i.e., on the same campus) and the emerging broadband ISDN (B-ISDN) technology, an extension ISDN into the multi megabit transmission range, can provide solutions for interactive video services. The basis for B-ISDN is the asynchronous transfer mode (ATM), a novel and efficient *fast packet* switching technology.

The Next Generation of Hospital Information Systems

In his keynote address at the Fifth World Congress on Medical Informatics (MEDINFO 86) in Washington, DC, Professor Feigenbaum (1986) of Stanford University quoted Professor Marvin Minsky of MIT: "Can you imagine that they used to have libraries where the books didn't talk to each other?" With this question, he visualized the Library of the Future as a place for active *knowledge servers* that replaced the passive books and journals of today's libraries. In the context of the next generation of hospital information systems (HISs), we may rephrase the quotation as follows: "Can you imagine that they used to have hospitals in which the medical records didn't speak up?" Again, in this futuristic sense, we may view medical records as active objects that remind, suggest, and perhaps even seek out advice. This Hospital of the Future is a place in which health care providers have access to all information about a patient in a timely fashion and are actively supported by medical knowledge servers regardless of where they reside in the organizational setting (Reinels and Shortliffe 1987; Shortliffe 1991). A communication system within the hospital must be able to cope with all information modalities including voice, text, image, video, and telemetry data in order to use the new generation of file servers, image servers, voice servers, knowledge servers and so forth. These servers will be essential components in the next generation of HISs. The operation of hospitals will be supported with transaction processing services, clinical care and nursing care supported with management control systems, diagnosis and therapy are aided with clinical decision support systems and access to the clinical literature and national reference databases, and the fiscal management of hospitals will be supported with executive decision support systems (Malec 1991; Hammon and Pickton 1991).

Requirements and Geographic Extent

The communication requirements in the next generation of hospital information systems must be comprehensive and include not only textual information but also dynamic three-dimensional images and voice. The communication system must be able to transmit information from a variety of databases and, in the future, also knowledge, experiences, and perhaps even wisdom. The information must be transmitted reliably and securely at speeds that match the intellectual capacity of its users so that their trains of thought are enhanced. Thus the full power of the next generation of medical and clinical knowledge servers can truly extend the human mind. In order to accomplish this, it is important that information be presented in a focused and relevant manner. More information alone will overload the users, with the consequence of introducing anxiety and even hostility toward information systems. Intelligent provision and packaging of information, perhaps tailored and formatted to the situation at hand (e.g., a complex diagnostic problem) and to the individual's training and background (e.g., whether medical student or expert physician) will allow users of the next generation of HISs to manage their data more effectively and turn it into useful information and productive actions.

The communication system must also be extensive and reach all personnel in the hospital, from the nurses and physicians on the patient floors, to the technicians in various laboratories and the security guards at the doors. In an academic hospital, the educational and research enterprises, as well as the medical library, must also be included in order to arrive at a truly integrated information management system (Matheson and Cooper 1982). Since the patient is the focus of the hospital, we may want to give the families and close relatives of patients (or former patients for continued care) some consideration and include them in the circle of communication. Given the current trend of the health care industry to vertically integrate, we may also consider enlarging the circle of communication to include satellite clinics and physician office practices of affiliated health care providers; occupational health departments of nearby companies and industries; emergency and disaster support organizations such as fire, police, rescue squads, and the Red Cross; and public health offices of the local administration (Yamamoto 1974). Telecommunication and information services can be used to increase the local community's allegiance to the hospital and thus increase its competitive position within the health care delivery arena. This enlarged circle of communication has the side effect of increasing the risk of breaching the confidentiality and protection of patient information (Griesser 1988; Sauter 1988). However, the new telecommunication technologies will permit the implementation of much more efficient and effective security measures (Weinstein 1990).

Organizational Structure

It has been said that effective information systems will change the organizational structure, which in turn will change the use and requirements of the information systems. This statement is especially true for medical and clinical information systems, which need to adapt to frequent administrative reorganizations and external pressures for more information. For example, in the 1970s the hospital information systems tried to optimize order entry tasks in order to capture charges that could be passed on to third party payers. In the 1980s the emphasis shifted toward patient classification according to diagnostic criteria in order to maximize reimbursement under the diagnostic related group (DRG) procedures, and, in the 1990s, the focus is shifting to quality assurance and outcome research of clinical services. The external pressures from insurance and governmantal agencies for detailed documentation of patient care is increasing at an alarming rate. It is therefore instructive to examine the impact that comprehensive and intelligent communication networks will have on the management and the organizational structure of businesses (Clemons 1991). Based on interviews with senior executives of large information processing corporations, Carlyle (1987) writes:

> Present trends suggest that the next three decades in information processing will be as revolutionary as the last three. The combination of peer networks, a MIPS glut, and artificial intelligence will remake the structure of corporations and redefine the meaning of work.

While this statement was made in the context of a business environment, it should apply to hospitals and academic medical centers as well. Writes Carlyle,

> Current hierarchies and vertical chains of command are out of tune with the information economy of tomorrow. Information networks hold the key to knowledge in the twenty-first century and an elite new class of information workers will replace a whole middle tier of clerical, supervisory, and administrative staffs.

Academic medical centers are actually ahead of this development since they are to a large extent already administratively decentralized. However, the electronic networks are often incomplete, missing, or uncoordinated and therefore these institutions cannot capitalize on or take full advantage of their decentralized structure.

Telecommunications Technologies

Frequency Division Multiplexed Systems (FDM)

The telephone industry has been remarkable in providing worldwide connectivity. Analogue voice signals of 4 kHz bandwidth are transmitted over long distances using various media such as wire pairs, coaxial cables, microwave links, optical fibers and the like. The collection of telephone switching centers constitutes a network that spans the entire globe. The centers are connected via wideband communications links that combine many voice channels. As shown in Table 1, the communication links form a hierarchy of voice channels called groups (Saltzberg 1990). The end result is a point-to-point connection allowing two persons to converse freely, interactively, and privately.

The methods of transmitting analog signals over long distances involves a number of techniques such as multiplexing several voice channels onto a single carrier and repeated amplification (regeneration) at regular intervals. In the early analog telephone network, the predominant method of multiplexing was based on frequency shifting, whereby 4 kHz base-band voice channels are electronically shifted to higher frequency bands and mixed together. This mode of multiplexing is called narrow-band frequency division multiplexing (FDM). The composite signal of the FDM switches is transmitted over coaxial cable pipes, and because of attenuation the signals must be regenerated at regular intervals. For example, in AT&T's L5E coaxial cable system, which can transmit 13,200 voice channels through one coaxial cable pipe, the signal is amplified every mile, or in the TAT-7 submarine cable, which provides telephone connections under the Atlantic, the signal is amplified about every 6 miles (Pierce and Noll 1990). It is not uncommon that a voice signal is amplified several thousand times before it reaches its destination and the total amplification (over all regeneration units) may reach 1 million decibels (an extremely large power ratio). Unfortunately, analog amplifiers always add noise to the signal and, when the distance is very long (e.g., between continents), the noise level will be too high for comfortable conversations.

In summary, voice communication using analog signals is very effective for limited distances and FDM is an effective and bandwidth efficient multiplexing method. However, the repeated amplification and regeneration of the analogue

Table 1. Frequency division multiplexing (FDM) carrier standards in North America.

Name of group	Level	Channels	Bandwidth
Voice channel		1	4 kHz
Group	L1	12	48 kHz
Supergroup	L2	60	240 kHz
Mastergroups	L3	600	2,520 kHz
Jumbogroup	L4	3,600	17 MHz
	L5	10,800	57 MHz
	L5E	13,200	62 MHz

signals along the transmission paths increases the noise to unacceptable levels unless very high quality analogue amplifiers and multiplexers are used. These very high quality analog amplifiers and multiplexers are expensive to manufacture and practically impossible to maintain (many of them are built into the submerged cables). A cost-effective solution to this problem is the transmission of the analog voice signal in digital form.

Time Division Multiplexed Systems (TDM)

The pressure to move to digital communication systems comes not only from the desire to maintain high quality voice connectivity, but also from the increasing demand to transport data that is already in digital form. For example, it does not make sense to convert a word processing document in a PC into a sequence of audible beeps (as it is done in your modem) in order to send it via the telephone to your colleague. We should be able to access the telephone network in such a way that it takes advantage of the digital nature of computer-based data.

Today, all long distance and most intermediate distance voice communication is performed digitally in most telephone exchanges of the United States. Digital signals can be regenerated without adding noise which is especially advantageous for long distance communications. In addition, digital amplifiers and multiplexers are less costly to produce and maintain. The method of multiplexing is called time division multiplexing (TDM). It is a method that allows several lower speed digital channels to be interleaved onto a higher speed channel. By agreement with the International Telephone and Telegraph Consultative Committee (CCITT), the international standards-setting body for the telephone industry, each voice channel is digitized at 8,000 samples per second with a resolution of 8 bits per sample. This provides a digital stream of bits with an aggregate bit rate of 64 kb/s ($8,000 \times 8$ bit per second). This 64 kb/s digital signal stream is called DS-O. It is the basic unit of a one-way (i.e., unidirectional) telephone connection. As is done with analog voice channels, several DS-O channels can be combined into a higher speed channel. For example, in North America the TDM hierarchy combines 24 digital voice channels into one DS-1 channel (see Table 2). This DS-1 channel is the widely deployed T1 carrier system in the United States. It has a total data rate of 1.536 Mb/s (24×64 kb/s) and a bit rate of 1,544 kb/s, i.e., 8 kb/s are needed for signalling functions. (Note: In Europe the T1 carrier system operates at 2,048 kb/s providing 32 channels).

Table 2. Time division multiplexing (TDM) carrier standards in North America.

Stream	Carrier	Channels	Data rate
DS-0		1	64 kHz
DS-1	(T1)	24	1.544 MHz
DS-2	(T2)	96	6.312 MHz
DS-3	(T3)	672	44.736 MHz
DS-4	(T4)	4032	274.176 MHz

Broadband Fiber Optics and Photonic Switching

Research in using fiber optics technology for digital communications has made enormous progress in the last decade. The fabrication of low loss, single mode fiber optic waveguides (i.e., cables) makes it now possible to transmit light pulses in the multi Gb/s (gigabit per second) range over a distance of more than 100 km using low noise photodiodes (Li 1987). With photonic amplifiers (i.e., amplifiers that boost light intensity without the need for conversion to electronic energy), this distance can be boosted to over 350 km (AT&T 1987). Currently, AT&T's commercial lightwave transmission systems in the Washington to Boston corridor transmit at the OC-36 rate (1.8 Gb/s), an international standard rate for optical carriers that represents about 24,000 simultaneous telephone conversations (Rogalski 1987) and the recently proposed trans-Pacific cable connecting Japan and the U.S. and the trans-Atlantic cable connecting Germany and the United States will use the OC-48 rate (2.4 Gb/s). At the present time national data networks in the United States (e.g., NSFNET) use 1.5 Mb/s (T1 channels), but upgrades to 45 Mb/s (T3 channels) are being installed in the 1990s (Walsh 1988). Plans call for the development of hardware and software for a National Research and Education Network (NREN), that would transmit and switch data in the 3 Gb/s range by the year 2000 (Bell 1988; Fisher 1991; Gore 1991).

Some claim that the transmission capacity can be boosted to 13 Gb/s using fundamental photon packets that exist in fiber optic materials and perhaps even into the 20 Gb/s to 30 Gb/s range by using tuned lasers and wave length multiplexing techniques (Bachus et al. 1986; Kahn 1987). It is obvious that the fields of material science and optics have given us opportunities to transport data as never before. In summary, there is no shortage of transmission capacity in sight. The only question is how one can get the information on and off an optical fiber at these incredible speeds and how we can build switches that can direct these data streams to the places where we need them? Photonic and electronic switches using GaAs solid state or superconducting materials may form the first stage. This would be followed by a demultiplexing stage that converts the high speed lightwaves to multiple lower speed channels that can then be used by host computers, superminis, or workstations.

Wireless Communication Systems

Wireless communication systems using radio waves go back to the nineteenth century when Marconi transmitted his first message between Europe and Newfoundland, Canada. While most of the useful frequency spectrum is consumed by the broadcast industry (e.g., radio, television), bidirectional radio communication is as old as the radio itself (e.g., Ham radios, CBs or citizen bands, and walkie-talkies). Since the communication uses an open shared medium, interference is avoided by consensus, regulations, and international agreements. Basically, each country regulates and controls the usage of the electromagnetic spectrum by assigning frequency, bandwidth, transmission power, and location, taking into consideration the propagation characteristics of radio waves at various frequencies and, of course, past usage and prior commitments.

With the move toward higher quality audio and video distribution systems within the broadcasting industry, especially compact digital audio (CD disc) and high definition television (HDTV), the demand for more bandwidth has increased. However, the spectrum of usable and available frequencies is limited, forcing the industry to develop methods that allow reuse of frequency bands and more efficient use of bandwidth. For example, the same frequency can be reused in different geographic areas by limiting the power of transmission of a single radio or television tower. In order to use bandwidth more efficiently, digital communications and packet switching concepts are now also considered by the broadcast industry.

For bidirectional radio communication the citizen band radios (CBs) and the amateur radios have been popular in the United States, especially in the trucking industry where CBs are used for communication among truck drivers. For the most part, however, the community using two-way radio communication has been small compared with the number of telephone users. An exception to this is the cellular telephone. When the telephone industry entered the wireless communications mode with cellular telephones, the demand soared quickly beyond all expectations. This shows that the linkage to an existing ubiquitous network is an important factor for the acceptance of a new telecommunications technology. Using cellular telephones, for example, physicians can stay in contact with their office, colleagues, and patients while on the road. Since the time of commuting to and from work or driving between different places of work seems to increase every year, having a cellular telephone in the car saves personal time. The total amount of time that the cellular telephone can save is great considering that the average commute time is more than an hour in any metropolitan area in the United States. The large demand for cellular telephones has caused access problems during rush hours because the number of users is limited by the current analog systems (e.g., in Los Angeles). New methods employing digital techniques and packet switching will increase the number of users who can be served simultaneously within a cell.

While cellular telephony has been designed to fit the pattern of streets and roads, the cells are quite large (up to several miles). Several companies promote ideas to create wireless communications systems within a single building using microcells (Eglowstein 1991; Freeburg 1990). A microcell has the size of an office suite or wing of a building. It is controlled by a low power central transmitter and sensitive receiver that interacts with the individual user stations such as PCs, telephones, fax machines, and the like. In turn, the central microcell transceivers communicate with the corporate communication facility either via coaxial or optical fibers (e.g., PBX, mainframe, etc.). The users are free to position their workstation anywhere within the microcell. Also, if people move around with portable computers, they still can maintain connection with the corporate databases. In the hospital this has practical implications since physicians, nurses, and students move from patient to patient. Often they need to access a patient information database and a wireless access mode could be handy. Physicians, nurses, and students with portable computers can access information resources wherever they are—in the lounge, the laboratory, the hallway, the conference room, or the library cubicle.

Wireless communication systems will enable true personal communication systems. These systems attach a unique identifier to a telephone set which, in turn, is carried by a person. The network keeps track of where the person is located. These systems can be viewed as extensions to the popular peeper systems. Hospitals are installing care terminals in patient rooms, but with this technology one might consider installing patient care terminals mounted to the patient's bed that can be moved around with the patient. In the future, we might even think of sending this personal patient care computer home with the patient for follow-up monitoring, education and support.

Recently Motorola Inc. announced several breakthrough technologies (Eglow-stein 1991; Freeburg 1990) for a wireless data communication system that has the potential to significantly change how we look at the wiring of health care facilities. Motorola, a leader in telecommunication and solid state semiconductor technology, brings digital cellular telephony into the building while extending its data trans-missions capacity to exceed those of traditional local area networks (Ethernet, tokenring, etc.). Motorola's in-building microcellular communication system elim-inates the "last 100 feet" of wiring to office desks and equipment. As we all know, this is the most troubling and most expensive section of a building's wiring plan because people constantly rearrange their desks, PCs, workstations, and so on.

In order to achieve such a wireless in-building communication system that has a capacity and reliability exceeding those of local area networks, Motorola needed to advance the state-of-the-art of several technologies and integrate them into a working system. First, an appropriate carrier frequency needed to be selected. Not all frequencies have properties that are useful for microcells. For example, frequen-cies in the infrared range (IR) are too high because these waves act more like light rays and require *line-of-sight* paths. Radio waves in the upper UHF band are too low because they cannot be contained within buildings since they propagate through solid walls (i.e., the size of the microcell is difficult to control). An ideal frequency band provides sufficient bandwidth to allow high data transmission rates and uses microwave signals with propagation characteristics to allow microcells to be configured to typical office suites. Such a frequency range has been recently released by the Federal Communications Commission (FCC) in the United States. They opened up ten 10-MHz-wide frequency bands in the 18 and 19-GHz micro-wave range. Frequencies in this range pass through interior drywalls and office partitions but are reflected by solid objects such as concrete floors and metal grids. Since the attenuation of the signal with the distance from the transmitter is sufficiently large, the same frequency can be reused within a short distance. Also, each of those 10-MHz-wide channels has enough bandwidth to enable very high two-way digital transmission rates with sufficient signal separation to ensure reliable performance and integrity.

Motorola announced four technologies that make it practical to build high performance communication systems within buildings (Freeburg 1990):

- An intelligent six-sector microwave antenna operating in the 18 GHz and 19 GHz frequency range
- A high performance RF (microwave) digital signal processor to modulate a bidirectional bit stream of 15 Mb/s (mega bits per second) onto a microwave carrier frequency
- Several GaAs-based ICs (gallium arsenide-based integrated circuits) that operate in the 18–19 GHz range
- A private branch exchange (PBX) on a chip that supports true packet switching, circuit switching, and fast packet switching

All four technologies are integrated with novel system software. The latter permits simultaneous voice and data communication. Motorola's technology will have a higher performance than current local area networks that are based on coaxial or twisted pair cables (Ethernet or tokenring), but future enhancement, they claim, will push data rates into the 100 Mb/s range. Key to the high performance is the integrated design combining traditional packet switching, circuit switching, and fast packet switching. Regular packet switching supports current local area networks, circuit switching supports voice and dedicated 64 kb/s data transport (e.g., for fax and still images) used in narrowband ISDN (see below). The fast packet switching mode opens the door to the implementation of efficient methods to transfer data in burst mode (e.g., single high resolution color images). This fast packet switching technology is perhaps the most significant breakthrough since this communication network technology does not waste bandwidth when no data is transmitted (as is the case for circuit-switched networks) nor does it have to process complex network protocols (as is the case for the traditional packet-switching protocols). Motorola's integrated design is a true enabling technology that promises many uses in the health care industry.

Satellite Communications

Ever since the first man-made satellites were shot into orbit, the communications industry took advantage of the enormous *view* that satellites have over the earth. Being in direct view allows the use of microwaves to beam data up to and down from the satellites. Long terrestrial distances can be covered this way with only three signal amplification stages (two in the earth stations and one in the satellite). To cover such long terrestrial distances on the surface of the earth would require a large number of microwave towers and as many signal amplification stages. Today nearly 60% of all intercontinental communications traffic uses geo-synchronous satellites that orbit earth at about 35,800 km above the equator.

Satellite communications can provide effective means to reach areas that have no or only very poor connectivity to the public-switched network. For example, rural health care facilities can linkup with tertiary care centers that are usually university based and located in a metropolitan area (House 1990; Nymo and Engum 1990). The linkage can be used for videoconference-based tele-education programs, access to national databases, and expert medical advice. NASA's Advanced

Communications Technology Satellite (ACTS) program is preparing for several major test and demonstration programs. Key technologies include: transmitters and receivers operating in the 20/30 GHz frequency range; high performance antennas capable of producing fixed spot narrow (1°) beams; power augmentation on demand to respond to rain attenuation; on-board signal processing, switching and storing of signals for broadband ISDN applications at the DS-3 or 45 Mb/s rate, and integration of these services with the public-switched network (Pelton 1990).

The concept of a personal communication system based on satellite technology was recently proposed by Motorola, Inc., and named IRIDIUM. About 77 satellites would circle the earth in a geo-stationary orbit. Since these satellites are in line-of-sight with each other, they can communicate with each other and also with the area below them. The entire surface of the earth could be covered in this manner and anybody with a small microwave dish and a low power transceiver operating in the 30 GHz range could connect with the satellite above. The satellite in turn would establish a link with other satellites until a downlink to an earth station is found that provides the connection to the desired telephone number. Clearly, this is a futuristic concept but the technology to accomplish it is basically available. The potential benefits of bringing health education programs and if necessary up-to-date clinical information from large areas into developing countries of the third world are great and should be of interest to the World Health Organization.

The Worldwide Telephone Network

One of the greatest technical achievements in this century has been the creation of a worldwide communications network that permits private and personal voice communication using the telephone. The network that established the connections consisted initially of human-operated switchboards, then electromechanical relay banks activated by the current pulses produced in the rotary telephone sets (pulse dialing). Today the network consists of electronic switches that are activated by signals produced in the touchtone telephone set (touchtone dialing). While touchtone dialing speeded up the dialing process, it also has side effects—the signals that establish connection and disconnection travel within the same channel as the human voice (this mode of signaling is called inband-signaling). For example, an expert whistler who can produce a sound at exactly 2,600 Hz for a certain amount of time could trick the local exchange so that it would accept other touchtone number (e.g., a long distance number) and redirect the call to this number without disconnecting. Thus, for the cost of a local call, the expert whistler could reach the entire world (Flory 1990). Sophisticated thieves produced electronic boxes, called blue boxes, that made use of this technical loophole. This resulted in large losses for AT&T, especially after international operator-assisted dialing to Europe was introduced in 1963. The blue box users could already dial international numbers in 1965 while regular telephone subscribers had to wait until about 1970. The proven cost of this fraud amounted to about $20 million per year in the early to mid-1970s, but some estimates claim it was substantially higher (as high as $100 million per year). The solution to the blue box problem came, when the control structure of the telephone network was changed from an in-band signaling to an out-band signaling method. The latter method uses a separate channel to carry control information (e.g., connect, disconnect, telephone number, etc.) and business information for the telephone company. This channel uses different lines and a different routing network between the telephone exchange and thus the telephone subscribers do not have direct access to the computer-controlled switches of the telephone network. The switch to out-band signaling is a significant advance in telephone network architecture because it separates the flow of user data from the flow of control information.

During the 1950s the electromechanical switches were replaced with electronic switches, and in the 1960s it became clear that the emerging digital electronics would displace the analog circuitry in the telephone switching centers of AT&T. By the early 1970s the decision was made to digitize the entire telephone network with the goal of achieving an all-digital network by the end of the century. In fact, AT&T had already achieved this goal (from a business and tax perspective) by 1988 when it took a huge tax write-off of all analog switching equipment on its long distance service. The tax write-off does not include the local loops (i.e., the connections from the central office to the residential subscriber) since they are now the responsibility of the regional bell operating companies (RBOCs). For the most part, the local loops are still used in analog mode but the conversion to an all-digital connection is in progress.

Integrated Services Digital Network (ISDN)

In the past 20 years, the telephone industry achieved much progress in the worldwide interconnectivity for individual voice communication. This was possible because significant technical advances were made in the transmission and switching of voice signals through the replacement of the mechanical relays with computer-controlled electronic switches and migration from analog to digital transmission facilities. In spite of this progress, the access to this worldwide digital network remains very poor and is essentially limited to a 3 to 4-KHz analog voice channel (Newell 1985). For various reasons, including tariffs and governmental regulations, the customer loop (i.e., the telephone wires that come into homes and residences) have not been included in the modernization of the telephone network.

Similarly, the data processing industry has made remarkable progress in the last two decades. It has moved from mechanized accounting with punch card equipment to distributed processing using workstations and artificial intelligence techniques to support decision making. In the area of telecommunications, however, the data processing (DP) industry minimized the use of the communications channels provided by the telephone industry. If it was necessary to use a telephone link, expensive modems and statistical multiplexers were used to overcome the limitations imposed by the analog voice channels. As a rule, the data processing departments preferred to install their wire pairs and coaxial cables rather than rely on the internal telephone department or local telephone company. The result was a myriad of local networks each with its own proprietary communication protocols. In part, these proprietary protocols were used to capture and control business markets. Therefore these protocols were entrenched in the data processing industry and a move to more open systems is only a recent phenomenon.

The farsighted and pioneering work of the Advanced Project Agency of the U.S. Department of Defense (DARPA) led to a national computer network (the ARPA-NET) in which data is transmitted using the packet-switching concept (Kahn 1987). This packet-switching technology is now accepted internationally. The International Organization for Standardization (ISO) adopted a seven-layer open system interconnect model (OSI) that became the universally accepted reference model for international standards dealing with information interchange. All major computer vendors have adopted this ISO-OSI model and have agreed to eventually incorporate the international standards into their products.

The packet-switching concept and its associated protocols impose a large overhead on data communications that is transaction oriented. However, just consider the case of a simple transaction such as the request to look up the demographic information of a patient. A short message (e.g., a medical record number or social security number) is sent from the terminal (or workstation) to the database server. As this short message (a few bytes long) moves (logically) through each OSI layer, header and trailer bytes are added. Eventually a physical record, perhaps 100 percent to 500 percent longer, is transmitted over the physical medium (e.g., twisted wire pair or coaxial cable). At the database server these header and trailer bytes must be removed and finally the look-up program receives the short message. The (traditional) packet-switching technology consumes a lot of bandwidth on communications channels and requires a lot of central processing unit (CPU) cycles to process protocols. However, it is an elegant solution when a single dedicated physical communications channel needs to be shared by many users.

Today, there is an alternative which is made possible by three fundamental changes in the telecommunication industry: (1) total digital communication, (2) time-division multiplexing, and (3) out-of-band signaling (i.e., using a separate channel network for dialing, signaling, and billing purposes). The Integrated Services Digital Network (ISDN) makes use of these changes and attempts to bring the packet switching and digital circuit switching technologies together (Roca 1986). ISDN preserves the elegance of the packet switching technology for multiplexing many short messages over a single channel with the efficiency of dynamic circuit switching for bulk transfers of large amounts of data. The goal is to provide a standard approach for universal digital interconnectivity regardless of modality (i.e., voice, data, video) from potentially every telephone in the world that exists today (Aldermeshian 1986; Carney and Prell 1986; Cummings et al. 1987; Higdon et al. 1986; Neigh and Spindel 1986).

ISDN will overcome the 4 KHz limitation that current analog voice channels impose, and provides a full-duplex digital interface with a user capacity of approximately 144 Kb/s in both directions (2 × 64 Kb/s + 16 Kb/s) for each basic rate ISDN access port (BRI) and 1.5 Mb/s for each primary rate ISDN access port (PRI). The BRI interface requires only a single twisted wire pair and thus can be installed in all places where an analog telephone is used today. The PRI interface requires coaxial cables (or twisted wire pairs for short distances) and is available at most business locations. Data rates above 100 Mb/s are available when broadband ISDN (B-ISDN) is introduced; it typically requires fiber optic cables.

The ISDN technology will have profound implications for businesses and consumers alike. A large impact is also expected on the networking industry, especially on those making modems and related equipment, as well as software companies that are involved in networking. ISDN eliminates the use of modems, and the network protocols for packet switching can be greatly simplified since error control and routing information is handled in a different fashion (Falek and Johnston 1987).

Basic Concepts of Narrowband ISDN

ISDN is based on the concept of utilizing a single user interface to the existing conventional telephone network to furnish end-to-end connections in digital form as easily as the telephone set does for voice (ISDN Planner's Guide 1987). Users who have an ISDN interface in their home or business have access to all network services regardless of information modality such as voice, text data, or image. An important characteristic of ISDN is the separation of user information from network information into separate logical channels (out-of-band signaling) (Falek and Johnston 1987). This separation has the advantage of increasing the transmission capacity to the information bearing channels (B-channels) and achieving greater flexibility and control over the telephone switches via the signal channel (D-channel). The latter is necessary for network control such as dialing, maintenance, and error control, but also to deter fraud and illegal use of the telephone network (Flory 1990; Orthner 1991). Advanced features such as calling party identifications, multiple simultaneous message types (e.g., voice-annotated text), remote device status information, and the like are possible with this new signal channel (D-channel) that uses messages in the form of data packets instead of touchtone signals.

Each ISDN interface has one D-channel that is used for network signaling and control and two or more B-channels for carrying customer information. Each channel is designed for full duplex communication at 64 Kb/s. All channels are then digitally time-multiplexed onto the same physical channel (i.e., a pair of copper wires). Currently, two interfaces are defined and approved by CCITT: The basic rate interface (BRI) intended for individual users in residences or small business offices and the primary rate interface (PRI) intended for businesses with database servers, private branch exchanges (PBXs), or local area networks (LANs) (Falek and Johnston 1987).

The Basic Rate Interface (BRI) of ISDN

The basic rate interface (BRI) consists of two bidirectional B-channels at 64 Kb/s each and one bidirectional D-channel at 16 Kb/s called 2B+D. Since the D-channel is used for signaling and other network functions, only 16 Kb/s are available to the user for data transmission. The D-channel provides packet-switched data transfers only (e.g., X.25); it cannot be used for regular voice. Thus the effective bandwidth totals 144 Kb/s but the signaling bit rate is 192 Kb/s.

All three channels (2B+D) may be used independently; that is, they may be connected to different telephone numbers at the same time. For example, one B-channel can be used for voice communication with a patient at home, while the other B-channel connects on the attached PC (or workstation) to a patient database, and the D-channel receives telemetry data collected by patient monitors in the patient's home. Since ISDN provides only one interface to the digital telephone network all three connections (2B+D) can be setup and dynamically changed without human intervention. For example, the following scenario is feasible. A physician with an ISDN workstation at home can use one B-channel (B1) to talk to a patient while, simultaneously, the patient's most recent summary data is retrieved from the patient record system via the D-channel and the latest laboratory results are downloaded from the clinical laboratory system via the second B-channel (B2). As the physician interprets and discusses the laboratory results with the patient, the second B-channel (B2) is redirected to the radiology PACS system (Picture Archive and Communication System) and a low resolution image is downloaded to the workstation. The physician may ask the patient to "hold" for a few seconds, freeing up this first B-channel (B1) to double the bandwidth to 128 kb/s by combining both B-channels (B1 + B2) in order to accelerate the downloading of the image in higher resolution. After the high resolution image is transferred, the first B-channel (B1) is reconnected to patient on "hold" and the conversation can continue.

The BRI interface supports also a "passive bus" at the endpoint which allows the interconnection of up to eight devices (e.g., data terminals, facsimile) on a single B-channel. Again, the D-channel signals will control the time division multiplexing of the data from the attached devices and the connections will appear totally transparent to the terminal operators. The baud rates of the devices need not be the same but the aggregate bandwidth of all active devices can obviously not exceed the total bandwidth of 64 Kb/s (ISDN Planner's Guide 1987).

The physical interface of the BRI access consists of two twisted-wire pairs for full duplex transmission but only one nonloaded twisted-wire pair needs to enter into the residence or business office if electrical power is available. The ISDN interface box will split the single wire pair into two wire pairs—one for transmission, the other for receiving.

The Primary Rate Interface (PRI) of ISDN

The primary rate interface (PRI) is intended for connections to a large PBX, a local area network (LAN), or a database server. In the United States and Japan the PRI access supports 23 B-channels and one D-channel (23B+D) at 64 Kb/s each. The effective bandwidth is 23×64 Kb/s (1,472 Mb/s). The D-channel is dedicated to signaling and controlling the 23 B-channels; no user data is transmitted on it. The basic bit rate of the PRI channel is 1.544 Mb/s which is the standard T-1 carrier rate in the United States and Japan. In Europe, the PRI access provides 30 B-channels and one D-channel. A framing channel is also necessary because the D-channel cannot carry all signal and control information for 30 B-channels.

The PRI has three advantages in a hospital or business environment (Newell 1985).

1. It provides a speed multiplexed full duplex interface between colocated systems using the convenient medium of simple twisted-wire pairs;
2. PRI can be used as a high speed multiplexed access point to a public or private branch exchange; and
3. The PRI can be used to create public switched networks in which the basic channel is the 64 Kb/s B-channel carrying only end user information (i.e., the B-channel is not burdened with signaling overhead that reduces the data rate to 56 Kb/s).

It must be said, however, that these advantages have little meaning if the major computer systems vendors do not provide the appropriate interface hardware and operating system support. For example, if two DEC VAX computers are collocated in one computer room it is currently cheaper and easier to link them with ethernet hardware and DECNET software. It is available and it works. Also, a clear B-channel of 64 Kb/s is too slow for a typical LANs which typically use bit-rates in the order of 10 Mb/s (ethernet) or 4 Mb/s (tokenring).

Again, the physical interface of the PRI is one twisted-wire pair at the NT1 interface and two twisted-wire pairs at the NT2 interface (one for receiving and one for sending) for full duplex communication at a signalling rate of 1.544 Mb/s. Additional wire pairs are needed if auxiliary electrical power needs to be provided by the telephone company.

Broadband ISDN (B-ISDN): A Revolution to Come

The rapid advances in reliable, high speed communications using fiber optics and the widespread deployment of fiber optic cables within the telephone industry and corporate world forced the telephone industry to extend the ISDN concept to much higher data rates than the BRI and PRI access permits. The change is driven by the expectations of future interactive video communication needs and the potential profits that can be made by offering such services. In 1988, the CCITT Study Group VIII outlined the broadband ISDN (B-ISDN) with a series of draft recommendations for the study period 1988–1992. It will push the transmission speeds into multiples of 140 Mb/s to the 1.7 Gb/s range using optical fibers. For some applications such as the transmission of uncompressed high resolution dynamic color images data, rates in the order of 100 to 600 Mb/s may be necessary (Kahn 1987). When fiber optic lines reach the residential subscribers, B-ISDN will permit video conferencing and movie distribution with far better quality than is possible with today's VCRs and video tapes. Standards for broadband ISDN have not been formulated yet but one may assume that they will provide compatibility with the existing narrowband ISDN standards (Falek and Johnston 1987). Also, one may safely assume that packet-switching technology will also be employed for voice communication. This opens the door to many other innovative uses of this national digital communication network. For example, automatic detection of pauses that occur naturally during conversations may be used to conserve bandwidth since these (silent) voice packets need not be transmitted. In addition, voice and video packets may be given transmission priority over datapackets to assure a continued smooth flow of high fidelity voice and video in a packet-switching environment. Techniques to "playback" voice faster than it is spoken may increase the efficiency of "reading" voice-annotated text or images. We may be able to increase the quality of care by combining several information modalities.

ISDN Software Protocols

Current standards are limited to the BRI and the PRI. In addition, protocols have been defined for the interconnection of ISDN switches between different vendors of the telephone industry. In the United States, the common channel signaling System #7 (SS7) protocol defines a structure of layered communication protocols that follow the principles of the CCITT open system interconnect (OSI) model (Falek and Johnston 1987). Some vendors of ISDN technology combine some of OSI layers to remove the artificial layering that is unnecessary in an circuit-switching environment. This makes the protocol substantially leaner and more efficient. It is quite clear that this technology can provide efficient communication systems for transaction oriented distributed systems. Many activities in the hospital have a transaction-orientation (e.g., order entry).

In spring 1991, several major ISDN vendors and user organizations in the United States agreed to a common ISDN protocol called National ISDN 1 (Barron 1991; Green 1991). This agreement aims to standardize some of the interfaces, protocols, hardware and software, whose compatibility is essential to making the use of ISDN ubiquitous and transparent in the United States. It is hoped that this industry consensus will speed up the deployement of ISDN technology across the United States. *Network Interface Description and Terminal Guidlines for National ISDN-1* (FR-NWT-000660), available from Bellcore, the Bell Communications Research Corporation: Customer Service, 60 New England Avenue, Piscataway, NY 08854–4196, 80522673.

Current Status of Narrowband ISDN Technology

The Integrated Services Digital Network requires that the communications system be an all digital network. The conversion of the analog telephone network to an all-digital one is now complete in many metropolitan areas of the United States. Therefore, we should see a major push by the telecommunications industry for the ISDN. Several PBX vendors have advertized switches with ISDN capabilities (Herman and Johnston 1987). For the local loop interface, a number of electronic circuit manufacturer are producing chip sets for the ISDN interfaces (e.g., Intel, AT&T, Siemens, Rockwell, AMD). Some modem vendors (e.g., Hayes Microcomputer Products, GA) are readying PC boards for the BRI interface; Intel is selling a kit that includes a printed circuit board, a chip set, and software (for OSI layers 1, 2, and 3) that can be used to build a BRI interface for the IBM PC.

Several Bell operating companies (BOCs), AT&T, Northern Telcom, and Siemens are holding field trials in the United States (Herman and Johnston 1987; Kemezis 1987), and in West Germany the Deutsche Bundespost is implementing ISDN with Siemens switches. Estimates for the widespread acceptance of this technology varies considerably. Some believe it will take until the mid-1990s, others estimate it will be in the late 1990s. Considering that this technology is offering so much to the medical community, one might be very optimistic and see this technology applied in the early 1990s in some medical centers.

The ISDN Standard Setting Process

In order for ISDN (i.e., narrowband and broadband ISDN) to become as ubiquitous and simple to use as the telephone, international standards must be recommended, adopted, and accepted worldwide. In addition, the technologic foundation for ISDN (i.e., hardware and software) must be incorporated into the telephone plants of the world in an incremental fashion so that existing equipment for voice and fax services are interoperable with ISDN. Considering that the total investment of the telecommunications plant in the United States alone is well above a trillion dollars, such a conversion is not a simple process. From the fiscal and human resource perspective alone, such a process will require decades.

At the global, worldwide level, the International Telecommunications Union (ITU) and the International Organization for Standardization (ISO) are involved with defining and approving standards for telecommunications and information systems respectively. Most work in ISDN involves the International Telegraph and Telephone Consultative Committee (CCITT), a body of the ITU. The CCITT consists of a Plenary Assembly that meets every four years and scores of study groups established by the assembly. The last plenary asssembly that convened in Melbourne, Australia, in November 1988. There are eight CCITT study groups for the 1989–1992 working period and Study Group XVIII is the focal point for most ISDN activities (Rutkowski) but Study Group VII (Data Communications Networks) and Study Group XI (Switching and Signaling) are also involved. In addition, the International Radio Consultative Committee (CCIR) is involved through a joint CCITT/CCIR Study Group addressing radio and television transmission networks.

The process of standards adoption within CCITT has been slow in the past, but since the 1988 plenary assembly a much faster process has been established for adopting new and amending old recommendations. For example, the new broadband-ISDN/asynchronous transfer mode (B-ISDN/ATM) recommendations were adopted in less than 24 months. During the 1985–1988 study period, Study Group XVIII received more than several thousand contributions for consideration and many related to the emerging broadband-ISDN (B-ISDN) standard was seen.

Considering the complexity of the material, it showed a new level of international cooperation on the broadband aspects of ISDN.

The standards formally adopted by the general assembly of the CCITT are called recommendations and the set of volumes are known by the color of the outer cover. For example, the recommendations of the Eighth Plenary Assembly in 1984 are called the red books, those of the Ninth Plenary Assembly in 1988 are referred to as the blue books. The color of the books containing the Recommendations of the Tenth General Assembly in 1992 is not known yet. Most likely they will be disseminated in electronic or optical formats.

Each recommendation is classified into a series and coded with an upper-case letter. For example, the letter I is reserved for standards pertaining to ISDN (e.g., I.121 Broadband Aspect of ISDNs, I.441 ISDN user-network, interface, data, link, layer, specification, etc.), the letter Q is used for telephone switching and Signaling (e.g., Q.921 ISDN user-network, interface, data, link, layer, specification, etc.), and the letter X is used for data communications networks (e.g., X.25, X.400, X.500). Some recommendations have several classifications if they address topics of several working groups (e.g., the I.441 and the Q.921 are the same).

The International Organization for Standardization (ISO) is a specialized international agency of the United Nations comprising the national standards bodies of more than 90 countries with, The American National Standards Institute (ANSI) represents the United States. ISOs is a large organization supported by more than 2200 technical committees and 20,000 experts from all over the world. To date over 4,900 ISO standards have been published. Most standards related to the information technology are the responsibility of the Joint Technical Committee 1 (JTC1), which was previously known as the Technical Committee 97 (TC97). With regard to ISDN, two subcommittees of JTC1 are important: (1) Subcommittee 6 (SC6), dealing with standards for telecommunications and information transfer, has four working groups involved with the first fours layers of the open system interconnection (OSI) reference model and (2) Subcommittee 21 deals with open system support services including the OSI reference model. This seven-layer OSI reference model has been adopted by the CCITT for the integration of telecommunication and informations systems.

ISO has a formal process for adopting standards consisting of four phases: WD (working draft), DP (draft proposal), DIS (draft international standard), and IS (international standard). A ballot procedure is used to elevate each standard to the next higher level, which typically takes about 2 to 3 years.

The United States is represented in CCITT and ISO formally through the Department of State but it has defered to the Exchange Carriers Standards Association (ECSA) and ANSI. The work, however, is done by many parties in many private and public organizations such as the National Institute of Standards and Technology (NIST), the Federal Communications Commission (FCC), the Federal Telecommunications Standards Committee (FTSC), Institute of Electrical and Electronic Engineers (IEEE), Corporation for Open Systems (COS), and others.

Clearly, the ubiquitous and transparent nature of ISDN coupled with the capabilities and elegance of a user-controllable information network has excited many strategic planners in academia, business, and government. The potential payoff of such a universal network lies not only in an increased academic and commercial productivity, but also as a pillar for safeguarding democracy. I agree with Luderer (1990) that the establishment of a global ISDN network would be one of the greatest cultural accomplishments in human history. A vision for a national network has been articulated by U.S. Senator Albert Gore (1991) and efforts are currently underway to create a high performance network for research and education (Fisher 1991). The efficient ISDN and B-ISDN technologies will play a role in these efforts and, with its potential, every school and library can link to this fiber optic data highway as proposed by Senator Gore.

Local Area Networks

Ethernet and Token Ring Networks

With the appearance of local area networking, technology many medical informatics professionals started building departmental systems (Hammon and Pickton 1991; Simborg et al. 1983; Tolchin et al. 1988) that were integrated with main frames that typically provided support for the financial system of the hospital. Even before the arrival of PCs, rather complete clinical HISs were implemented using proprietary network technology and distributed databases (Safran et al. 1990; Safran and Porter 1988). This technology is now applied to off-the-shelf PCs and industry standard local area networks (Beaman and Althouse 1989; Schuller 1990). For example, a large effort is currently underway at Brigham and Women's Hospital in Boston. All administrative, financial, and clinical functions will be integrated using off-the-shelf PCs and local area networking technologies, and all character-oriented terminals will be phased out. The design calls for the integration of more than 100 departmental tokenring networks with a hospital-wide backbone, also a token ring but configured. Each departmental network consists of two MUMPS server/routers (one is a live backup) each with 2 Gb disks storage, one DOS or OS/2 server for standard DOS packages, and up to 40 PC-based diskless workstations. The total network will serve approximately 2,000 PCs, but the design can support up to 4,000 PCs without network bottlenecks. The functionality calls for each PC to be able to access any MUMPS-based server in a totally transparent way (provided access is permitted). In total, the database will have about 140 Gb of disk storage, which is distributed over 140 servers. The software to support this network is based on the integrated HIS originally developed by the Beth Israel Hospital in Boston (Bleich and Slack 1989; Bleich et al. 1989; Safran and Porter 1988; Safran et al. 1989; 1990). This MIIS-based software system is being converted to ANSI Standard MUMPS by the information systems group of the Brigham and Women's Hospital.

The move to downsize mainframes will continue and LANs will play a vital role in this process. As the management of these networks improves (including access security, backup, etc.), the construction of these large networks becomes a viable and cost-effective alternative for hospitals. However, as graphic user interfaces and multimedia systems are demanded, the bandwidth of these LANs may become the bottleneck and higher speed networks (e.g., FDDI), and/or other network architectures (e.g., B-ISDN) may be needed.

Fiber-Distributed Data Interface (FDDI)

In the LAN arena the development of broadband fiber optic technology and the specification of the fiber distributed data interface (FDDI) standard (ANSI X3T9.5, ISO 9314) (Stallings 1991) are exciting developments and commercial products are available from several vendors. The FDDI standard is a tokenring architecture featuring two counter-rotating rings for bidirectional communications and fault tolerance. The ring has a bandwidth of 100 Mb/s and can carry data packets from several nodes simultaneously for greater speed and capacity. The FDDI tokenring network fills a need for interconnecting high volume file servers (mainframes, superminis, etc.), low speed LANs (e.g., IEEE 802.3, Ethernet, IEEE 802.4 tokenbus, or IEEE 802.5 tokenring), and imaging workstations. This network technology could form a platform for private networks linking corporate databases that are relatively close (e.g., within a campus). Since the bandwidth of the FDDI ring matches or even exceeds the typical bus bandwidth of superminis (e.g., the CI bus of a VAX cluster has a bandwidth of about 70 Mb/s), LANs users would not even realize that they are served by a computer housed in another building. The rapid progress of the FDDI standardization surprised many in the industry, and extensions to the standard are already being discussed (FDDI-II) to boost transmission capacity to 200 Mb/s in order to overcome shortcomings for interactive voice-video applications. However, other approaches such a the broadband ISDN (B-ISDN) standard and the metropolitan area network (MAN) standard (IEEE 802.6) (Luderer 1990) may make the FDDI technology obsolete faster than we think. The latter two standards use a common fast packet technology (known as the asynchronous transfer mode, or ATM), which is not only an extremely efficient technology but also an international CCITT recommendation (i.e., standard).

Summary and Conclusions

This chapter reviews and speculates on new communication technologies for hospitals and academic medical centers. It is clear that the next generation of HIS will be decentralized in the computing architecture but integrated in its functionality. The emergence of intelligent communication networks will play a vital role in the linkage of the many functions, databases, file servers, and knowledge servers (Rennels and Shortliffe 1987; Shortliffe 1991). Also, the circle of communications will expand beyond the physical boundaries of the hospital to include the offices of referring physicians and perhaps close relatives of patients. The structure of organizations may change as sophisticated computing technology reaches every workplace. Some executives believe that the number of administrative levels will decrease with increasing use of electronic mail and intelligent message switching.

One of the emerging technologies for hospital communication systems is the very high speed "fast packet" switching technique (e.g., ATM) using fiber optic cables (Barron 1988). This technology is highly applicable for linking different computing system in such way that they appear as one system to the users of the HIS. Examples of such an approach is available when a homogeneous software environments such as MUMPS is used (Beaman and Althouse 1989; Bleich et al. 1986; Munnecke and Kuhn 1988; Schuller 1990; Slack 1987). In a heterogeneous computing environment, a packet-switching technology can enable the linkage of different systems (Tolchin et al. 1987), but the level of effort needed to integrate and make the various communications protocols work across all hardware and operating systems can be substantial (Orthner 1988, Orthner and Pendelton 1987).

The integrated services digital network (ISDN) is an exciting technology for medium speed communication (e.g., up to 1.5 Mb/s) between users and various database servers. This technology is very effective and extremely efficient when the geographic location of the users precludes the use of fiber optic cables for a local area network (e.g., FDDI). In fact, this circuit-switching technology avoids the overhead of having to process all the protocols that the seven-layer OSI model prescribes. This is especially important in transaction-oriented applications and there are many of those in the hospital environment. For high speed networks the B-ISDN solution with its basis in the fast packet or cell-switching technologies are promising. This technology enables true interactive video applications.

Acknowledgment

This chapter is based on presentations given at a Working Conference of the IMIA Working Group 10 in May 1988, a meeting of the Institute of Medicine Technology Subcommittee on March 17, 1990, and the IMIA TELEMED Working Conference, November 1990 (Orthner 1991).

References

Aldermeshian, H. 1986. ISDN standards evolution. *AT&T Technical Journal*, 65:19–25.

Annual Report 1987. AT&T 17.

Bachus, E.J. et al. 1986. Ten channel coherent optical fiber transmission. *Electronics Letters*, 22:1002–1003.

Barron, J.J. 1988. FDDI and integrating packaging cast new light on future of fiber optics. *Comp.Design* 46–52.

Barron, L.L. 1991. ISDN: Is it or isn't it? *BYTE*, 16:166–167.

Beaman, P.D., and J. J. Althouse 1989. An efficient MUMPS distributed database using a high level LAN interface. *MUG Quarterly* 19:31–34.

Bell, C.G. 1988. Gordon Bell calls for a U.S. research network, *IEEE Spectrum*, February 54–57.

Bleich, H.L., R. F. Beckley, G. L. Horowitz, et al. 1986. Clinical computing in a teaching hospital. *New England Journal of Medicine* 312:756–764.

Bleich, H.L., C. Safran, and W. V. Slack 1989. Departmental and laboratory computing in two hospitals. *MD Computing* 6:149–155.

Bleich, H.L., and W. V. Slack 1989. Clinical computing. *MD Computing,* 6:133–135.

Carlyle, R.E. 1987. Reaching 30 years toward 2017. *Datamation,* September 142–154.

Carney, D.L., and E. M. Prell. 1986. Planning for ISDN in the 5ESS Switch. AT&T Technical Journal 65:35–43.

Clemons, E.K. 1991. Evaluation of strategic investments in information technology. *Communications of the ACM* 34:22–36.

Cummings, J.L., K. R. Hickey, and B. D. Kinney. 1987. AT&T network architecture evolution. *AT&T Technical Journal* 66:2–12.

Eglowstein, H. 1991. Full Ethernet networking without a wire in sight. *BYTE,* 16:229–230.

Falek, J.I., and M. A. Johnston 1987. Standards makers cementing ISDN subnetwork layers. *Data Communications,* October 237–255.

Feigenbaum, E. A. 1986. Autoknowledge: From file servers to knowledge servers. In *MEDINFO 86: Proceedings of the Fifth Conference on Medical Informatics, Washington, October 26–30, 1986,* eds. R. Salamon, B. Blum, and M. Jorgensen. Amsterdam:Elsevier/North Holland, XLIII - XLVI.

Fisher, S., 1991. Whither NREN? *BYTE,* 16:181–189.

Flory, D. 1990. The great blue box phone frauds. *IEEE Spectrum* 127:117–121.

Freeburg, T.A. 1990. Technical white paper: Wireless in-building networks. Arlington Heights, Ill.:Motorola Inc., Radio Telephone Systems Group.

Green, R. 1991. Remote connections. *BYTE* 16:161–168.

Griesser, G. 1988. Data protection in hospital information systems: 1. Definitions and overview. In *implementing health care information systems,* eds. H.F. Orthner and B.I. Blum. Springer-Verlag New York:222–253.

Gore, A. 1991. A national vision. *BYTE* 16:188–189.

Hammon, G.L., and R. J. Pickton. 1991. A local area network solution to information needs: The Moses H. Cone Memorial Hospital experience. In *Health care information management systems: A practical guide,* eds. M.J. Ball, J.V. Douglas, R.I. O'Desky, and J.W. Albright. New York:Springer-Verlag 273–282.

Herman, J.G., and M. A. Johnston. 1987. ISDN when? What your firm can do in the interim, *Data Comm.,* October, 222–233.

Higdon, M.L., J. T. Page, and P. H. Stuntebeck. 1986. AT&T communications ISDN architecture. *AT&T Technical Journal* 65:27–33.

House, M. 1990. Telecommunications for health care: An international perspective. In *The expanding role of telecommunications in health* ed. B. Kerlin. McLean, Va.: MITRE Corporation and the Agency for Health Care Policy and Research (AHCPR).

ISDN Planner's Guide. 1987. AT&T Network Systems and Marketing Communications.

Kahn, R.E. 1987. Networks for advanced computing. *Scientific American,* 257: 136–143.

Kemezis, P. 1987. What price ISDN? First cost details bared. *Data Communications,* August 51–54.

Li, T. 1987. Advances in lightwave systems research. *AT&T Technical Journal,* 66:5–18.

Luderer, G.W.R. 1990. Evolution of ISDN. *In ISDN systems: Architecture, technology, and applications,* (ed.) P.K. Verma. Englewood Cliffs, NJ:Prentice-Hall, Inc., 305–347.

Malec, B.T. 1991. Cost justifying information systems. In *Health care information management systems: A practical guide,* eds. M.J. Ball, J.V. Douglas, R.I. O'Desky, and J.W. Albright. New York:Springer-Verlag, 221–231.

Matheson, N.W., and J. A. D. Cooper. 1982. Academic information in the academic health sciences center: Roles for the library in information management. *J. Med. Educ.* 57(suppl):pt 2.

May, R.T. 1990. A high performance model for block level sharing of MSM databases across different hardware platforms, and operating systems. *MUG Quarterly,* 20:31–36.

Munnecke, T.H., and I. M. Kuhn. 1988. Large scale portability of hospital information system software. In *Implementing Health Care Information Systems,* eds. H. F. Orthner and B. I. Blum. New York:Springer-Verlag, 133–148.

Neigh, J.L., and L. A. Spindel. The role of ISDN in AT&T information systems architecture. *AT&T Technical Journal,* 65:45–55.

Newell, J.A. 1985. ISDN networks for business applications. In *Proceedings of ISCAS 1985.* Washington, D.C.: IEEE Computer Society Press, 711–714.

Nymo, B.J., and B. Engum. 1990. Telemedicine to improve the quality, availability, and effectiveness of the health services in rural regions. In *Seminar on the Regional Impact of Advanced Telecommunications Services, Kiruna, Sweden; June 19–21, 1990.* Kjeller, Norway:Norwegian Telecom.

Orthner, H.F. 1990. Impact of new communications technologies on the architecture of health information systems. In *Proceedings of the IMIA Working TELE-MED Conference,* eds. J. Duisterhout and J. van Bemmel. Amsterdam:Elsevier Science Publishers,

Orthner, H.F. 1988. New communications technologies for hospital information systems. In *Towards new hospital information systems,* eds. A.R. Bakker, M.J. Ball, J.-R. Scherrer, and J.L. Willems. Amsterdam:Elsevier Science Publishers.

Orthner, H.F., and N. Pendelton. 1987. A high-speed packet switching network for heterogeneous minicomputers. In *Proceedings: 1987 Workshop on Computer Laboratory Health Care Resources,* eds., Jarzembski, W.B. and B. A. Rowley. Lubbock, Tex.: Department of Biomedical Engineering and Computer Medicine, Texas Tech University School of Medicine.

Pelton, J.N. 1990. An overview of ISDN and satellite communication issues. In *The North American ISDN users' forum (NIU-Forum) August 6–9, 1990,* ed. S.

Wakid. Gaithersburg, Md.:National Systems Laboratory, National Institute of Standards and Technology.

Pierce, J.R., and A. M. Noll. 1990. Signals: The science of telecommunications. New York:W. H. Freeman, 85–96.

Rennels, G.D., and E. H. Shortliffe. 1987. Advanced computing for medicine. *Scientific American,* 257:154–61.

Roca, R.T. 1986. ISDN architecture. *AT&T Technical Journal* 65:5–17.

Rogalski, J.E. 1987. Evolution of gigabit lightwave transmissions. *AT&T Technical Journal* 66:32–40.

Rutkowski, A.M. 1990. The ISDN standarization process. In ISDN systems: Architecture, technology, and applications, ed. P.K. Verma. Englewood Cliffs, N.J.:Prentice-Hall, 156–184.

Saltzberg, B.R. 1990. Theoretical foundation of digital communication. In *ISDN Systems: Architecture, technology, and applications,* ed. P. K. Verma. Englewood Cliffs, N.J.:Prentice-Hall.

Safran, C., and D. Porter. 1988. New uses of a large clinical data base. In Implementing health care information systems, eds. H.F. Orthner and B.I. Blum. New York:Springer-Verlag, 123–132.

Safran, C., D. D. Porter, C. D. Rury et al. 1990. ClinQuery: Searching a large clinical database. *MD Computing,* 7:144–153.

Safran, C., W. V. Warner, and H. L. Bleich. 1989. Role of computing in patient care in two hospitals. *MD Computing,* 6:141–148.

Sauter, K. 1988. Data protection in hospital information systems: 2. Software methods. In *Implementing health care information systems,* eds. H.F. Orthner and B.I. Blum. New York:Springer Verlag, 254–273.

Schuller, G. 1990. Distributed systems. *MUG Quarterly,* 20:17–29.

Shortliffe, E.H. 1991. The networked physician: Practitioner of the future. In *Health care information management systems: A practical guide,* eds. M.J. Ball, J.V. Douglas, R.I. O'Desky, and J.W. Albright. New York:Springer-Verlag, 3–18.

Simborg, D.W., M. Chadwick, Q. E. Whiting-O'Keefe, S. G. Tolchin, S. A. Kahn, and E. S. Bergan. 1983. Local area networks and the hospital, computers in biomedical research, 16:246–259.

Slack, W.V., 1987. The soul of a new system. *Massachusetts Medicine,* November, 24–28.

Stallings, W. 1991. Data and computer communications, (3rd ed.) New York: Macmillan.

Tolchin, S.G., W. Barta, and K. Harkness. 1988. A hospital information system network. In *Implementing health care information systems,* eds. H.F. Orthner and B.I. Blum. New York:Springer-Verlag, 149–163.

Tolchin, S.G., E. S. Bergan, M. Arseniev, P. Kuzmak, R. Nordquist, D. Siegel. 1987. Transaction processing using remote procedure calls (RPC) for a heterogeneous distributed clinical information system. *Comp. Methods and Programs in Biomedicine* 25:193–208.

Walsh, J. 1988. Designs on a national research network. *Science,* 239:861.

Weinstein, S.B. 1990. ISDN multimedia services. In *ISDN systems: Architecture, technology, and applications,* ed. P.K. Verma. Englewood Cliffs, N.J.:Prentice-Hall, 262–304.

Yamamoto, W.S. 1974. Planning technology in health services development: Uses of the telephone. In *Computers in biomedical research,* eds. R.W. Stacy and B.D. Waxman. New York:Academic Press, 17–30.

12
System and Data Protection

Gretchen Murphy

System reliability and security data integrity and confidentiality are universally recognized patient computer-based record (CPR) system attributes (Bleich et al. 1987). Originating in the ethical relationship between patient and physician and in the legal and professional policies and standards applicable to medical practitioners, these essential elements of a sound—that is, a properly (and *only* properly) structured, maintained, and used—CPR SYSTEM have evolved in other settings throughout history and most recently in the computer context. Requirements that these essential elements be present have been extended throughout U.S. health care, regardless of setting, by current federal and state legislation, as well as by institutional and professional association policy. The scope of these related terms encompasses programs within hospitals and other health care organizations that use paper medical record systems (Lavere 1982; Privacy Protection Study Commission 1977; Waters and Murphy 1982). Organizations using CPR systems face these same problems, but at a higher level of complexity. Basic methods used to maintain patient information reliability, security, and integrity, and safeguard confidentiality are therefore folded into formal goals and objectives for organizations, regardless of the system they use.

> Health records are used to provide a medium of communication for current and future patient care. . . . the patient must be assured that the information shared with health care professionals will remain confidential. Without such assurance, the patient may withhold critical information which could affect the quality of care provided, the relationship with the provider, and the reliability of the information maintained (American Medical Association 1985).

These organizational policies and procedures are currently being adapted in order to accommodate the increased automation of patient information in departmental and institution-based computer systems in hospitals and ambulatory care settings. These, by design or by evolution, are becoming basic building blocks of CPR systems (Blum 1986). To satisfy this need, clearly defined criteria must be agreed upon and built into the functionality of future CPR systems to ensure that clinical information for each patient is protected in collection, processing, storage, and use.

To accomplish this, CPR system designers, developers, and managers must address the appropriate application of human roles through legal, organizational and professional policies, standards, and procedures; they must address technical roles through appropriate utilization of hardware, software, and communications resources. CPR systems are desperately needed to assist practitioners in providing clinical care as effectively and efficiently as possible. Widespread application of such systems is dependent on resolution of current expectations from providers and patients on system reliability and security, and on data integrity and confidentiality. The challenge is to steadily develop and employ computer technology to provide improved access, legibility, adequacy, and clinical utility of patient information through automated patient care record systems. Furthermore, the patient care systems need to maintain maximum protection to patients in information integrity and confidential use, given that computer-based systems, by their very nature, are at slightly increased risk in this area over paper-based systems.

Composition of Patient Computer-based Record Systems

All computer-based patient record systems consist of the following:

Hardware equipment: central processing unit, mass storage devices, communication channels and lines, and remotely located devices (like terminals or microcomputers [personal computers] with or without local area networks [LANs]) serving as human/computer interfaces

Software: operating system, database management system (including data definition language), communication system, and application programs

Data: databases containing patient demographic, administrative, legal, and/or clinical data documenting medical services and personal data

Human beings: as originators and/or users of the health care data, such as health care professionals, paramedical personnel, clerical staff, administrative personnel, and computer staff (e.g., manager, organizers, system analysts, programmers, and operators) (Griesser 1989).

The purposes of CPRs need to be carefully identified so that adequate planning for the above attributes can be accomplished. This includes identification of the care environment, personnel involved, content of patient information and proposed information flow within the environment. A thorough review of risk and liability issues should be addressed as well (Griesser 1989).

Questions to Determine Future Direction

Consideration of system reliability and security and of data integrity and confidentiality will focus on a discussion of these essential questions:

- What are the current system reliability and security provisions; data integrity and confidentiality features for major CPR systems in place today? Are risks and liability issues clearly known?
- What is the optimal and practical CPR system for 1991–92 given the projected state and availability of computing and communications technology?
- What are feasible alternative technology specifications, designs, and configurations for the optimal 1995 CPR system and what are the comparative costs?

Exploration of these questions involves several perspectives. Initially, definitions are made in order to provide basic vocabulary and define the scope and relationship of common terms used in data security discussions. What are system reliability and security features? Where does data integrity and confidentiality fit? Does the concept of patient privacy create special needs? To address this we have assembled the following lexicon to define our key system-related and data-related terminology.

System reliability: Accuracy and dependability of data collection, processing, and maintenance secured through appropriate system design, including use of physical security measures that are directed toward protection of environment and equipment (Griesser 1989). Today's computer systems achieve solid reliability. Clinical systems are designed to assure 100 percent backup in many environments.

System security: Protection from unauthorized access, including provision for hardware, software, communications, and system users and uses determinations based on organizational computer security programs (Martin 1983).

Data security: The protection of data from accidental or intentional disclosure to unauthorized persons and from unauthorized alteration. Techniques for security include software and hardware features, physical measures such as locks and badges, and an informed, security conscious staff (Schraffenberger 1988).

Data integrity: The soundness or completeness of the data that are being used. Data integrity may be maintained by implementing security measures, by implementing procedural controls, by assigning responsibility, and by establishing audit trails (Schechter 1988).

Usage integrity: Implementing protection measures against unauthorized access to programs and data, including measures against unintentional or deliberate misuse of patient care data or hospital business data (Griesser 1989).

Program integrity: Assurance that computerized programs are the same as those in the source documents and that they have not been exposed to accidental or malicious alteration, unauthorized copying, loss by theft and destruction by hardware failures, software deficiencies, operating mistakes, or physical damage by fire or water (Griesser 1989).

Privacy: The right of the individual to be left alone, to withdraw from the influence of his environment; to be secluded, not annoyed, and not intruded upon by extension of the right to be protected against physical or psychologic invasion or against the misuse or abuse of something legally owned by an individual or normally considered by society to be his or her property (Westin 1976).

Confidentiality: Status accorded to data or information indicating that it is sensitive for some reason, and that therefore it needs to be protected against theft or improper use and must be disseminated only to individuals or organizations authorized to have it. Confidentiality is the professional and/or contractual duty of physicians, nurses, midwives, secretaries, medical technicians, paramedical staff, social workers, hospital managers, computer staff, research investigators, and the like in hospitals . . . to safeguard the privacy of their patient/client information regardless of how it is acquired, collected, stored, processed, generated, retrieved, or transmitted in a health care institution (Waters and Murphy 1979; Griesser 1989).

Within this lexicon, key definitives need to be proposed as standard reference points for emerging CPRs. An adequate understanding of the proposed users of CPR systems is also important. They may be viewed from alternative perspectives according to their relationship with the patient and/or services provided. As documentation of health care and medical services shifts from paper to computer, practitioners will necessarily transfer responsibility to document within the computer systems. Legal, professional, and accrediting standards will be retooled to specify computer system roles and responsibilities. The nature of data collection and retrieval may change, but principles of professional documentation will not. The user roles listed below reflect this point.

Initiator: The person who identifies the purpose of the CPR, decides what data area is needed, what processing procedures are to be used, and what data are to be retrieved (and for whom).

Originator: The person who generates information is responsible for the correctness and completeness of the data and the proper use of the system at that point. Health care practitioners, system operators, and administrative users are included in this group.

Custodian: The person or organization who owns the CPR and is responsible for processing, storing, transmitting and retrieving the confidential data. The custodian is also responsible for the correct performance of information handling according to legal and organizational data security program provisions. Health record professionals administer patient record systems in health care organizations.

User: Those persons entitled to the information for a specific task. They are responsible for the correct use and interpretation of the information. The term *authorized users* reflects the context of both manual (preautomated paper-based medical records) and automated CPRs. Users range from clinical to administrative to clerical and clearly can be categorized on a *need to know* or *access* basis. Griesser (1989) proposes access rights to a hospital information system in his discussions of data protection in health care information systems.

Each health care organization will need to identify and qualify access rights for its setting based on legal and professional standards. Emerging system linkages will call for significant policy extensions to today's environment.

Confidentiality and the CPR

Originators of landmark CPR systems have grappled with the problem of how to ensure their systems will provide high levels of clinical access and utility for clinical personnel and yet keep patient information secure as well. Being well-established systems, these landmark CPRs employ alternative system access strategies to address the issue. All use some form of password security. In hospital environments, several of these institutions agree that, because it is not possible to predict which physician or nurse will need to see a patient's records, clinical personnel should be allowed to access the records of all patients while they are in the hospital. For practical purposes, systems originators allow all clinical personnel access to the computerized medical record of all patients in the hospital. Restriction occurs only after the patient is discharged (Gardner 1989). A major goal of CPRs is met—to provide better access to more complete patient data for clinical care.

It should be noted that this consensus and the practice referenced is based on the human role in CPR systems management rather than the technical options available. Furthermore, this refers to access for clinical use and does not address the other aspects of access in which extended users are involved. In such cases, specific patient authorization will continue to be required as it is in paper-based systems to provide the data for express purposes such as reimbursement or legal support.

> The proliferation of computers as an integral part of daily business has resulted in a ready acceptance of "convenient" data exchange to carry on everyday business. Information specialists concerned about security and proposing limits on access are often viewed as "roadblocks" in effective user acceptance of such systems. There is growing evidence that the majority of data security problems arise from human errors such as omitting data, sharing passwords, and signing onto a system and then leaving it unattended (Bissen 1988).

In a discussion of full automation of hospital medical records, Benjamin and Baum (1988) indicate that a literature review of confidentiality issues demonstrates that data security remains a focal issue. The fact is that many computer-based systems pose comparable confidentiality risks to those experienced by manual records systems. Some of these are:

- Personnel errors that inadvertently alter, release, or lose information
- Natural disasters such as fire or water damage that destroy information
- Misuse of data by legitimate users
- Malicious use of medical information
- Unauthorized break-ins to the system
- Uncontrolled access to patient data (Benjamin and Baum 1988)

Furthermore, a specific data security program may be lacking in the organization that owns and operates the system.

These risks illustrate both the human and the technologic aspects of this problem in a general way. Effective understanding of today's CPRs requires a detailed survey of a representative sampling of CPR systems. Investigators will be challenged to identify a current profile of these features as employed in the current environment (Westin 1982). New technology and expanded system expectations that are sought by users contribute to the *moving target* status of these features. Yet concern for this topic continues to inhibit clinical system implementation in health care today.

Risk and Liability Issues

Risk and liability concerns range from consideration of hardware and software features to policy and procedure breakdowns that fail to prevent unauthorized user access and/or manipulation of patient data. Moreover, an increasing emphasis on effective clinical alerts or reminder features that are designed to work with patient CPR systems will provide diagnostic and care expectations that will eventually have an impact on medical practice standards. Thus the issue of developing a new legal code that will assign liability for system, program, and/or data failures must be explored.

> If technical problems with the network should lead to the delivery of inaccurate information to the physician, who would be held responsible for resulting mis-steps in management—the manufacturer, the programmer, the medical personnel, or all three? . . . what will be the liability of health-care specialists and nurses led into error by their use of the information systems? (Schwartz 1987)

As yet, this is largely unexplored territory. Griesser (1989) notes specific risks that must be considered in the implementation of hospital information systems (HISs), as follows:

Risks mainly related to usage integrity can be caused by

- Illegal access to computer rooms, data archive(s), medical records library, documentation of programs, remote devices, programs opening trapdoors
- Illicit use of data-communication facilities through hacking, electromagnetic pickup, concealed transmission, infiltration through active communication channels, masquerading, and piggyback entry
- Illegal modification of programs
- Illegal modification (i.e., falsification) of data
- Illegal inspection of programs
- Illegal inspection of data by browsing through the database
- Use of programs other than allowed
- Use of data other than allowed
- Theft of recording media

- Illicit copying of the contents of recorded media
- Inspection of wastepaper baskets (e.g., in computer center or the ward areas)
- Inspection of output in user's offices
- Disregard of organizational rules
- Disregard of ethical conduct by breach of professional discretion
- Operational errors

Risks mainly related to data and program integrity can originate from

- Hardware failures or errors
- Data-communication error
- System program error (new version)
- Application program deficiency (new version)
- Operational error at console input, disk handling, tape handling, and printer handling
- Missed alarm message
- Incorrect reaction to alarm
- Damage to data during acquisition, input, processing, storage, output, and distribution
- Simultaneous updating of records
- System failure during updating
- Incorrect restart after system failure
- Insufficient check on data consistency
- Insufficient check on plausibility
- Allocation of correct data to another patient (Griesser 1989)

An Optimal and Practical CPR System for 1991–1992

Perhaps the most sensitive issue surrounding the practical implementation of the CPR is to resolve the problem of confidentiality and the computer.

Recent research in medical confidentiality has proposed a three-zone confidentiality model, with an inner zone having extreme sensitivity and an outer zone lesser. The moderate area between the two zones would utilize traditional medical confidentiality requirements (Gabrieli 1989).

Statutory protection of the CPR data and correct indoctrination of the technical data processing community to develop awareness to the sensitive nature of medical data and assurance to patients/consumers that they will control the release of their own records will need attention (Gabrieli 1989). One simple provision for patient confidentially would be to provide patients with copies of audit trails of the names of users who access their CPR.

Obtaining an optimal and practical CPR system for 1991–1992 will depend on development and acceptance of an effective patient data security program that will consist of organizational policy and procedures, hardware, software, and communications protection, and a reconsideration of the organization of patient data within computer systems to reflect this information zone perspective. Today, state legislation on sensitive HIV testing has placed specific limitations on patient data collection, storage, and use within clinical systems. Federal legislation is also in place that sets boundaries for patient data handling for selected categories of patients.

Today, system reliability requires dual processing and 100 percent backup provisions. Technical security ranges from

- Hardware from key locks to terminal devices to secured rooms
- Software provisions to identify, authorize access, and audit individual users by specific functions
- Personnel restrictions on the use of the system
- Reduced system efficiency resulting from use of various identification, authorization, and audit procedures

> Medical records (computerized) should . . . be secure against improper alteration or destruction. Security risks posed by networking that involve a providers medical records system will require careful research and resolution to avert situations which could have catastrophic legal consequences. The only currently reliable way to prevent infection of a computerized medical records system by viruses from the outside is to close the system and eliminate networking and electronic data sharing with outside computer systems (Waller et al. 1989).

Individual system designers will need to identify and apply precise and consistent controls over selective access to data. These controls, coupled with personnel, procedures, and physical measures taken by management can greatly reduce an organization's exposure to potential data security problems. There will be a need to assure that efficient system user identification techniques are embedded into the applications to minimize costly overhead in technical protection features. Furthermore, system reliability may require use of technology such as WORM (write-once-read-many) and patient-carried CPR cards with updating from visit to visit to assure that reliability.

Institutional Data Security Program

A formal institutional data security program should be designed as a component of the developing CPR system. An effective data security program includes organizational and system provisions. Organizational provisions include formalization of a data security committee with oversight responsibility for an institution-wide program. Better programs

- Provide a foundation in ethics and education
- Include organizational policy structure
- Involve professionals practicing in the facility
- Build in maximum physical security for hardware use
- Provide comprehensive software support

As previously introduced, procedural and practical protections within the institution must provide for physical security of hardware and enactment of operational procedures related to data entry, systems operations, and data retrieval. Protection of organizational systems includes adequate focus on prevention, detection, and recovery. Prevention requires appropriate location, trained personnel and effective procedures. Detection involves maintaining and verifying physician access as well as system access. Backup facilities adequate for providing patient data protection are essential to the program (Waters and Murphy 1983).

Clear responsibility for data protection and designation of retention for computer-stored patient data must rest with high level line management. The challenge will be to propose policies and adopt effective technical measures that will effectively meet needs. There must be assurance that authorized persons can access their data easily without being uncomfortably aware of the data security provisions, yet that unauthorized persons cannot access restricted data.

Immediate notification to a designated computer operator when unauthorized data access attempts are being made is an essential component. Notification can be a message that identifies the user and the data set with a comparable message sent to the user to discourage access. Maintenance of a record of all unsuccessful data access attempts will enable data security personnel and system managers to track patterns. Technical protective measures should be based on the probability of a potential breach of information, the value of what is being protected, and the probable effects of loss. Potential breach is anticipated in designing the technical data security program. Value of what is being protected and probable effects of loss are determined by the health care professionals and users of the data (Waters and Murphy 1983). Patient data have clear guidelines within the context of privacy and confidentiality previously discussed (Griesser 1989).

Feasible Alternatives for 1995

By 1995, feasible alternatives will include the following:

- Clearer guidelines for the use of CPR outlined by professional associations, vendors, providers, and consumer groups
- More precise technical security features for 100 percent redundancy/backup for clinical data in use
- Model CPR systems that have created an industry standard for data security features
- More effective user recognition of the need for an overall program
- More effective and efficient data entry linked with user recognition
- Organizational data security programs tailored to CPR system functions

The need to balance efficient, user friendly CPR systems with effective data security to assure patient confidentiality will continue to be a challenge and a barrier to CPR systems acceptance and diffusion in 1995.

Conclusions

System reliability and security can be generally assured through hardware and software tools available today, although LANs and systems linkages still pose some problems. Yet, because these provision may be expensive and can inhibit ease of use, these are not consistently applied in today's CPRs. It is clear that questions around patient confidentiality have not yet been solved and new clinical systems developers continue to see this issue surface from users. The legal code has not evolved enough to buttress the work that has been accomplished. Generally, privacy and confidentiality standards in paper systems will need to be retooled for the emerging CPRs. Organizations embarking on CPR developments can plan on greater accountability demands in this critical area. Strong institutional data security programs will be needed to set policy and oversee technical practice. Major components of these programs will be professional inservice for all system users and provision for increased patient roles in the control and/or monitoring of access and dissemination of CPRs. Technology will offer greater opportunities for patient care information use. Wise stewardship will be needed to implement and manage responsible data security systems.

Acknowledgments

As chair of Working Group 8, I acknowledge the contributions of all the group members, especially the assistance of John Norris, who acted as assistant chair, and Elemer Gabrieli, who served as advisor to the group.

References

American Medical Record Association. 1985. Confidentiality of patient health information. Position statement of the American Medical Record Association, Chicago.

Benjamin, C.D., and B. Baum. 1988. The automated medical record: A practical realization? *Topics in Health Record Management* 9(1):5–6.

Bissen, C.A. 1988. Data security: Protecting a corporate asset. *Topics in Health Records Management* 9(1):14.

Bleich, H.L. 1987. Clinical computing in a teaching hospital: Use and impact of computers in clinical medicine, ed. J.G. Anderson and S.J. Jay. New York: Springer-Verlag.

Blum, B.I. 1986. *Clinical Information Systems.* New York: Springer-Verlag, chaps. 7–8.

Gabrieli, E.R. 1989. Electronic ambulatory medical record. *Journal of Clinical Computing* 18(2):27–53.

Gardner, E. 1989. Computer dilemma: Clinical access vs confidentiality. *Modern Healthcare* 19(44):32–34,38,40–42.

Griesser, G. 1989. Data protection in hospital information systems: I. Definition and overview. Implementing healthcare information systems. New York: Springer-Verlag.

Lavere, G.J. 1982. The ethical aspects of medical privacy, computers and medical privacy. Workshop Manual, Computers and Medical Privacy Conference, San Diego.

Martin, J. 1983. Managing the database environment. Englewood Cliffs, N.J.: Prentice Hall, 587.

Personal privacy in an information society. July 1977. The Report of the Privacy Protection Study Commission, Washington, D.C.

Schechter, K.S. 1988. Conversion issues and data integrity: A consultant's perspective. *Topics in Health Record Management*, December.

Schraffenberger, L.A. 1988. Practice bulletin, data security. *JAMRA* 59(8):46–47.

Schwartz, W.B. 1987. *Medicine and the computer: The promise and problems of change. Use and impact of conflicts in clinical medicine.* New York: Springer-Verlag, 332.

Waller, A.A., S.N. Chernoff, and D.K. Fulton. 1989. Automated medical records: Legal questions and risks. *Computers in Healthcare*, November.

Waters, K., and G. Murphy. 1979. *Medical records in health information.* Silver Spring, Md.: Aspen, 260.

Waters, K., and G. Murphy. 1983. *Systems analysis and computer applications in health information management.* Silver Spring, Md.: Aspen.

Waters, K., and G. Murphy. 1982. *Systems analysis and computer applications in health information management.* Silver Spring, Md.: Aspen Systems.

Westin, A. 1976. *Computer, health records and citizen rights.* National Bureau of Standards Monograph 157. Gaithersburg, Md.: National Bureau of Standards, 348.

Westin, A.F. 1982, Patients' rights: Computers and health records. In *Managing computers in health care*, ed. J.A. Worthley. Arlington, Va.: AUPHA Press, 201.

Statutes

Federal Statute, Drug and Alcohol Treatment & Rehabilitation Act 42C.F.R., Part 2.

Washington State Statute, Sexually transmitted disease information, R.C., 10. 70.24.110.

13
Medical Text Processing: Past Achievements, Future Directions

Carol Friedman and Stephen B. Johnson

Natural language plays a central role in medicine. It is by far the most convenient means for health care personnel to convey medical information, particularly in terms of the amount of time required, the ease of use, and the completeness of representation. As a partial consequence of this, much crucial medical information is not available in any other form: The patient chart in most institutions consists largely of unstructured text, as does the vast majority of the medical literature. Moreover, natural language is unequaled as a general means of expressing complex meanings (Blois 1984).

These properties point strongly to the utility of natural language processing in the medical domain. Systems based on a such an architecture could capture medical data in natural language form, structure it in various ways, store it as a permanent record, retrieve it through natural language queries, and present data to users in natural language, if desired. Although no such system currently exists that performs all these functions in an integrated manner spanning all areas of biomedical endeavors, many of the necessary functions can be accomplished with today's technology in specific domains of biomedicine.

We will first present a survey of the state of the art in natural language processing systems in general, outlining the principal techniques that have been explored and discussing the principal research goals. Then, we will give an overview of medical applications that utilize elements of this technology. We will conclude by considering future directions for the field.

Current Text Processing Systems

Evaluating a text-processing system is not a straightforward task. One reasonable evaluation method would be to see how well a system performs on a body of text. Although performance is very important, considering it singularly without other criteria may be misleading because the underlying methodology may have serious flaws that would be manifested only when the system was extended to handle a larger variety of text. This is discussed in more detail in Allen (1987). Many researchers try to achieve high performance with very limited domains as an experimental first step (e.g., Dyer 1982; Hayes and Carbonell 1981; Hayes and Mouradian 1981; Kwasny and Sondheimer 1981). Evaluation of these systems, however, must include insights as to complexity if the domain were significantly expanded and as to how the performance would be affected. Thus, competence is also important in evaluating text-processing systems. By competence, we refer to the amount of knowledge the system contains that encompasses features of human language processing: this includes knowledge about the language of the domain, its structure and semantics, and knowledge about the domain itself. Therefore, an important research issue in language processing is to investigate and correctly characterize human processing in order to improve upon the functionality and interrelationships of syntax, semantics, commonsense knowledge and specialized domain knowledge in computerized natural language interfaces (Bobrow and Webber 1980; Schank and Birnbaum 1981).

Another issue closely related to natural language processing concerns the problem of knowledge representation, which is fundamental to those applications that subsequently use the information contained in the unstructured text. The language processor must be capable of extracting and transforming the relevant text information into a formal model of information. Although this issue is not discussed in our survey, a comprehensive collection of articles concerning research in knowledge representation can be found in Brachman and Levesque (1985).

Semantic Systems

This technique utilizes semantic information to process natural language text, and ignores syntax entirely. There are several variations of this methodology which will be described below.

Pattern Matching. One method for handling text is based on a pattern matching technique that is a variation of a keyword search. The text is scanned for certain pattern combinations, which when found are translated into standard encoded forms. This method has had some success in certain medical subareas; for example, it is being used by a SNOMED microcomputer software system (Rothwell et al. 1982) to automatically encode pathology diagnoses from natural language text.

This method has several serious limitations. It is useful for texts which are naturally very structured such as pathology diagnoses, but not for text containing complex narrative such as the descriptive section of pathology procedures, patient history, and discharge summaries. In narrative, the same information may be expressed in such a large variety of ways that it would be impractical, if not impossible, to capture all the correct pattern combinations.

A more serious limitation to this method is the fact that the pattern matching methodology completely ignores the structure of language and therefore cannot capture many significant relations between terms. This may lead to a serious misinterpretation of information. An example of this problem involves negation: Without syntactic relations, it is difficult to extract the difference between *no pain*, *no relief of pain*, and *no symptoms except pain*. Another significant limitation is that this method cannot be easily ported from one subarea to another. For example, the heuristics that are successful for pathology diagnoses will not be successful for analyzing descriptive findings from pathology procedures.

Script-based Systems. Another method for handling text that has had a significant impact on natural language processing combines keywords and scripts. A script is a formal representation of the possible courses of events that may occur in a given stereotypical situation. A particular script is selected from a collection of predefined scripts by scanning a text for certain keywords. The script is subsequently used as a guide for the remainder of the processing of the text. The script defines various roles that have to be filled and it describes the properties of the entities that can fill them. When an entity in the text is found that contains the appropriate properties, the corresponding role is filled. Cognitive Systems has built two systems based on this methodology: ERIK is used by the Coast Guard to process messages about ship movements, and ATRANS is used by banks to process transfer of electronic funds. More details of this methodology can be found in the literature (Rieger 1974; Schank and Riesbeck 1981; Schank et al. 1980).

Although this technology is useful in some applications, it has the same limitations as those described above for pattern matching systems. An additional shortcoming is that it is limited to very narrow domains where the text clearly describes one typical situation and where the information is expressed in typical ways. Even in simple text, these criteria are not easy to satisfy. Often the text cannot be narrowed down to only one stereotypical situation because it contains elements of several situations, and frequently the information is expressed in unforeseen ways. Another limitation within the clinical field is that in patient documents it is often the atypical rather than the typical situation that is important to capture.

Semantic Grammars and Frame-based Systems. One approach to text processing is to use a grammar that describes the text using semantic relations rather than syntactic ones. The rules of a semantic grammar resemble those used in syntactic parsing except that semantic categories (e.g. body part, diagnosis, procedure) are employed for both terminal and nonterminal symbols instead of syntactic parts of speech (noun phrase, verb phrase, etc.). Semantic grammars tend to be much larger than syntactic grammars because there are usually many more semantic categories and relations between categories than there are syntactic categories and relations. In addition, syntactic information usually has to be added in order to reasonably handle complex sentences such as those containing conjunctions and embedded clauses.

Early systems using semantic grammars are SOPHIE (Brown and Burton 1975), which is an electronic circuit tutorial system, and LIFER (Hendrix et al. 1978) and PLANES (Waltz and Goodman 1977), which are both interfaces to database management systems.

Semantic grammars are often combined with frames designed for a specific application in order to provide domain-specific contexts. The frames are templates containing slots for specific semantic categories that are filled in the process of parsing the text. This technique has been used by Canfield (1989) to develop a prototype system to process echocardiogram textual findings. The shortcoming of using only semantic knowledge is that although the semantic grammar technology itself is portable, a new semantic grammar would have to be written for each new domain. Additionally, semantic grammars are usually not easy to deal with because they are generally larger than syntactic grammars. Moreover, a new set of templates and mapping procedures would have to be constructed, and the heuristics would be different. The absence of syntactic information causes the same performance problems as those of the other strictly semantically based systems discussed in this section.

Syntactic and Semantic-based Systems. These systems have separate syntactic and semantic processing stages, allowing for a more robust model because the syntactic component is independent of domain. Since syntax is complex, this offers a significant advantage over the purely semantic approaches because the same syntactic component can be utilized for all domains.

The Linguistic String Project, one of the pioneer efforts of text processing, developed a comprehensive English grammar (Sager 1981), as well as a methodology for text-based sublanguage analysis (Friedman 1986; Sager 1986) in specialized domains, which influenced several other text processing systems. The domains chosen were mainly within the field of clinical patient documents. This system's approach utilizes semantic patterns corresponding to particular syntactic relations to map clinical information into structured frames that are used to create a structured database from patient documents.

The Logicon system (Montgomery and Glover 1986) also contains syntactic and semantic components. It analyzes reports of space events and also contains frames specially designed for this particular application. The Logicon system contains a sophisticated discourse component so that it can successfully identify complex object and temporal references to preceding material. However, the message-processing component contains domain-specific code that would not be easy to port to another domain.

Another system that interweaves syntactic and semantic analysis is SHRDLU (Winograd 1972). However, it is difficult to separate the semantic and syntactic components in this system. RUS (Bobrow and Webber 1980), and the DIAGRAM system (Robinson 1982) also use semantic and syntactic components which are interleaved. A more detailed analysis of this methodology is provided by Woods (1980). Other more recent systems have similar functional components, but use different grammar formalisms which are based on logic. These are described in several articles (Kaplan and Bresnan 1982; McCord 1985; Pereira and Warren 1980; and Rosenschein and Shieber 1982).

All these systems have the limitation that they are fragile and cannot handle unexpected input. Some also have considerable domain-specific code that performs the construction of the frames and the mapping of text terms to the slots.

Syntactic, Semantic, and Knowledge-based Systems. Quite a number of other text-processing systems contain syntactic and semantic components, but they also contain additional components that provide pragmatic, commonsense, and domain knowledge. These systems attempt to integrate several functionally different components used by humans for text processing and are all prototype systems that have not been used yet in production.

The PROTEUS system at New York University has been used to process several different types of text messages (Grishman and Sterling 1989; Ksiezyk and Grishman 1989), for example, messages concerning the failure of naval equipment. One of the aims of this system is to combine different types of knowledge into the system in a way that facilitates the separation of domain-specific information from general language information.

The TACITUS system developed by Stanford Research Institute analyzes messages from various domains, such as reports of terrorism in the news and also naval equipment failure reports (Hobbs et al. 1988). It is also concerned with the issue of how commonsense and domain knowledge is used to interpret information in text. It has components for acquiring new knowledge and for experimenting with different processing strategies.

PUNDIT, the UNISYS message-processing system, also processes messages in limited domains (Lang and Hirschman 1988; Palmer et al. 1986; Weir 1988). This system produces a discourse representation of messages that can be used to populate databases or generate summary reports. General solutions to several difficult processing problems, such as recovering implicit information, have been demonstrated by porting the system to several different domains.

The above systems are also all very delicate and usually do not perform well when presented with a new situation, such as a new lexical term, a new syntactic structure, or a new semantic pattern. They also only contain relatively small knowledge components. A significant extension of the knowledge components would be difficult and time consuming to achieve, and it is not clear whether these systems would perform efficiently if the knowledge components were substantially extended. Some research addressing the issue of robustness is described in Hayes and Mouradian (1981), Kwasny and Sondheimer (1981), and Weischedel and Sondheimer (1983).

Applications in the Medical Domain

Natural language-processing techniques have been incorporated into a wide variety of medical applications. The processing techniques employed by these applications range in complexity from simple lexical procedures for manipulating medical terms, to pattern matching algorithms for indexing longer medical phrases, to sophisticated systems that employ syntactic, semantic, and pragmatic knowledge to analyze large medical discourses.

Modes of Input

Before examining how medical language has been used in applications, it is important to consider the various ways in which medical language data can be captured for input to medical systems. There are essentially three modes of entry: the medical language input may be typed directly by the user, dictated by the user then typed by a transcriptionist, or spoken directly into the system. Keyboard entry works well when the input consists of single words or short phrases and when users have basic typing skills. Applications that enable physicians to search the medical literature provide one example of this scenario, in which physicians enter medical terms to indicate the topic of interest. Transcription is effective when the amount of natural language input is large and when some delay in the availability of the data can be tolerated. Many hospitals use transcription services to capture discharge summaries and departmental reports dictated by physicians. Direct speech entry is feasible for highly structured scenarios in which single words or short phrases are elicited in specific contexts. Systems using this technique are essentially a collection of prompts and menu choices in which voice replaces the use of a keyboard or mouse to make selections (Joseph 1989; Swett et al. 1989). Recognition of continuous speech is still beyond current technology, although a number of experimental systems that integrate speech recognition with natural language processing techniques are under development.

Natural Language Interfaces

In the following section, we will not take into consideration the mode by which natural language is captured by an application and made available as machine-readable text. Instead we will focus on the use of natural language as an interface between a medical user and a database, knowledge base, expert system, textbook, the medical literature, or some other information resource. There are three ways in which an application can use natural language as an interface:

- Natural language input submitted by a user to the system may serve as new information to be stored in a database or knowledge base.
- Natural language terms or sentences input by a users can be interpreted as a query for information to be retrieved from such resources.
- The information retrieved by a system may be converted into natural language for presentation to the user.

Although a few systems perform two or more of these functions, we will consider each of these uses of natural language separately below.

Processing Medical Language Input. We will first survey applications that convert machine-readable, free text into some structured representation suitable for further computer processing such as storage in a database. These applications can be divided into two types, depending on the complexity of the structured representation obtained by the system: those that map natural language into a predefined indexing vocabulary and those that generate more complex structures (e.g., relational database tables). The more complex structures have richer semantics and can accommodate such features as modifiers of medical terms, negation, uncertainty, duration, repetition, change information, relations between terms (e.g., anatomic relationships), and relations between events (e.g., causality, time sequencing).

Many applications employ an indexing vocabulary developed specifically for that system or for the institution where the application is used. Increasingly, national standards have emerged for controlled vocabularies for medicine. One of the most utilized vocabularies for automated indexing in clinical domains is the Systematized Nomenclature of Medicine (SNOMED). SNOMED is a simple frame-like structure, with slots ("axes") for topography, morphology, etiology, function, disease, occupation, and procedure. Each slot can be filled with an index term from one of seven disjoint classification hierarchies (Cote 1986; Rothwell et al. 1989). Medical subject headings (MeSH) is the de facto standard for systems indexing the medical literature. MeSH has a polyhierarchic classification scheme and a secondary vocabulary of subheadings that are used to provide contextual information about main terms (National Library of Medicine 1989). The Metathesaurus of the Unified Medical Language System (UMLS) combines the strengths of SNOMED, MeSH, and other vocabularies by establishing mappings between terms in different vocabularies (Lindberg 1990; National Library of Medicine 1990). Tuttle et al. (1989) give an overview of the methods used to implement the UMLS Metathesaurus. The lexical techniques that were applied to help automate the mapping between controlled vocabularies (identification of inversions, permutations, coordinations in medical terminology) are described by Sheretz et al. (1989).

Various critiques have been made of SNOMED and similar taxonomies, discussing the limitations of strict hierarchical classifications, the need for explicit semantic links between medical terms, the difficulties with semantic overlap between the slots, and problems resulting when concepts belong to multiple categories (Dunham et al. 1984; Graitson 1985). A general critique of SNOMED, MeSH, UMLS, and other controlled vocabularies for medicine and requirements for a proposed vocabulary can be found in Cimino et al. (1989).

Quite a number of systems have been developed to extract clinical information from the medical record and encode it in an indexing vocabulary. The simpler indexing systems use pattern matching algorithms for indexing medical terms and phrases. Diseases, side effects, and symptoms are indexed into SNOMED in Wingert (1985; 1986). A combination of menus and natural language input is used for the automatic encoding of medical records in Cristea and Mihaescu (1988).

More complex indexing systems combine pattern matching methods for identifying medical terms in text with knowledge-based techniques. Medical knowledge is used to guide the overall processing of a medical text by defining the possible sequences of topics and subtopics characteristic of the domain (this is the script technique described under *Script-based Systems* above). Often knowledge about the classification hierarchy of terms is incorporated to enhance the term-matching process. Domains in which these methods have been attempted include the history and physical sections of a patient chart (Archbold and Evans 1989), echocardiography reports (Canfield et al. 1989), discharge summaries (Gabrieli and Speth 1987, 1985), case histories of liver disease (Obermeier 1985), radiology reports (Ranum

1988), coroner's reports (Tong 1989), and diagnoses (Wagner et al. 1988). Syntactic parsing techniques and morphologic analysis can be used in place of the pattern matching approach and effectively combined with knowledge-based techniques (Evans 1987).

A different approach to the processing of medical discourse is the progressive regularization of medical text from its surface form through various intermediate forms into a normalized, structured form. The output of systems based on this approach may be frame structures or relational database tables. These systems exploit the sublanguage properties of medical discourse, that is, the fact that medical language is used in highly restricted ways compared with the language of everyday speech. Domains of application include radiology reports (Hirschman et al. 1976), discharge summaries (Sager et al. 1987), journal articles on lipoprotein kinetics (Sager 1986), and pharmacology reports (Sager 1978).

Systems based on the sublanguage approach process medical narrative in several stages: syntactic analysis; identification of sublanguage semantic patterns; syntactic regularization (e.g., converting passive sentences into active sentences); and mapping into a frame structure. The resulting representation can then be mapped into a relational database, for instance, a database of rheumatoid arthritis encounters generated from progress notes (Chi et al. 1985). Early use of semantic knowledge (sublanguage patterns) improves grammatical analysis (Friedman et al. 1983). The sublanguage patterns also facilitate the handling of the fragmentary sentences so common in clinical reports, enabling the recovery of implicit information (Marsh 1983). The modular design of these systems enables refinement of individual system components in relatively independent fashion and facilitates portability to other domains, particularly because domain-specific knowledge is separated from domain-independent knowledge (Hirschman et al. 1989).

An important aspect of systems based on the sublanguage approach is that they are founded on a rigorous methodology for developing semantic representations of medical discourse, based on analysis of corpora of real medical texts (Grishman and Kittredge 1986; Harris et al. 1989; Kittredge and Lehrberger 1982). A structured methodology contributes the following benefits to the development of natural language processing systems: it becomes possible to assign a precise meaning to the notion of verifying that the system does what was intended; large systems are easier to maintain because they are less ad hoc; it is more realistic to consider extending the function of a system; the system is easier to port to other domains (Johnson 1987). Sublanguage methods can also be used to develop or expand controlled medical vocabularies (Johnson and Gottfried 1989).

Processing Medical Language Queries. Having examined how natural language input to an application may be processed, we now turn to the use of natural language as a means of querying databases and knowledge bases. As with systems that process natural language input, these applications range from processing simple search terms to full natural language questions and commands. Several programs for searching the medical literature provide simple lexical techniques for transforming free text entry of search terms into the controlled vocabulary used to index journal articles. These include Grateful MED (Haynes and McKibbon 1987), PaperChase (Horowitz et al. 1983), and MicroMeSH (Lowe et al. 1987). Some expert systems use similar methods to match a clinician's input with terms used in description of diseases. For example, the medical diagnosis system DXplain uses word stemming, spell-checking, and synonyms to map entry terms into its controlled vocabulary (Barnett et al. 1987). Obermeier (1984) presents a more sophisticated natural language interface to a medical exert system, using knowledge-based parsing techniques. Expert systems for teaching students medicine greatly benefit from a natural language interface. Examples include two different systems for teaching medical diagnosis and gross anatomy that employ the same interface software (Hagamen and Gardy 1986), and another system that simulates patients (Harasym and McGeary 1987).

There are many commercially available interfaces to database management systems that incorporate natural language-processing techniques—indeed, too many to survey here. Examples of experimental systems developed specifically for medical purposes include

- A natural language interface to provide medical personnel access to a clinical database containing kidney failure therapy data, which uses a combination of syntactic and contextual analysis (Woodyard and Hamel 1981)
- A system for the automated indexing of free text pathology and radiology reports for information retrieval purposes (Gell 1982)

Much effort has been directed to providing users access to the medical literature. These applications involve classifying (indexing) documents, usually by assigning one or more keywords. The assigned keywords can then be used to query a database of documents information retrieval from clinical reports. Because manual indexing is highly labor intensive, various attempts have been made to help automate this process. For example, statistical analysis of vocabulary usage has been used to classify book chapters and journal articles as to medical speciality and also by level of description (e.g., molecule, cell, organ (Cole et al. 1987, 1988). Another important research area is improving on the accuracy and precision attainable by keyword-based retrieval systems. More effective retrievals are possible when semantic relations between terms are considered. For example, it was found that coding semantic relationships in a bibliographic retrieval system as well as the index terms they relate helps to partition the literature, which improves the effectiveness of searches (Miller et al. 1988; Powsner et al. 1987).

Extensive study of science sublanguages has shown that particular sciences are characterized by particular sets of relations among words and that these relational structures are shared by discourses (e.g., journal articles) in a single field irrespective of national language. An excellent example can be seen in the highly detailed analysis of the sublanguage of immunology in English and in French (Harris et al. 1989). Moreover, it is possible to exploit the similarities of syntax and semantics of clinical narrative in Indo-European languages (e.g., English and French) in order to development a single language processor that can be adapted for different languages (Nhan et al. 1989). This work and similar studies suggest a foundation for a computer-based solution to the problem of international communication in science (Harris and Mattick 1988). The sublanguage approach was explored in an experimental system for processing the content of articles on lipoprotein kinetics into a relational database that would be used for validating and refining mathematical models of metabolic systems (Sager and Kosaka 1983). Related techniques were applied to develop a retrieval system for a textbook of hepatitis. This system used syntactic analysis, sublanguage semantics, and hierarchical links in the text, reflecting the refinement of topics, in order to focus user searches (Walker and Hobbs 1981).

Generating Medical Language Output. In addition to its use as input to medical applications and as a means of posing queries, natural language is also a convenient mode for the output of applications. Natural language text is useful in providing explanations, critiques, or advice for users of expert systems and computer-aided instruction. Result texts for clinical laboratory tests were generated based on answers made by laboratory technicians to a series of predefined questions. The text was composed from predefined text segments using an augmented transition network (Kuzmak and Miller 1983). An expert system for instructing students in medical diagnosis used a natural language interface to generate explanations of its reasoning (Hagamen and Gardy 1986). A rule based expert system produced a textual critique of radiology diagnoses by combining prose fragments. The critique served as an explanation of the expert system's reasoning process (Mutalik et al. 1988). The Roundsman expert system uses templates to construct a literature-based recommendation for treatment of patients (Rennels et al. 1989).

Future Directions

It is noteworthy that the text-processing systems which presently perform very well are those which have been developed with limited language competence. Because of this shortcoming, they do not offer a methodology for obtaining significantly improved competence.

Therefore, we cannot look to them to provide the generalized solutions needed for comprehensive text processing. However, these systems provide an essential service in that they are the only current means whereby textual information can be automatically extracted and encoded for subsequent use by other computerized processes. Therefore, any such system that performs well in a subarea of medical text processing will continue to be very valuable in the near future.

At the same time, systems developed by natural language researchers have concentrated on language competence and therefore have produced systems which currently do not perform well, but instead, contain generalized language-processing capabilities. These systems have advanced to the point where they promise to show results in the very near future. In particular, many of these systems are developing techniques which will make them more robust. However, much work still remains to be done. This work involves solving difficult problems in all areas of knowledge relevant to text processing. The syntactic analysis of simple sentences is presently well developed. Techniques have yet to be developed for the handling of sentences containing complex and ill-formed structures. The semantics of simple statements is also well defined presently. However, work is needed on temporal semantics, on the semantics of uncertainty, and on a semantics which deals with recovery of implicit information and referential identity. Work in both commonsense and domain knowledge is just beginning to be addressed.

The issue of joining the pragmatic efforts of medical applications with theoretic achievements in computational linguistics points to the need for collaboration among groups working on different aspects of medical language processing and to the need to establish various standards for representing linguistic information. Computer-readable dictionaries are one example of such a standard. Appropriately structured dictionaries can be shared by many research groups, despite differences in methods of parsing, knowledge representation, and the like. For example, the *Longman Dictionary of Contemporary English* (*LDOCE*) is a comprehensive machine-readable dictionary that contains 60,000 entries with a wealth of syntactic information and even some semantic content (Boguraev and Briscoe 1987). A lexicon for biomedical text processing should contain single and multiple word entries with information about syntactic categories, morphology, allowed complements of verbs, syntactic transformations in which a word participates, and links to a national semantic coding scheme such as UMLS (McCray et al. 1987). A small portion of this information might be obtained from medical dictionaries such as *Dorland's Illustrated Medical Dictionary*, which is available in machine-readable form for research purposes (McCray and Srinivasan 1990). A single resource that relates conceptual and linguistic information, such as the model proposed by the MedSORT-II project (Evans 1988) would contribute significantly to the development of future medical computer systems that integrate textual and structured data.

Although the above natural language problems are difficult, principled and generalized solutions offer the promise of a comprehensive text processing facility that can be applied using one uniform methodology to all texts within the medical domain. We therefore look to these systems for a long-range solution to text processing. When this task is accomplished it will represent a major advancement, for then virtually all information embodied in medical text will become interpretable by a computer.

References

Allen, J. 1987. *Natural language understanding*. Reading, Mass.: The Benjamin/Cummings Publishing Co. Inc., 2–20.

Archbold, A., and D. Evans. 1989. On the topical structure of medical charts. In *Proceedings of the Thirteenth Annual Symposium on Computer Applications in Medical Care*. Washington, D. C.: IEEE, 543–547.

Barnett, G., J. Cimino, J. Hupp, and E. Hoffer. 1987. DXplain: An evolving diagnostic decision-support system. *Journal of the American Medical Association* 258:67–74.

Blois, M. 1984. *Information and medicine*. Berkeley: University of California Press.

Bobrow, R.J., and B.I. Webber. 1980. Knowledge representation for syntactic/semantic processing. In *Proceedings of the First Annual Conference of the AAAI, Stanford University, California*, 316–323.

Boguraev, B., and T. Briscoe. 1987. Large lexicons for natural language processing: Utilizing the grammar coding system of LDOCE. *Computational Linguistics* 13:203–218.

Brachman, R.J., and H. Levesque, eds. 1985. *Readings in knowledge representation*. Palo Alto, Ca.: Morgan Kaufmann.

Brown, J.S., and R.R. Burton. 1975. *Multiple representations of knowledge for tutorial reasoning*. In *Representation and understanding*, ed. D. G. Bobrow and A. Collins. New York: Academic Press.

Canfield, K., B. Bray, S. Huff, and H. Warner. 1989. Database capture of natural language echocardiography reports: A unified medical language system approach. In *Proceedings of the Thirteenth Annual Symposium on Computer Applications in Medical Care*. Washington, D. C.: IEEE, 559–563.

Chi, E., M. Lyman, N. Sager, C. Friedman, and C. Macleod. 1985. A database of computer-structured narrative: Methods of computing complex relations. In *Proceedings of the Ninth Annual Symposium on Computer Applications in Medical Care*. Washington, D. C.: IEEE, 221–226.

Cimino, J.J., G. Hripcsak, S.B. Johnson, and P.D. Clayton. 1989. Designing and introspective multipurpose, controlled medical vocabulary. In *Proceedings of the Thirteenth Annual Symposium on Computer Applications in Medical Care*. Washington, D.C.: IEEE, 513–518.

Cole, W., P. Michael, J. Stewart, and M. Blois. 1988. Automatic classification of medical text: The influence of publication form. In *Proceedings of the Twelfth Annual Symposium on Computer Applications in Medical Care*. Washington, D.C.: IEEE, 196–200.

Cole, W., P. Michael, and M. Blois. 1987. Distinguishing man from molecules: The distinctiveness of medical concepts at different levels of description. In *Proceedings of the Eleventh Annual Symposium on Computer Applications in Medical Care*. Washington, D.C.: IEEE, 117–120.

Cote, R. 1986. Architecture of SNOMED—Its contribution to medical language processing. In *Proceedings of the Tenth Annual Symposium on Computer Applications in Medical Care*. Washington, D.C.: IEEE, 74–80.

Cristea, D., and T. Mihaescu. 1988. Combining menus with natural language processing in recording medical data. *Journal of Clinical Computing* 16:156–166.

Dunham, G.S., D.E. Henson, and M.G. Pacak. 1984. Three solutions to problems of medical nomenclatures. *Methods of Information in Medicine* 23:87–95.

Dyer, M. 1982. In-depth understanding: A computer model of integrated processing for narrative comprehension. Research Report No. 219. New Haven, Conn.: Yale University. Department of Computer Science,

Evans, D. 1987. Final report on the MedSORT-II project: Developing and managing medical thesauri. Technical Report No. CMU-LCL-87- 3. Pittsburgh, Pa.: Carnegie Mellon University. Laboratory for Computational Linguistics.

Evans, D. 1988. Pragmatically structured, lexical-semantic knowledge bases for unified medical language systems. In *Proceedings of the Twelfth Annual Symposium on Computer Applications in Medical Care*. Washington, D.C.:IEEE, 169–173.

Friedman, C. 1986. Automatic structuring of sublanguage information. In *Analyzing language in restricted domains: Sublanguage description and processing*, ed. R. Grishman and R. Kittredge. Hillsdale, N.J.: Erlbaum, 85–102.

Friedman, C., N. Sager, E. Chi, E. Marsh, C. Christenson, and M. Lyman. 1983. Computer structuring of free-text patient data. In *Proceedings of the Seventh Annual Symposium on Computer Applications in Medical Care*. Washington, D.C.: IEEE.

Gabrieli, E., and D. Speth. 1985. Automated analysis of the discharge summary. *Journal of Clinical Computing* 15:1–28.

Gabrieli, E., and D. Speth. 1987. Computer processing of discharge summaries. In *Proceedings of the Eleventh Annual Symposium on Computer Applications in Medical Care*. Washington, D.C.: IEEE, 137–140.

Gell, G. 1982. Free text processing in clinical documentation. *Journal of Clinical Computing* 10:170–179.

Graitson, M. 1985. SNOMED as a knowledge base for a natural language understanding program. In *The role of informatics in health care coding and classification systems*, ed. D. Cote, D. Protti, and J. Scherrer. New York: Elsevier Science Publishers.

Grishman, R., and J. Sterling. 1989. Analyzing telegraphic messages. In *Proceedings of the DARPA Speech and Natural Language Workshop*. Palo Alto, Ca.: Morgan Kaufmann.

Grishman, R., and R. Kittredge, eds. 1986. *Analyzing language in restricted domains: Sublanguage description and processing*. Hillsdale, N.J.: Erlbaum Associates.

Hagamen, W., and M. Gardy. 1986. The numeric representation of knowledge and logic-two artificial intelligence applications in medical education. *IBM Systems Journal* 25:207–235.

Harasym, P., and J. McGeary. 1987. Microcomputer assisted patient simulation (MAPS): An intelligent computer assisted instructional system. In *Proceedings of the International Conference on Computer Assisted Learning in Post-Secondary Education, University of Calgary, Calgary, Alberta, Canada*.

Harris, Z., M. Gottfried, T. Ryckman, P. Mattick, A. Daladier, T. Harris, and S. Harris. 1989. The form of information in science—Analysis of an immunology sublanguage. Dordrecht, The Netherlands: Kluwer Academic.

Harris, Z., and P. Mattick. 1989. Science sublanguages and the prospects for a global language of science. *Annals of the American Academy of Political and Social Science* 495:73–83.

Hayes, P.J., and J.G. Carbonell. 1981. Multi-strategy parsing and its role in robust machine communications. CMU-CS-81-118. Pittsburgh, Pa.: Carnegie Mellon University.

Hayes, P.J., and G.V. Mouradian. 1981. Flexible parsing. *American Journal of Computational Linguistics* 7:232–242.

Haynes, R., and K. McKibbon. 1987. Grateful Med (search software). *MD Computing* 4:47–49.

Hendrix, G.G., E. Sacerdoti, D. Sagalowicz, and J. Slocum. 1978. Developing a natural language interface to complex data. *ACM Transactions on Database Systems* 3:105–147.

Hirschman, L., M. Palmer, J. Dowding, D. Dahl, M. Linebarger, R. Passonneau, F. Land, C. Ball, and C. Weir. 1989. The PUNDIT natural language processing system. In *Proceedings of the Annual AI Systems in Government Conference.* Washington, D.C.: IEEE Computer Press.

Hirschman, L., R. Grishman, and N. Sager. 1976. From text to structured information: Automatic processing of medical reports. *AFIPS Conference Proceedings.* Montvale, N.J.: AFIPS Press, 45:267–275.

Hobbs, J., M. Stickel, P. Martin, and D. Edwards. 1988. Interpretation as abduction. In *Proceedings of the 26th Annual Meeting of the Association for Computational Linguistics*, Buffalo, N.Y., 95–103.

Horowitz, G., J. Jackson, and H. Bleich. 1983. Paper chase: Self-service bibliographic retrieval. *Journal of the American Medical Association* 250, No. 18.

Johnson, S. 1987. Mathematical building blocks. *AI Expert*, May, 42–50.

Johnson, S., and M. Gottfried. 1989. Sublanguage analysis as a basis for controlled medical vocabulary. In *Proceedings of the Thirteenth Annual Symposium on Computer Applications in Medical Care*, Washington, D.C.: IEEE, 519–556.

Joseph, R. 1989. Large vocabulary voice-to-text systems for medical reporting. *Speech Technology* 4:49–51.

Kaplan, R.M., and J. Bresnan. 1982. Lexical-functional grammar: A formal system for grammatical representation. In *The mental representation of grammatical relations*, ed. J. Bresnan. Cambridge, Mass.: MIT Press.

Kittredge, R., and J. Lehrberger, eds. 1982. *Sublanguage—Studies of language in restricted semantic domains.* New York: De Gruyter.

Ksiezyk, T., and R. Grishman. 1989. Equipment simulation for language understanding. *International Journal of Expert Systems.*

Kuzmak, P.M., and R.E. Miller. 1983. Computer-aided generation of result text for clinical laboratory tests. In *Proceedings of The Seventh Annual Symposium on Computer Applications in Medical Care.* Washington, D.C.: IEEE, 275–278.

Kwasny, S.C., and N.K. Sondheimer. 1981. Relaxation techniques for parsing grammatically ill-formed input in natural language understanding systems. *American Journal of Computational Linguistics* 7:99–108.

Lang, F., and L. Hirschman. 1988. Improved portability and parsing through interactive acquisition of semantic information. In *Proceedings of the Second Conference on Applied Natural Language Processing*, Austin, Tex.

Lowe, H., G. Barnett, J. Scott, R. Eccles, E. Foster, and J. Piggins. 1988. Remote access microMeSH: A microcomputer system for searching the MEDLINE database. In *Proceedings of The Twelfth Annual Symposium on Computer Applications in Medical Care.* Washington, D.C.: IEEE.

Marsh, E. 1983. Utilizing domain-specific information for processing compact text. In *Proceedings of the Conference on Applied Natural Language Processing*. Santa Monica, Calif.: Association for Computational Linguistics.

McCord, M. 1985. Modular logic grammars. In *Proceedings of the Association for Computational Linguistics*. Santa Monica, Calif: Association for Computational Linguistics, 104–117.

McCray, A., J. Sponsler, B. Brylawski, and A. Browne. 1987. The role of lexical knowledge in biomedical text understanding. In *Proceedings of the Eleventh Annual Symposium on Computer Applications in Medical Care*. Washington, D.C.: IEEE, 103–107.

Miller, P., K. Barwick, J. Morrow, S. Powsner, and C. Riely. 1988. Semantic relationships and medical bibliographic retrieval. *Computers and Biomedical Research* 21:6–77.

Montgomery, C.,and B. Glover. 1986. Reporting and analysis of space events. In *Analyzing language in restricted domains: Sublanguage description processing*, ed. R. Grishman and R. Kittredge. Hillsdale, N.J.: Erlbaum.

Mutalik, P., P. Fisher, H. Swett, and P. Miller. 1988. Structuring coherent explanation: The use of diagnostic strategies in an expert critiquing system. In *Proceedings of the Twelfth Annual Symposium on Computer Applications in Medical Care*. Washington, D.C.: IEEE, 26–31.

National Library of Medicine. 1989. *Medical subject headings*. Bethesda, Md.: Library Operations.

National Library of Medicine. 1990. *UMLS knowledge sources—Experimental edition*. Bethesda, Md.

Nhan, N., N. Sager, M. Lyman, L. Tick, F. Borst, and Y. Su. 1989. A medical language processor for two Indo-European languages. In *Proceedings of the Thirteenth Annual Symposium on Computer Applications in Medical Care*. Washington, D.C.: IEEE, 554–558.

Obermeier, K. 1985. GROK—a knowledge-based text processing system. In *Second Conference on Artificial Intelligence Applications*. Miami Beach, Fla: IEEE.

Obermeier, K. 1984. Design and implementation of natural language front ends for expert systems. In *Proceedings of the SPIE International Society for Optical Engineering* 485:99–103.

Palmer, M., D. Dahl, R. Passonneau, L. Hirschman, M. Linebarger, and J. Dowding. 1986. Recovering implicit information. In *Proceedings of the 24th Annual Meeting of the Association for Computational Linguistics*, Columbia University, N.Y.

Pereira, F.C.N., and D.H.D. Warren. 1980. Definite clause grammars for language analysis—A Survey of the formalism and a comparison with augmented transition networks. *Artificial Intelligence* 13:231–278.

Powsner, S., K. Barwick, J. Morrow, C. Riely, and P. Miller. 1987. Coding semantic relationships for medical bibliographic retrieval: A preliminary study. In *Proceedings of the Eleventh Annual Symposium on Computer Applications in Medical Care*. Washington, D.C.: IEEE, 108–112.

Ranum, D. 1988. Knowledge based understanding of radiology text. In *Proceedings of the Twelfth Annual Symposium on Computer Applications in Medical Care*. Washington, D.C.: IEEE, 141–145.

Rennels, G., E. Shortliffe, F. Stockdale, and P. Miller. 1989. A computational model of reasoning from the clinical literature. *AI Magazine* 10:49–57.

Robinson, J.J. 1982. DIAGRAM: A grammar for dialogues. *Communications of the ACM* 25:27–47.

Rosenschein, S.J., and S.M. Shieber. 1982. Translating English into logical form. In *Proceedings of the Association for Computational Linguistics*, 1–8.

Rothwell, D., F. Wingert, R. Cote, R. Beckett, and J. Palotay. 1989. Indexing medical information: The role of SNOMED. In *Proceedings of the Thirteenth Annual Symposium on Computer Applications in Medical Care*. Washington, D.C.: IEEE, 534–539.

Rothwell, D., L. Hause, and C. Frey. 1982. Lab management memo. *Pathologist*, May.

Sager, N., C. Friedman, and M. Lyman. 1987. *Medical language processing— Computer management of narrative data*. Reading, Mass.: Addison-Wesley.

Sager, N. 1986. Sublanguage: Linguistic phenomenon, computational tool. In *Analyzing language in restricted domains: Sublanguage description and processing*, ed. R. Grishman and R. Kittredge. Hillsdale, N.J.: Erlbaum.

Sager, N., and M. Kosaka. 1986. A database of literature organized by relations. In *Proceedings of the Seventh Annual Symposium on Computer Applications in Medical Care*. Washington, D.C.: IEEE, 692–695.

Sager, N. 1981. *Natural language information processing: A computer grammar of English and its applications*. Reading, Mass.: Addison-Wesley.

Sager, N. 1978. Natural language formatting: The automatic conversion of texts to a structured database. In *Advances in Computers*, ed. M. Yovits. New York: Academic Press, 17:89–162.

Schank, R., and L. Birnbaum. 1981. *Memory, meaning, and syntax*. Research Report No. 189. New Haven, Conn.: Yale University, Department of Computer Science.

Schank, R., and C. Riesbeck. 1981. *Inside computer understanding*, chap. 2. Hillsdale, N.J.: Lawrence Erlbaum.

Schank, R., M. Lebowitz, and L. Birnbaum. 1980. An integrated understander. *American Journal of Computational Linguistics* 6, No. 1.

Schank, R., and C. Rieger. 1974. Inference and the computer understanding of natural language. *Artificial Intelligence* 5:373–412.

Sherertz, D., M. Tuttle, N. Olson, M. Erlbaum, and S. Nelson. 1989. Lexical mapping in the UMLS Meta-Thesaurus. In *Proceedings of the Thirteenth Annual Symposium on Computer Applications in Medical Care*, Washington, D.C.: IEEE, 494–502.

Swett, H., P. Fisher, P. Mutalik, P. Miller, and L. Wright. 1989. The IMAGE/ICON system: voice activated intelligent image display for radiologic diagnosis. In *Proceedings of the Thirteenth Annual Symposium on Computer Applications in Medical Care*. Washington, D.C.: IEEE, 977–978.

Tong, R., A. Appelbaum, and L. Balcom. An automated injury coding system. In *Proceedings of the Annual AI Systems in Government Conference*. Washington, D.C.: IEEE.

Tuttle, M., D. Sherertz, M. Erlbaum, N. Olson, and S. Nelson. 1989. Implementing Meta-1: The first version of the UMLS Meta-Thesaurus. In *Proceedings of the Thirteenth Annual Symposium on Computer Applications in Medical Care*. Washington, D.C.: IEEE, 483–487.

Wagner, J., R. Baud, F. Borst, C. Kohler, and J. Scherrer. 1988. A knowledge-based system for interactive medical diagnosis encoding. In *Expert systems and decision support in medicine: 3rd Annual Meeting of the GMDS EFMI Special Topic Meeting*. Peter L. Reichertz Memorial Conference, Hannover, West Germany.

Walker, D., and J. Hobbs. 1981. Natural language access to medical text. In *Proceedings of the Fifth Annual Symposium on Computer Applications in Medical Care*, Washington, D.C.: IEEE.

Waltz, D.L., and B.A. Goodman. 1977. Writing a natural language data base system. *Proceedings of IJCAI*, 144–150.

Weir, C. 1988. *Knowledge representation in PUNDIT*. Unisys Technical Report (October). Paoli, Pa.: Unisys.

Weischedel, R.M., and N.K. Sondheimer. 1983. Meta-rules as a basis for processing ill-formed output. *American Journal of Computational Linguistics* 9:161–177.

Wingert, F. 1985. Automated indexing based on SNOMED. *Methods of Information in Medicine* 24:27–34.

Wingert, F. 1986. An indexing system for SNOMED. *Methods of Information in Medicine* 25:22–30.

Winograd, T. 1972. *Understanding natural language*. New York: Academic Press.

Woods, W.A. 1980. Cascaded ATN grammars. *American Journal of Computational Linguistics* 6:1–12.

Woodyard, M., and B. Hamel. 1981. A natural language interface to a clinical data base management system, *Computers and Biomedical Research* 14:41–62.

14
Essential Technologies for Computer-based Patient Records: A Summary

Richard S. Dick and Elaine B. Steen

Summary

The purpose of this summary is to convey an overall view of the technologies that are relevant to or are exhibited in today's computer-based patient record (CPR) systems and also to highlight those technologies that will be required to build the state-of-the-art CPR systems of the near future. The needs of users of systems are the most important consideration in the design and development of any computer-based system. It is important that the designers and implementers of systems understand not only the users, but also how they will use the system and what demands they will place on the system to meet their evolving needs. Some of these users and uses have specific technologic implications of which designers of CPR systems need to be cognizant. In general, current CPR systems do not address the information needs of many of these users.

We hope that designers and developers of CPR systems and, in particular, CPR vendors will make use of the information contained in this book as they commence their design of future CPR systems. The recommendations section, especially, should be considered by CPR designers and developers. It is intended that CPR designers will use this document as a resource for gaining insight into features that are most needed and desired by the health care community. Furthermore, we hope that this document will assist designers of CPR systems to anticipate the scope of future CPR systems, and that appropriate plans will be made early in the design process to accommodate the vast array of data and system linkages required to support the extensive requirements of all of the users of the CPR. The major design challenge will be the task of integration, that is, of building CPR systems using existing modules, subsystems, and components that address portions of, or individual applications among, the multitude of capabilities that need to be included in future CPR systems.

The following themes have emerged from this study. There is no single comprehensive CPR system available today that might serve as a model for emulation for future CPR systems as defined herein. CPR systems are, or should be, the heart of the entire health care information system, since all other peripheral systems (e.g., laboratory, pharmacy, or billing) feed data into or rely on data retrieved from the CPR. Today's CPR has rarely been, but should be, a longitudinal (lifelong) record, that is, it should have all patient data for all time the patient is cared for within a health care program. As a lifelong record, the CPR must be transferrable and even transportable (portable data carrier, laser card, smart card, etc.) so that crucial data concerning the patient is readily available regardless of where the patient seeks care. Database management systems (DBMS) and database technologies have evolved to the point where they are essential for storage and integration of the CPR. The CPR is so complex that no single database can accommodate all of its data, and an integrating DBMS is essential. A distributed database environment (with its attendant advantages and disadvantages) with broadband, high speed communications networks is implied in future CPR systems. Terminals and workstations will be the primary tools used by health care professionals to interact with the CPR systems. At a minimum, to satisfy the clinical requirements of health care professionals, the terminals must support text and graphics and the workstations must support high quality images, mouse-type data selections, windowing, graphics, and sound, while providing subsecond response times to most queries. Data acquisition is perhaps the most crucial element to be addressed in the future CPR systems. Clearly, the systems must be so easy to use and unobtrusive that health care professionals can enter data in an amount of time comparable to or less than the time used for paper-based patient records. Productivity gains should be sought, but CPR systems of the future should not require more time than the health care professional is now accustomed to use in the course of providing care. Voice input or voice recognition is an important element of future CPR systems. Display technologies will also be important to the success of future CPR systems. Flexible displays tailored to the specific needs of clinical care users are likely to be crucial. The patient record is a complex mix of information containing high quality images from radiology, as well as from other departments that use images as diagnostic tool for patient care. These high quality images present some significant challenges to the CPR system of the future, but technologies will soon be in place to make all types of images from the CPR available throughout a health care facility.

Both data and system communication standards for transmitting complete or a partial patient records are of prime importance to the realization of the CPR. Significant efforts are now underway to support record format standards development, but much more needs to be accomplished in this area before the whole of the CPR can be shared within and across institutions. A tougher problem is the standardization of vocabularies (data terms and items) that appear in many portions of the patient record. This is a content rather than a format issue that has only recently begun to be addressed in any substantive way. Vocabulary control in the CPR is an issue of immense importance to patient care, and it will require great efforts on the part of many organizations over a period of years before adequate uniformity is finally realized in the CPR. The universal use of communication standards, such as Fiber Distributed Data Interchange (FDDI-II) and Integrated Services Digital Network (ISDN) will make it possible to transmit the CPR or selected portions of it across fiber optic and other high speed, high bandwidth networks. The CPR, and especially high definition images from the CPR, will be among the first applications to test these new communications technologies that are now emerging.

Among the highest priorities for growth in the 1990s is the further development of data protection technology to ensure fully the privacy and confidentiality of patient data contained in the CPR. There are societal and legal concerns related to these issues that should be resolved satisfactorily before the CPR can be more broadly realized. Much of the technology to assure the CPR security and integrity exists presently, but generally these technologies have not been adequately deployed or embedded in present CPR systems. CPR systems require a two-way linkage with other relevant primary care CPR databases. CPR systems also need to provide realtime linkages to clinical research databases, medical knowledge bases, and bibliographic databases to support care providers with timely, relevant, patient-specific information that facilitates more scientifically based, clinical decision making. In the other direction, the CPR must be capable of being used to create secondary research databases from which experiential knowledge (medical knowledge bases) can be derived.

There are no monumental or breakthrough technologies required to realize a CPR in the 1990s. Instead, what appears to be needed are more concerted efforts to focus existing and emerging technologies on building more effective and more clinically acceptable CPR systems. Examples of model centers—sites that have excelled at demonstrating various facets of the CPR—need to be established, and their progress highlighted as soon as possible. Similarly, demonstrations of advances in health care made possible by the CPR should be initiated promptly to accelerate the realization of the optimal CPR.

Current State of CPR Systems

Description of the Technology

The majority of clinically relevant computer-based information systems in health care today have evolved primarily from efforts to automate the functions of a single department such as the laboratory or pharmacy, and they are not examples of CPR systems. The more noteworthy examples of operating CPR systems today use data that go well beyond the routine collection and communication of data provided by one or more department systems. It is important to remember that the CPR system is only one module in a larger medical information system, whether it is within a hospital, a clinic, or a large medical center, yet the CPR system is always the integrating module for all patient care data for all other departmental systems. For example, all laboratory systems require data from the CPR about the patient—an identifier or perhaps additional stored data within the patient record—but, more importantly, the results of the ordered laboratory tests should be inserted into the CPR. All modules (laboratory, pharmacy, billing, etc.) of the health care system such as a hospital information system (HIS) should be either reading data stored in the CPR or conveying data to the CPR for storage.

The definition of a CPR system, therefore, is restricted to computer-based systems designed for the management of the entire patient care record. Such a design could involve a system with physically distributed computers and their databases with logical central control of the entire record or a centrally located complete CPR within a single computer stored database. The key requirement is that through some mechanism there is central knowledge, control, and organizational integrity of the entire record for each patient. This central control should allow a single terminal located anywhere in the information system to access the entire integrated record regardless of the location of any other departmental subsystem where the various data items may have originated. The central controlling system should provide integrated and coordinated use of the data, which is impossible as a function of any originating subsystems. Examples of this extended use include integrated reports, generation of alerts/reminders as to clinical conflicting or interacting orders, and complex data searches across data elements from multiple departments.

While the distributed design has gained support from networking technologies, currently most systems that qualify as CPR systems use a central integrated physical database design. CPR systems today do not yet provide all of the necessary applications for acquisition and retrieval of patient care data. Today's CPR consists of data transmitted to the CPR system via interfaces with departmental subsystems and then entered into the CPR with applications programmed on the CPR system. One of the major differentiating factors between current CPR systems is the extent of their use of communication networks to departmental subsystems.

A few academic systems that clearly can be described as CPR systems have been developed in academic environments and share several common traits. First, they maintain a large data dictionary to define the contents of their CPR. The design of the data dictionary is sufficiently flexible to incorporate the continually expanding base of medical data required for new medical technologies and innovations. Second, all patient data recorded in the CPR is tagged with the time of the transaction, thus making the CPR a continuous chronologic history of the patient's medical care. Third, the systems provide rich research tools for using with the CPR data. This feature makes primary patient data in the CPR not only of value in direct patient care, but also as (1) a repository of secondary (derived) research data on which to perform clinical research, perform outcome evaluations, and assist in continuous quality improvement studies in the hospital, or (2) a source of data for collection in secondary research databases. Fourth, the systems should be able to retrieve and report the data in the CPR in a flexible manner. Because of the comprehensiveness of the data, it no longer should be viewed only in the specialized formats reported by the departmental subsystems, but should be capable of being reported with all other data from the CPR in all the various ways required by all users of the CPR.

Although these common traits exist among some CPR systems, many differences are also evident. How they have achieved these traits is very system specific.

The actual designs of these databases are unique and the tools for working with the database all appear to be system dependent. What one is able to conclude is that while there may be unanimity about many of the goals of a CPR, there is no common approach to reaching those goals. Although the CPR is the core or central feature of the more sophisticated health care information systems since all other system components interact with it, most CPR system developers had to compromise with a partial CPR system because of the magnitude of the total task and economic constraints.

Comparative Strengths and Weaknesses

No single health care information system operational in 1990 captures the entire CPR, yet the distinguishing feature of those that can be designated as CPR systems is the structure of their database design. In all cases, they use an approach wherein a data dictionary can be expanded to accommodate new data elements to be captured in the CPR. Such flexibility sets these systems apart because their databases are neither fixed nor is significant reprogramming needed to meet the continuing CPR demands for system innovations and enhancements.

Unfortunately, no single database structure or data dictionary is common to the current efforts in this field. Those that have been successful in implementing the most robust CPRs to date have used their own individual designs, and therefore do not conform to any particular standard. This has resulted in the evolution of disparate systems that cannot exchange information easily. It is precisely this situation that precipitated the interest in evolving standards such as HL7, Medix, ACR/NEMA, and others. Even among these, none yet address in a robust manner a comprehensive vehicle for exchanging an entire CPR. When standards for exchange of patient data are adequately developed there will be no need for standardizing the database structures of individual CPR systems, but all CPR systems will have to accept records in the standard communications format as input and as output.

Future CPR Systems

The CPR systems of the 1990s will be designed and built with the objective that the CPR is the central integrating component of the entire health care information system. It is important that future CPR systems be designed from the outset with this crucial requirement. Future CPR systems will either (1) offer the CPR in a physically centralized single computer database accessible to all other system components, or (2) provide a logical representation of complete and integrated CPRs, with portions of the CPR physically distributed among the databases of several networked computers. Each of these scenarios has advantages and disadvantages that are described in subsequent sections of this chapter. Furthermore, it is expected that in the next few years sets of standards will evolve that permit CPR systems to communicate normalized data (i.e., meaningful content in the record using terminology that has been preprocessed for vocabulary control) via a common exchange format with the flexibility to transmit any part or all of the CPR.

Databases and Database Management Systems

Description of the Technology

It is important to distinguish the database (the computer-based patient record or CPR) from the database management system (the CPR system). The CPR functions relate to data content (patient's medical problems, diagnoses, and treatments; data from surgeons, pediatricians, psychiatrists, etc.); the proper implementation of this data content is usually an educational requirement for health care professionals. The CPR system functions relate to capacity, response time, reliability, security, cost, and the like. The proper implementation of these functions is usually a technical/engineering design requirement, independent of the database content.

The CPR database should contain detailed information about each care transaction, synthesize information from all facilities in the medical center providing care for the patient, and cover the patient's lifetime of care within the health care program. Multiple values for static and time-oriented data must be supported, and the status of the record at any point in time must be accurately reconstructible (i.e., preserving the data integrity). The patient record must provide an integrated source to data about the patient including image (e.g., x-ray films) and sound (voice input/output and auscultations). Distribution of subsystem application functions and data storage (e.g., in specialized departments) must be accommodated, but through a mechanism that guarantees synchrony and integration of data. Access to data in the patient record will need to be limited to individuals with a legal right to know; their access to the data will be routinely logged, with a record of who has accessed what. Response time requirements for terminals will vary according to what is being done with single data item entries and retrievals at the subsecond level; complex interactions or search queries may take several seconds to one or more hours.

The data structure underlying the patient record is characterized as an integrated distributed database. Individual records will require multiple data structures (or data files) for retrieval optimization and a variety of patient care applications will be responsible for generating and using data. Data synchrony must be guaranteed at both the applications level and the database management system level. Patient identification procedures must be standardized; and a comprehensive dictionary of data item definitions must be developed. Avoiding obsolescence of terminology in the data dictionary will require a progressive separation of the application from the underlying terminology database.

There is no one or "right" database structure. In selecting the most desirable database for the CPR, we must be careful to select the database technology that most completely satisfies the needs of the users of the CPR. In truth, multiple databases may be necessary since no single database structure is likely to be optimal for each of the various retrieval requirements of the CPR.

Several database architectures have evolved in recent years. Among them are the following: (1) hierarchical, (2) relational, (3) text-oriented, and (4) object-oriented databases. Each of these architectures has its own particular sets of strengths and weaknesses. Current CPR systems use primarily hierarchical, relational, and text-oriented models.

Comparative Strengths and Weaknesses

Problems with the hierarchical database structure come to the forefront when the data are needed for more then one purpose. Then multiple hierarchies have to be superimposed on a single data structure or the data have to be copied. The multiple hierarchy approach is exemplified by IBM's IMS system, now used for many hospitals as the foundation for their patient care systems (PCS). It is complex and requires an expert programming staff for its maintenance. The copying approach is exemplified by the use of MUMPS-based systems for patient care and research at Brigham and Women's Hospital in Boston. Since the access hierarchy is based in the first case on the patients and in the second case on medications, procedures, and diagnoses, the research databases are created by periodic copying.

The tree structure, the most logical implementation of a hierarchical relationship, is an effective database structure only as long as the levels of the hierarchy are limited. Retrieving involves retrieving the root record and following pointers to the record in the next lower levels, which in turn contain pointers to the level below it. This process is inefficient when the structures have to be mapped sequentially onto disks; each step requires a disk access. New data storage devices may overcome this limitation, thus enhancing the desirability of this database structure.

The popularity of the relational database management system (RDBMS) may in large part be attributed to the personal computer and individual use of small relational databases. To use relational database concepts appropriately, one needs to understand precisely what a relational database represents. The relational model of data has a flat, two-dimensional view of the world with all data expressed in the form of tables. These tables must obey a set of normalization rules. The tables have unique rows and columns; their cells are single valued. If these conditions are met, the models, mathematical operations and logic will provide provable correct transformations. Consistency and integrity of database content is supported by having minimal redundancy in the normalized relations. This tabular structure is simple and familiar, hence the RDBMS' popularity. It is general enough to represent many types of data and clearly is adequate for many medical applications.

RDBMS has the problem of poor retrieval response times when the databases become large and the retrieval requires examination of many data elements. In addition, fourth generation languages (4GL) tools that are part of the RDBMS do not provide general programming capability. They provide convenient direct retrieval and limited update, but processing for deep data analysis is not supported.

At best, result files can be extracted for subsequent processing. Therefore, although these structures may be utilized into an overall scheme of data storage, none of these RDBMS is capable of being the sole approach to a CPR.

The latest approach to database development is built on the concept that the database reflects the meaning or semantics of the objects being described; and the database is a collection of object descriptions that belong to classes which have certain characteristics. In the object-oriented database model, an object is a member of an entity that has its own internal storage of values and a public interface. Messages are used to instruct the object to report or alter its private memory and to carry out procedures. The set of characteristics and rules that describe the object is called that object's entity class.

Object-oriented databases have grown out of object-oriented languages with some added characteristics to control, manage, and query the database. The data structure and the programming languages are closely related in this model. Again, while object-oriented databases will not be the total solution, tools and concepts introduced by this approach will be a key ingredient of database structures used to support the CPR.

The strengths of database technology are that new DBMS deal more effectively with voluminous amounts and increased complexity of data than previous database technology did. However, as databases grow in size and complexity and as the number of simultaneous users increases significantly, whether an acceptable response time can be provided remains unclear, even with state-of-the-art DBMS technology. Major problems with existing database management systems include

- The direct tie between programming language and database structure
- Specialization in design to optimize certain functions at the cost of others
- The difficulty in mapping complex logical structures onto physical media

The strengths of the CPR systems include a growing awareness of the need to have at least a view of a complete centralized CPR. If the CPR is physically distributed among several diverse computers in a network, then this view must be assembled from each computer on the network. Although the latter scenario has several advocates and some advantages, it also has several severe problems, as will be noted later. For example, strengths of the distributed CPR scenario include (1) the ability to house selected portions of data for the CPR at the source (e.g., workstation/server on the network in a pulmonary laboratory); (2) a potentially faster response times for queries because the load of servicing those queries is distributed across multiple computers, each of which serves a fairly specific function; (3) the fact that failure of one system or node on the network does not take the entire system down; and (4) the fact that the cost of the system may be less than if a central system were utilized. The weaknesses of such a distributed scenario include (1) significant overhead for collecting all the diverse and distributed pieces of information about a patient each time a provider places a query that requires the assembly of diverse information residing in several places; (2) duplication of several portions of the CPR because some demographic and other information about the patient will be required and duplicated on each node in the distributed network; (3) an increasing chance for errors in the CPR due to inconsistent policies in various departments where the data is collected and stored; (4) an increasing chance that portions of the CPR are out of step (not synchronized) with other parts of the CPR on the network, making it difficult to present a cohesive view of the CPR; (5) the difficulty of implementing a consistent retrieval and data entry protocol because of variations in the various nodes on the network; and, most significant of all, (6) the increased chance for breach of security of the CPR because multiple systems entry points significantly increase the opportunity for penetrating the *integrated* system's security measures. With the exception of the last issue (security), a distributed system might provide a "view" of the virtual record in another way. Given the downward trends in the price of hardware, one could overcome most of the objections noted above by dedicating a node on the network to the continual aggregation of distributed elements of the CPR onto one node that has the entire CPR resident, while also providing consistent retrieval and display for the care provider. However, the tougher issue of security for all the distributed nodes on the network that in some instances contain very sensitive information from the CPR has not been addressed.

Potential Use in Future CPR Systems

The database structure must accommodate recording of transaction level detail if the CPR is to (1) be generated as an integral part of the care process; (2) be a resource for operations or clinical research; or (3) serve as the sole legal record. In other words, the set of data that are clinically relevant to care of the patient must be supplemented by who did what, where, when, and how.

Medication data can be taken as an example. Patient management decisions require a record of the daily dose, start date, stop date, and possible adverse reactions for any treatment. Support of the care process requires a record for each order containing the medicine: its strength, form, signum, prescribing physician, number prescribed, number of refills allowed, and the date the prescription was written. In addition, a dispensing record must be maintained for each prescription filled with the order information plus a prescription number, number of doses dispensed, manufacturer, lot, dispensing pharmacist, and cost. A medication administration record must include the amount, time, and person responsible for each dose administered. Use of the record as a legal audit trail requires the addition of the name of the individual entering the order, the individual validating the order, and date/time stamps of all actions.

The data structure must have the capability of dealing with multiple versions of the same data element. Two situations must be accommodated. The first case involves data that can change but are not thought of as being time oriented, for example, patient name; a full history of changes must be recorded together with index searches for both current and prior names. The second case involves collecting an audit trail of corrections to an entry. At a minimum, an audit trail must be made of changes occurring after a data element has been validated and made available for electronic access. It will probably also be necessary to record updates made before the validation step. For time-oriented data, valid intervals of observations and state as well as data entry and correction times are needed.

The data structure underlying the CPR must be designed to provide a single integrated source for data about the patient. This requirement has implications both for the way in which health care professionals interact with the CPR system and for the database architecture.

Each datum must be recorded at the earliest appropriate point in the care process. Subsequent interactions with the CPR would involve verification or update of existing information, together with addition of new information. Such a process would stand in stark contrast to current practices with paper-based records in which each new care provider records a new summary of facts together with an assessment in a unique pen and paper style. With each cycle of care, the CPR would become more accurate; consensus would be identified, and points of disagreement would be highlighted.

The architecture of the CPR must take advantage of distributed data processing. Distribution is necessary to permit (1) use of different types of processing resources, (2) sharing of common data with local data augmentation, and (3) integrated access to autonomous, remote information/knowledge databases.

Each of the available hardware alternatives has a place in the operation of a medical information system. Mainframe facilities may remain appropriate for storage of large databases. Workstations have an advantage in memory-intensive operations such as graphics or spread sheet/flow sheet manipulation. Intermediate processing nodes will be required to transform information from dissimilar nodes and make it accessible. These mediating nodes may also provide the required privacy protection.

In a given situation, the system mix may mandate use of a suboptimal technology for a specific task. The correct role for each structure underlying the CPR must be designed to function in a distributed system supported by a changing mix of hardware.

Thus, the appropriate architecture for a CPR will incorporate some aspects of both centralized and distributed database models. The CPR database will consist of multiple structures, all or portions of which may bs physically separated. At the applications level, there must be user/server concepts to guarantee database synchronization and validity. The CPR database supports data of general user interest. An individual user will extract a particular subset of that data of immediate interest. Programs for the manipulation of that data subset can reside on the user's workstation or be part of the server system. Data of interest to only one user can remain at the workstation, but changes in data originating from the server must be transmitted back to the server, where (subject to update algorithms) the server database is updated. The architecture of the CPR must permit control of access to data by both category of data and category of user. In some cases, it will be necessary to control access at the individual datum and user level. The data structure must permit notification regarding patient agreement to release individual data items to individual users. The data structure must permit retention of audit trails each time a particular datum is accessed.

The response time requirements for the CPR will depend upon the type of use. Retrieval response time can vary depending upon the complexity of the task. A physician retrieving a single laboratory result will be frustrated if more than 1 or 2 seconds are required. On the other hand, a request to graph changes in the results of two clinical variables over a year of a patient's follow-up of care can take 20 to 30 seconds without becoming frustrating.

At least five major structures will be required to record patient- or process-related data. Initial data capture should be into this transaction-oriented file containing both information about the patient and information about how that information was or is going to be obtained. A variety of transient indexes into this transaction file should support work flow management. Data should flow selectively from the transaction files to a summary record containing information of long-term significance. This latter information will be the subset of data available for interactive historical recall and transfer between facilities. Other process-related data should be archived to bulk offline storage. Research files containing interpreted data should be constructed from the transaction files and maintained for the duration of interest. The archiving mechanism for the transaction file should permit reconstruction of the state of the database at any point in time for legal purposes and reconstruction of the research files on demand.

Terminals and Workstations

Description of the Technology

Three general classes of workstations are emerging that seem likely to prevail in future CPR systems:

- Smart terminals
- Handheld or semiportable data entry devices
- Robust workstations

Smart terminals will have a cathode ray tubes (CRT) screen (color optional), keyboard and data entry/pointer/selector device (e.g., mouse, touchscreen, lightpen or voice), and a reasonably powerful (e.g., 80386) central processing unit (CPU). These smart terminals will use a graphic user interface (GUI) and communicate with the file servers, computer servers, and rule servers for decision support on the network. They will package input data for delivery over the local area network (LAN) to the CPR system, and they will process structured information retrieved from the CPR to display via the GUI.

Handheld or semiportable devices will consist of a liquid crystal display (LCD), an 80286 or more powerful CPU, and multiple communications capabilities to facilitate either manual or voice entry into the CPR. These portable or nearly portable devices will be used by the bedside nurses.

Fully configured, robust workstations will employ one or more state-of-the-art CPUs, large memory configurations, very large capacity rotating memory systems (including magnetic and multiple types of optical media); exhibit displays supporting high resolution imaging, text and graphic data, and a highly sophisticated GUI with windows; and provide voice input/output and access to intelligent gateways to burgeoning external sources of clinically relevant knowledge bases and literature retrieval. In the early 1990s these workstations will utilize 80386 or 80486 chips or possibly 68030 or 68040 general purpose processors. Reduced instruction set-computers (RISC) are certain to be the dominate CPU technology later in the decade, with upwards of 100 or more million instructions per second (MIPS) becoming available for the desktop computer. Additionally, special purpose hardware such as high performance, digital signal processors (DSP) for handling a multitude of clinically relevant tasks such as waveform analysis, voice recognition cards, graphic acceleration cards, and additional processors will enhance the performance and capabilities of these high end workstations.

The operating systems (OS) for the CPR workstations will be either UNIX (AT&T's version 5.x or a variation of it such as Mach, the multiprocessor version), the Apple MacIntosh OS, or the long promised OS/2 from MicroSoft. Exactly which of the windowing packages will be used will vary depending on the OS selected, and it is too early to predict which will gain dominance over the 1990s. Crucial to the workstation and its OS are the communications software and the database management system.

Comparative Strengths and Weaknesses

The strengths of the handheld or semiportable data entry device include its portability, its convenience for data capture while providing care, and the capability of nearly instant feedback in response to entering the patient's data as, for example, validity checks and limited decision support functions. Its weaknesses include the fact that full functionality and the power of a sophisticated workstation or terminal are largely missing, and the cost of such devices will rise dramatically as more sophisticated options are added.

The strengths of the smart terminals include their comparatively low unit cost while providing powerful GUI access to the CPR via the network. The smart terminal does not possess significant processing power and therefore can only be relied upon as an access tool for the health care professional. The workstation, on the other hand, may well become the most powerful tool ever devised for health care professionals and may ultimately come to be considered an indispensable tool. These workstations will probably be available for under $3,000 (1990 dollars). Perhaps its only shortcomings are its high cost and the fact that it is not portable. Further innovations may yet help both of these problems.

Potential Use in Future CPR Systems

Health care professionals will use workstations and terminals as an indispensable tool to perform tasks associated with charting and providing care. They may be located at the patient's bedside, nursing stations, clinical workrooms, or professionals' offices. Clearly, the workstations will utilize a GUI and the workstations will be connected to a LAN. Basic to this vision of the CPR is a distributed information-processing system interconnected via a broadband (probably fiber optic-based) high speed network. Two principal decisions will govern the acquisition and installation of these CPR workstations: selection of the GUI and how the workstations transmit and receive data over the LAN.

Data Acquisition and Retrieval for Patients and Health Care Providers

Description of the Technology

Data acquisition for the CPR is one of the most challenging topics in medical informatics. For automated data entry in one hospital, analog-to-digital converters are observed on nearly every conceivable device in the hospital, and these have been installed for the sole purpose of directly capturing patient data without human intervention insofar as it is possible. It is safe to say that there have been many more failures than successes in getting physicians engaged in (much less become an eager or active participant in) the data entry process. CPR systems present a broad spectrum of approaches to this problem from nearly eliminating the need for any physician input (i.e., do not ask the physician to change any practice habits and use clerical intermediaries) to extensive hierarchical menus directing data input selection by keyboard, lightpen, or mouse. Some systems have been installed that required house staff and other professionals to type, using what they thought were cumbersome data entry devices; not surprisingly, such systems have failed. Most systems today lie somewhere between these two extremes. One of the most prominent hospital information systems today uses the point and click lightpen method for data entry and it has had mixed (very significant use to very small amount of use) reception by physicians. A short (preferably subsecond) response time has proven to be one of the most important factors for successful CPR systems. This statement primarily refers to the retrieval of data but is equally important for the input of data. One of the most potent revolutions in computer technology, the GUI has only recently begun to be used in the health care setting for such features as icons and pull-down menus. The use of an off-the-shelf GUI system as a terminal for accessing older, established systems is now being explored.

Most CPR systems today are providing output data to CRT screens in textual, tabular, and some limited graphic forms. Much of the CPR can be presented to the health care professional using low cost monitors capable of high resolution graphics, because most of the record can be presented as text, tables, or graphs (e.g., trends in laboratory values). These displays can effectively support low resolution views of the patient (e.g., a facial identification) or other simple graphics, but not high definition images from radiology. Pictures (not simple graphics) from radiology and other imaging departments of a health care facility cannot be presented (see the subsequent section on images) except on much more complex and expensive displays. Health care professionals usually need to have records that can be carried about as desired; therefore, output from the CPR systems include hard copy of screens, graphs, or tables, and of signals such as electrocardiograms (EKGs). With a complete online CPR, there is less need to print multipart copies of these outputs. Nonetheless, outputs need to be printed on low noise devices such as inkjet or laser printers rather than on noisy impact printers.

Retrieval requests today can take the form of key words, coded strings, or Boolean logic. Standard query languages (e.g., SQL from database technology) are only now beginning to appear in a few CPR systems. Modifications specific to medical applications are being suggested that will make such standards more appropriate for the CPR. The retrieval needs of health care professionals vary with the specialty and other aspects of the services they provide. Special entry points for retrieval and specially designed data outputs customized to the needs of certain classes of health care professionals are being explored as new hardware capable of supporting such overhead becomes available. This emphasis on tailoring the CPR systems to more effectively meet the retrieval and display (output) needs of individuals or groups is a significant step in improving acceptability of the CPR. Significant new hardware, primarily optical media for archival storage of the CPR have recently been introduced. It is now possible to store from 250 to 550 megabytes on small approximately 4.75 to 5.25 inches) optical discs capable of storing a complete CPR. Low cost, high capacity jukeboxes have been introduced making it possible to store up to 130 or more gigabytes (billion bytes) using 240 CD-ROM disks; these could be accessible (in as little as 4 seconds) in a networked setting. Such a jukebox supports up to five CD-ROM disk drives so that multiple users could simultaneously access archived copies of records for many patients. This means that timely retrieval of vast quantities of local information (including the CPR) could now be made available in CPR systems.

Comparative Strengths and Weaknesses

It is generally agreed that data for the CPR should be captured only once and used by all portions of the system that use that particular data item. Although many believe that the data should be entered into electronic form by the primary user, this remains a sensitive issue with already burdened health care professionals who fear changes to their traditional mode of practice. Still, secondary data entry by an intermediary has the following disadvantages: (1) introduction of errors as part of the transcription process; (2) delays in the availability of information waiting to be entered that may be critical to other members of the care team; (3) lack of immediate feedback to physicians for editing alerts/alarms and error checking of orders; and (4) lack of the ability to use linked databases for assistance in the decision making process. Experience has revealed that the extent of involvement required of care professionals can be the most troublesome part of operating a CPR. There is a real attitudinal problem among many health care professionals, an attitude that data entry is "only a clerical function," unworthy of their time or consideration. Early systems introduced into health care did little to dissuade health care professionals of this attitude and, in fact, seemed to cement the attitude that data entry was little more than an exercise in advanced frustration. Therefore, the key to the success of next generation of CPR systems is the ease of use (including voice input via voice recognition systems) and incentives for data capture at the data source.

Potential Use in Future CPR Systems

It seems clear that future CPR systems will use GUI and that workstation technologies and terminals capable of fully integrated graphics will be distributed throughout the health care facility. Emphasis will be placed on improving the accessibility and availability of terminals for accessing the CPR at the site where care is given; this is especially true for nursing staff members. Future CPR systems will provide for both local and central clustering of data storage via multiple servers on the network. The emphasis will be on the accurate collection of primary data by health care professionals and as close to the actual care setting as possible. Table 1 is included to illustrate the extent of the data to be collected for the CPR, and it the shows the sources of such data. Not only are these data in the CPR important for serving the needs of the health care professional, they also will be required for realtime links with medical knowledge bases, bibliographic databases, and other relevant (and sometimes remote) information resources. Timeliness of retrieval is a crucial factor in successful CPR systems, especially in intensive or coronary care units and for physicians in emergency rooms. In this regard, it is likely that timely access to remote information resources will be a major challenge for system developers because of the overhead usually associated with such rapid access.

In future CPR systems it is likely that the retrieval, displays, and reporting of data will be user configurable. This means that the same data may be presented differently or in different combinations to different health care professionals with differing views or windows into the same CPR. There is also likely to be more patient interaction in the care process, both from the view of data entry (patient participation to collect the patient's history) and from health risk management. There will also be more participatory decision making in the selection among alternative care options.

Image Processing and Storage

Description of the Technology

Medical imaging today includes diagnostic images or pictures obtained by film scanners, computed radiography (CR), magnetic resonance (MR), computed tomography (CT), ultrasound, and nuclear medicine sources. Images acquired from each of these sources are being recorded digitally today. In the near future, digital images will be routinely available in most radiology departments. Medical images in today's medical record are typically two dimensional, still pictures. In digital form, the intensity resolution (number of measurable levels of gray) varies from 8 to 12 bits (from 256 to 4096 levels of gray) which permits the display of images with medium to high contrast. Their image definition (spatial resolution) varies from 64×64 pixels (picture elements) for nuclear medicine images to $4,000 \times 5,000$ (20 million total) for output on modern film scanners.

The amount of information associated with the storage of medical imaging dwarfs all other data fields commonly appearing in a patient record (e.g., text such as a patient's history). A single high definition chest image can require 25 megabytes for storage. To put this in context, 100,000 pages of text (of 300 words per page) occupy about the same amount of storage. The image definition for diagnostic and therapeutic decision making from an electronic image appears to be at least $2,000 \times 2,000$ pixels, while 10 to 12 bits will be required for intensity resolution. Less well-defined images for nondiagnostic purposes may well be adequate for some situations, but radiologists will feel comfortable only with images that are at least as good as film roentgenograms. A film image normally has an image definition of 5 to 25 million pixels and an intensity resolution of 256 to 4096 levels of gray. The 100 or more gray levels observable on a typical CRT monitor are inadequate unless contrast can be controlled by means of an adjustable intensity window. Such contrast control requires display buffers that store 9 or more bits (10 to 12 is preferable) per pixel.

New technologic developments are expected to lead to a new generation of picture archiving and communications systems (PACS) which will be installed in many radiology departments by 1995. PACS permit the electronic storage, transmission, and display of medical images throughout a medical facility. PACS consist of an archive for image storage, a network to distribute images, and multiple display systems for image display. Stored images are retrieved from the optical disk archive and transferred to a central magnetic storage device. From there images are transmitted over a broadband, high speed network to any of a large number of display stations capable of high definition presentation and interactive contrast control. PACS offer many advantages not available with conventional film. For example, two or more physicians can simultaneously examine exact duplicates of an image at their respective and sometimes distant locations.

Comparative Strengths and Weaknesses

Primarily, the strengths of imaging technologies include the ability to support high definition images as part of a totally digital electronic patient record and the capability to transmit images to providers at distant sites. Imaging systems in the near future will eliminate such concerns about the current status or location of an image as *missing* or *in transit*.

Medicine's requirements for high resolution (high contrast and high definition) press the technology beyond the state of the art for computer graphics workstations. Similarly, the data transmission requirements for medical images over that for computer graphics presents an additional problem. For example, Ethernet typically transmits at a peak speed of 1 megabyte per second, which is too slow for transmission of images of the quality required by medicine. Furthermore, internal computer architectures and disk storage do not support the data transmission speeds required for high quality medical images. It seems probable that by 1995 these problems will be addressed sufficiently to support the transmission and display of medical imaging

Potential Use in Future CPR Systems

The use of medical imaging is becoming increasing significant to satisfy modern health care. Imaging is not restricted to the radiology department, since images are routinely generated also by ophthalmologists, dentists, pathologists, dermatologists, and other specialists. Images have become an essential part of the patient record, and records without images are viewed as incomplete. This erodes confidence in the electronic record from a physician's viewpoint. Completeness of the patient record is essential, not only for diagnostic and therapeutic decision making, but also for evaluating the appropriateness and quality of those decisions.

PACS will have important implications for the future patient record. Text, graphs, handwritten copies of physician and nurse notes as well as images can all be made available interactively in a responsive windowing workstation. The complete patient record, including images, can be made available to all health care professionals using the tools developed for PACS.

Computers are being used to model microscopic and macroscopic views of the human body from molecules to organ systems. These models should increase our understanding of health and disease and many will be useful in the care of individual patients. Three dimensional renderings of shaded images allow the appreciation of spatial relationships not possible in two dimensional sectional data. The addition of motion pictures or motion graphics adds even more visual meaning to some images. It may take several more years to realize some of these capabilities, but it seems certain that computer generation and visualization of various models will evolve. These models include mechanisms for the action of pharmaceuticals, proteins, DNA sequences, cell physiology, ion channel dynamics, organ behavior, cardiac dynamics, brain metabolism, hip joint mechanics, facial reconstruction, and many other medically important processes. Parallel processing will probably be utilized for such modeling to provide the realtime responses that are required for clinical settings.

Data Exchange Standards and Vocabulary Control

Description of the Technology

Standards efforts for components of the CPR have only recently gained significant developmental momentum in the United States. Since so much is at stake in this sizable medical market, a market that remains largely untapped from the vendor's viewpoint, standards take on an even more prominent role in the required technologies. Many vendors seem hesitant to invest substantial sums in developing certain technologies until directions for the industry become clearer, and standards play an important role in this regard. HL7, Medix, ASTM, and ACR/NEMA, and other efforts are representative of the movement currently underway to develop standards for data exchange. Generally, each of these efforts (except as noted below) seems to focus on addressing a particular portion of the CPR. For example, HL7 effectively addresses the transmission of data from systems such as laboratory to hospital mainframe, but does not address the transmission of any image data. ACR/NEMA, on the other hand, addresses primarily the transmission of select sets of image data. Most of these data exchange standards have now evolved to the point of first implementations that show promise of practical use, but they are still emerging and are far from complete. The ACR/NEMA standard, for example, does not yet address the transmission of images from such practice settings as dermatology or dentistry. These standards might be classed as midlevel standards, because they are neither aimed at low level (e.g., levels 1–6 of the Open Systems Interconnect model) exchange, nor are they a high level standard addressing the exchange of the entire CPR. These midlevel standards are, for the most part, still immature, but they are evolving rapidly. The standard that purports to be the most comprehensive for the entire CPR is Medix (IEEE P.1157); yet being one of the youngest, it remains in its very early stages of development. Standards efforts for supporting the exchange of an entire CPR (or portions thereof) are critical to providing incentives for vendors to move ahead with developments essential to the CPR, while also sending a strong message encouraging a reduced emphasis on proprietary software and hardware.

Vocabulary control (which is similar in concept to *uniform vocabulary*) is a term commonly used by librarians. To a librarian, it implies that in order to achieve order and consistency for accessing materials in a library a set of common terminologies should be established for classifying and categorizing the library's holdings. The same is true for the CPR. In order to provide meaningful access and to convey precise meaning to all members of the health care team, a significant emphasis on consistency of terminology in the CPR seems warranted. The unified medical language system (UMLS) under development at the National Library of Medicine (NLM) is such an effort. The UMLS project has strong implications for the CPR, yet it addresses the broader issue of resolving terminology issues across other systems as well. The broad category of vocabulary is really a *content* issue that is much more complex and difficult to solve than the *format* issue discussed above.

Depending on the specific circumstances, the effective retrieval and use of information from the CPR is dependent on some level of consistency in the way the same findings, clinical problems, procedures, drugs, and the like have been named or described within a single patient record, across many patient records in a single CPR system, across CPR systems, and/or in other systems that contain data relevant to the understanding and treatment of patient problems. The greater the need for aggregation of data from many patient records (as in outcomes research, for example), the more important consistent description of clinical content becomes. The development of effective vocabulary control within and across CPR systems requires the existence of suitable vocabularies or classifications for describing the content of CPRs, the ability to relate the terms used in different vocabularies to denote the same concept, and cost effective mechanisms for using controlled vocabularies in CPR data acquisition and processing.

By 1990, statistical and billing requirements led to widespread use of the *International Classification of Diseases, 9th edition. Clinical Modification (ICD-9-CM)* and current procedural terminology (CPT) to code or classify diagnoses and physician controlled procedures in patient records. The numeric codes from these systems are therefore present in a variety of full or partial CPR systems and provide a measure of consistent content description across CPR systems. Unfortunately, ICD-9-CM codes are fairly general and sometimes do not discriminate among related but distinct patient conditions. Also since the ICD-9-CM is updated very infrequently, general codes may continue to be used even after a specific condition has become significant or prevalent enough to warrant its own code. In the case of CPT, the codes usually represent very complex combinations of procedures. Use of the codes for retrieval of all patients who have undergone one of the constituent procedures is therefore difficult. Assignment of CPT codes is often skewed by the pursuit of particular billing objectives. In many environments, alignment of ICD-9-CM and CPT codes occurs at a point and time distant from the actual provision of care and thus is conducive to coding errors. For these reasons, neither ICD-9-CM nor CPT codes are particularly useful for retrieving information from patient records.

Some developers of full or partial CPR systems have established a level of control over the actual terms that can be used in selected portions of the CPR. Core system dictionaries have been established, sometimes based on terms in independently maintained controlled vocabularies such as SNOMED (the College of American Pathologists' Systematized Nomenclature of Medicine), MeSH (NLM's Medical Subject Headings), or more specialty-specific lists, but generally relying heavily on locally developed terminology. Some of these systems include mechanisms for minimizing the number of unlinked synonyms entered in their dictionaries. Few, if any, are set up to eliminate the possibility of such entries. Some of these systems support automatic assignment of ICD-9 codes based on more specific vocabulary terms assigned to the CPRs. One reason why CPR system developers have not relied heavily on existing controlled vocabularies is that there is no single controlled vocabulary with adequate coverage of all aspects of clinical medicine. This is particularly true in the area of clinical findings. Another deterrent to the use of existing controlled vocabularies is their infrequent update schedules. In general, professional medical groups have been much better at developing vocabularies than they have been at maintaining and updating them on a regular basis. Perhaps the most significant deterrent, however, is that the use of reasonably specific controlled vocabularies for creating or indexing patient records can increase costs associated with ongoing record creation and maintenance.

There are numerous and promising vocabulary developments relevant to CPR systems. They include a planned new edition of SNOMED, the emergence of the Read Clinical Classification in Great Britain, the development of a clinical vocabulary base that conforms with ASTM E 1284–89 (Standard Guide for Nosologic Standards and Guides for construction of New Biomedical Thesauri), and National

Library of Medicine's UMLS project. The overall goal of the UMLS is to help users retrieve relevant biomedical information from multiple machine-readable sources, irrespective of the different vocabularies and classifications used in these sources. One of the new knowledge sources being developed in support of this goal is a Metathesaurus, which will link related terms and concepts from a variety of existing biomedical vocabularies and classifications. Meta-1, the first version of the Metathesaurus, was issued in 1990. It will contain all terms and concepts from MeSH and the Diagnostic and *Statistical Manual of Mental Disorders*, 3rd edition revised (DSM-IIIR) as well as some terms from SNOMED, ICD-9-CM, CPT, and the Library of Congress Subject Headings. Meta-1 and the subsequent versions of the Metathesaurus should be useful tools for the developers of the CPR systems.

Comparative Strengths and Weakness

Among the strengths associated with data exchange standards is the fact that there is now a definite momentum toward establishing midlevel standards for crucial components of the CPR. It is also apparent that vendors are cooperating in the formulation and implementation of the midlevel data exchange standards.

Unfortunately, a complete and well-defined data exchange standard for an entire CPR does not yet exist.

Inadequate support for the timely update and maintenance of clinical vocabularies remains an impediment to developing better vocabulary control of the CPR. Furthermore, there are few incentives for the use of reasonably specific controlled vocabulary that are strong enough to overcome both the one-time costs associated with switching to a new vocabulary system and the probable increased costs associated with ongoing record creation and maintenance.

Potential Use in Future CPR Systems

It now seems clear from the momentum which has developed that the level standards will continue to evolve at an accelerated pace, making it possible to aggregate major components of the CPR together from disparate and distributed systems. As significant as progress has been or will be among these midlevel standards, what is clear is that more attention now needs to be placed on evolving high level standards. It would be preferable to have a single, flexible (nearly infinitely extensible so as to accommodate all existing midlevel standards as well as unforseen data and tests that may evolve in coming decades) high level standard for exchanging the entire CPR. Success in achieving a reasonable level of vocabulary control in the CPR is dependent on the implementation of standards for the format and basic data elements of the CPR.

Strategy for Future CPR Systems

The establishment of a uniform set of CPR data elements and a format for transmitting them among CPR systems will be a valuable first step in achieving vocabulary control across CPR systems. Interpretation of uncontrolled vocabulary is much easier if its specific location within the patient record is designated uniformly and unambiguously. The next step will be to identify those CPR data elements with the highest priority for vocabulary control. The likely candidates are (1) the basic demographic elements (e.g., sex, race, geographic location) for which standard names or abbreviations are readily available, (2) the patient problem list and the names of procedures performed by direct care providers, both of which are already the subject of special coding procedures, and perhaps (3) a set of standard problem modifiers (e.g., acute, chronic). Controlled vocabularies with appropriate coverage of these elements exist today or will be available within the next few years.

In selecting one or more controlled vocabularies or classifications to be used in these data elements, CPR system developers should look for terminologies that (1) are updated at least annually; (2) allow automatic detection of changes or additions in new versions of the terminology; (3) facilitate the automatic update of affected data elements in existing CPRs when terms in the controlled vocabulary are modified; (4) can be converted automatically to ICD-9-CM or other appropriate schemes for billing and statistical reporting; and (5) are either currently incorporated in the UMLS or are included in UMLS development plans. It is not necessary that all CPR developers converge on a single standard vocabulary as long as all the vocabularies used are linked into the UMLS.

At least in the near term, portions of the CPR will continue to contain free text and uncontrolled terminology. To facilitate subsequent retrieval and use of these sections, care should be taken to include full terms and controlled acronyms in addition to, or in place of, codes or abbreviations in the indices to CPRs and in displays of patient data. A method for distinguishing the significant terms and bound phrases with medical meaning from the other language appearing in these portions of the CPR will also facilitate the use of text-processing and term-matching routines.

In the next 5 years, the most significant impediment to the implementation of effective vocabulary control within and across CPR systems will continue to be accompanying modest increases in CPR input and update costs. The use of controlled vocabulary should lead to a tremendous increase in the effective use of CPR data, however, and a reduction in the current costs associated with retrievals, and nonretrieval of information from patient records.

Systems Communications and Network Linkage Standards

Description of the Technology

By its very nature, that is, many individuals interacting to provide care for a patient, health care is information intensive. This implies a strong emphasis on the communication and transmission of that information to many people in diverse places. The information conveyed is complex and in all possible modalities including text, images, voices and sounds, and video. This broad array of information will need to be made available in such diverse locations as the bedside, ward, professional office, emergency setting including mobile units, and the home. Fortunately, technologies to support communications of all types are evolving at an unprecedented rate. Especially with the advent of fiber optic transmission, it now becomes feasible to transmit at high speed and at low cost the broad array of information contained in the CPR. For example, wide band, fiber optic transmission is now capable of supporting 1.7 gigabytes (1.7 billion characters) per second over a 100 km link. Today, through the Fiber Distributed Data Interface (FDDI) for which a standard is well established, systems can support two counter-rotating rings for bidirectional communication using a token ring architecture. Bandwidths of 100 to 200 megabits per second are common for support of up to 500 stations. Chipsets for the FDDI standard are now being produced by many companies. This technology has attainable distances measured in several miles and is quite adequate for a complex of buildings such as a large medical center or a campus. Perhaps of greater significance than FDDI is that of the Integrated Services Digital Network (ISDN). ISDN is the grand plan for providing an all digital network capable of high speed transmission of all modalities (data, voice, graphics, or video) over public telephone networks. The goal is to provide a standard approach for universal digital interconnectivity regardless of modality, from potentially every telephone outlet that exists today. ISDN will overcome the 4 KHz limitations that current analog voice channels impose and will provide a digital interface with an initial capacity of approximately 144 K bits per second for each basic rate ISDN port (i.e., potentially each telephone endpoint in a residence or office), and 1.5 megabits per second for each primary rate ISDN port at a business location with a computing facility. ISDN is made possible through a commitment to total digital communications (e.g., fiber optics), high speed digital switches, out of bound signalling (using a separate path for dialing, signalling, and billing), and worldwide acceptance of the ISDN standard. As part of ISDN, another standard, the asynchronous transfer mode (ATM), has evolved and will soon be adopted. Hospitals are primary candidates for using ATM-based switches because they make possible wide-bandchannels for transmitting radiologic images between hospitals.

Within the United States, a few communities are now fully converted to all digital switches that support ISDN. It is expected that between 1995 and the end of the century most of the transition from analog to fully digital switches will have occurred throughout most of the country. When complete, this transition to an all digital network will open a new era for communications of all types of information. This has immense implications for improving health care. The United States lags behind some of Europe in the implementation of ISDN primarily because the United States has been slow to replace analog switches with digital. An ISDN pilot project for health care has been in operation at a west German university since 1986. This pilot project utilizes a private branch exchange (PBX) with about 100 multifunction terminals. These terminals are located at several nursing stations, the clinical laboratory, and other key locations throughout the hospital. They are used to access the main databases on the hospital mainframe, laboratory data, and simultaneous voice communication with a health care professional, if necessary. For example, it is possible to simultaneously view laboratory result (including images) at a nursing station while also speaking with a remote clinical pathologist using a single ISDN instrument.

Comparative Strengths and Weaknesses

The advent of fiber optic communications links for both local area networks (LAN) and long distance transmissions makes it feasible to transmit a complete CPR in an acceptable time frame (subsecond for text or data and a only few seconds for a complex image). The rapid (faster than expected) realization of fiber optic technologies seemed to catch much of the industry by surprise; therefore, standards for broadband ISDN have lagged. The same holds true for FDDI-II, the evolving standard for wideband fiber. The cost of providing these additional communications services will undoubtedly come under scrutiny and may delay their utilization in health care.

Potential Use in Future CPR Systems

By the end of 1991, an ATM network will probably be operational in the St. Louis, Missouri, area. Among the first applications on this network will be the transmission, at 100 megabits per second, of high resolution medical images. The use of tuned lasers and wavelength-multiplexing could reasonably result in transmission rates between 20 and 30 gigabytes per second. Some have predicted higher rates of nearly 100 gigabytes per second. As present trends continue, the FDDI-II standard now evolving will make possible gigabyte transmission rates capable of transmitting uncompressed, high resolution color movies in a digital mode. We can expect that the next three decades in information processing will be as revolutionary as the last three have been. We can expect a MIPS glut for computers and a bandwidth glut in communication networks that will drive prices down. The coupling of these two events makes possible entirely new capabilities that seem certain to redefine how we work. The CPR may be viewed as a complex document, containing all types of information (visual, sound, and data) that will need to be transmitted at high speed to locations near and far in the natural course of providing care. There are no scientific breakthroughs needed for the transmission of all of the CPR; the technology is either in place or evolving to facilitate the transmission of the most complex portions of the CPR. A bill for establishing a high capacity, high speed *data superhighway* has been evolving which came before the United States Congress in 1990. Senator Gore, the bill's sponsor, has likened it to the interstates highway network which today crisscrosses America, only this data superhighway will be as essential to the fast paced activities of the twenty-first century as are today's interstates. Health care should benefit from the establishment of such a vision, and health care professionals and patients alike should encourage its establishment.

System Reliability and Security; Data Integrity and Confidentiality

Description of the Technology

System reliability relates to the availability of the hardware and software system for useful work in the clinical setting. System security relates to the appropriate measures taken to keep the computer-based information systems safe from unauthorized access. Data protection falls into two categories: (1) data integrity and (2) data confidentiality. Data integrity means the consistency and accuracy of the data stored in the CPR, whereas data confidentiality refers to the measures taken to ensure that data in the CPR are not divulged to anyone except those who are authorized or who have a *need to know* status.

System Reliability

CPR systems mandate the complete availability of the patient's record 24 hours a day for reading or updating—100 percent uptime, the system can never be down. System reliability is therefore an absolute requirement. The state of the art for reliability of computer-based information systems (for both hardware and software) has greatly advanced in the last two decades. In the not too distant past, users of large mainframe systems used to perform backups every few hours because experience had taught them that these complex systems could *go down* unexpectedly and all too frequently. Prudent programmers engaged in developing software on these systems would often save their work one or more times each hour. However, over the 1980s, many technologies have contributed to making today's systems so reliable that some users rarely consider making backup copies of their work. Disk drives, which used to account for the majority of system (hardware) failures, now commonly exhibit mean time between failures (MTBF) of 30,000 to 60,000 hours, with recent announcements as high as 100,000 hours. Similarly, there are now many systems on the market that are fault tolerant, meaning that a failure of one or more system components will not bring the entire system down. Therefore, it seems safe to assume that systems today and in the future will be extremely reliable. Systems are also very reliable with regard to accuracy and dependability of data routed through the various system components (e.g., parity bits in memory, check digits in barcodes, wands, etc.). The level of reliability for applications software in assuring the accuracy and dependability of data collected varies throughout the industry. In the United States, the Food and Drug Administration (FDA) has shown great concern about the reliability of patient data being transmitted from one medical device or system to another. Data integrity is of paramount importance to the CPR, and care must be taken to ensure that the CPR is 100 percent restorable upon recovering from any system failures. Most database management systems (DBMS) today dedicate considerable resources in addressing this issue.

System Security

In recent years, the Department of Defense (DoD) has established criteria for secure operating systems ranking them in three broad categories (A, B, or C), with the A category being the most secure. There are no modern operating systems in the DoD's A category, but in the next (lower level or B category) tier of secure operating systems, new versions of UNIX are beginning to be approved. Given the sensitivity of data contained in the CPR, it seems prudent to ensure that systems which contain or manipulate the CPR comply with at least the DoD's B level of secure operating systems. None of the major system vendors or universities that has developed or is developing CPR related software has done so under any highly secure (level A or B) operating systems as rated by the DoD. These DoD rated and approved operating systems are designed and tested, using a host of validation suites, to assure system security data and program integrity.

Today, systems that manipulate or build a CPR (or even a minimal patient record) typically have very limited security measures. For the most part, the developers of CPR systems have had to focus on more pressing issues such as building the basic CPR capabilities at the expense of adequately addressing CPR security issues. For example, to support remote access by providers, one CPR system makes use of the callback feature for remote access via modem. Yet it has been pointed out that such simple security measures may be easily foiled using something as simple as call forwarding. Properly implemented, audit trails can be a very effective tool in monitoring security of the data, programs, and the CPR. Audit trails may occur at three levels: the system level, the record level, or the data field level. At the system level, an audit trail is maintained for all who gain access to the system; at the record level, those who access a particular CPR are tracked; and at the data field level, a record is kept of who updates or examines a data field in the system. Many CPR systems currently use audit trails for tracking access to the system, especially for remote users requesting access. Few current CPR systems address audit trails in a more comprehensive manner, such as tracking every access and especially every update (at both the record and data field levels) to the CPR. Most CPR systems in use today utilize the traditional security method of soliciting an ID and personal password. Most of the vendors of CPR systems suggest that physical limitations on access (by placement of the terminals in areas usually restricted to care providers) offer a measure of security, but this alone is not enough. None of the current CPR systems seems to take advantage of the personal authentication devices now emerging that are designed to permit access to authorized individuals only. Data protection for CPR systems must guard against (1) personal errors that inadvertently alter, release, or lose information; (2) loss of data from fire or water damage; (3) misuse of data by legitimate users; (4) malicious use of data from the CPR; (5) unauthorized breakins to the system; or (6) uncontrolled or untraceable access to the CPR. In some cases the CPR system might be placed in a very physically safe environment similar to computers containing sensitive financial or defense data. CPR systems must exhibit at least the same safeguards as those provided for a person's financial data. Finally, CPR systems should adhere to established guidelines for use of the CPR, as outlined by professional associations, vendors, providers, and consumer groups, as well as by state and federal laws.

Data Privacy and Confidentiality

This section focuses largely on protecting information in the CPR related to the patient. However, all members of the health care team are to be protected in a similar manner. Therefore, all members of the health care team deserve the same level of protection against unauthorized access or abuse of information from the CPR as applies to the patient. Recent research in medical confidentiality has proposed a three-zone confidentiality model. This model incorporates an inner zone with extremely sensitive information and an outer zone concerning the least sensitive information. The area between these two zones is the area with the traditional medical confidentiality requirement at multiple levels. The model illustrates the need for CPR systems in the future to adequately address confidentiality at multiple levels. Patients must be permitted to take an active role in declaring those portions of their CPR that they wish to remain totally confidential (the innermost zone). Providers may also designate those elements of the CPR they wish to hold confidential (this might even include elements that are not divulged to the patient). Conceivably, there may be elements of such a confidential nature that they are not even entered into the CPR, but are only discussed privately between the patient and the provider (e.g., positive HIV test). One of the most important methods for ensuring not only confidentiality, but also data and program integrity, is to restrict access to the CPR system to only those with a need to know and then positively certify their identity before permitting access. Fortunately, this is not a problem restricted to medicine.

The CPR system must be capable of providing different levels of data confidentiality, as required by its users. For example, psychiatric data must be available only to the patient's psychiatrist. Sensitive data in the areas of drug abuse, alcoholism, or the like must be protected by legal and professional rules and regulations

Comparative Strengths and Weaknesses

Unfortunately, there are few strengths to extol in this section. The most notable strengths include the reliability of both hardware and most software systems (especially operating systems). Generally, these have matured to the point where they are quite adequate for CPR systems. CPR systems are now deployed on either a fault-tolerant system or on systems with one or more backups available (sometimes called a hot backup, meaning one that is ready to pick up where the failed one left off without the user's noticing there was a problem or failure) and experience shows very nearly 100 percent uptime. The weakness of systems which are not fault tolerant is that the process of going down and transitioning to the backup makes system failures more noticeable to users.

In 1991, CPR systems are vulnerable to unauthorized access both by computer hackers and by less sophisticated individuals with limited knowledge of software but great determination. System security is generally weak and is most often protected by only the use of a user identification number or code and password. Such an approach is inadequate, because experience shows that users often record their passwords in places accessible by others or even share their passwords with others, negating any security. Many CPR systems use audit trails, mostly at the system level, to discourage and track unauthorized access to CPR systems.

Today, data integrity within CPR systems is probably the weakest part of the system or gets the least attention from system developers. With the trend toward distributed computer systems supporting the CPR, this problem becomes even more critical. It is an issue that must be addressed more comprehensively before CPR systems can be trusted by users. This issue could prove to be the demise of an otherwise excellent CPR system. If users reach the point where they cannot trust the data in the CPR because of insufficient attention to data integrity, then the CPR system will be rendered useless by users.

Today, in the aggregate, CPR systems seem to represent limited measures for ensuring patient confidentiality, measures that are, on the whole, quite inadequate. Most CPR systems do not approach the levels of security or confidentiality that the airlines or the banks have installed to protect even less sensitive information.

Potential Use in Future CPR Systems

Technologic solutions are now emerging that address positive identification of persons requiring access to sensitive databases and systems. Restricting access to authorized individuals only, positively identifying such individuals, limiting the time it takes to verify such individuals, and maintaining confidentiality of patient data are related and conflicting goals for the CPR developer. For example, an inexpensive credit card size personal authentication device (PAD) is being marketed that is unobtrusive yet authenticates the identity of a person seeking access. Those requiring access to the CPR could use the PAD or a similar technology within the hospital or they might use it to authenticate their identity when requesting access from remote locations. Patients might have a similar card and use it in tandem with the care provider's card to assure even more privacy. This is modeled after the financial safe deposit box setting. A variety of mechanisms might be deployed to assure confidentiality, but it is certain that future CPR systems must take strict measures to protect confidentiality.

Text Processing and Query Language

Description of the Technology

To establish a diagnosis, some crucial information used is in textual form—specifically, the patient history and the physical examination. Nearly 20 years ago, researchers experimented with techniques for capturing these data in electronic form. As of today, we have not progressed much beyond those early experiments for capturing and storing electronically these crucial data.

Voice input and natural language understanding have been widely anticipated by both physicians and patients as a solution to this data entry problem. Since this problem is not unique to medicine, many people have been working on the problem of voice recognition. Voice recognition systems can accurately recognize most words spoken by an individual who has trained the system to recognize his or her pronunciation of words from a restricted vocabulary when spoken with a brief pause between each word. More sophisticated voice recognition systems are now emerging, many of which are capable of recognizing speaker-independent speech (i.e., no training of the system with a particular user's voice is necessary) in a limited vocabulary (i.e., 30,000 words). While these more sophisticated systems can recognize short phrases, longer stretches of speech require the speaker to pause between each word. There are enthusiastic reports of physicians who use commercially available technology to recognize and transcribe notes in radiology and emergency rooms. True voice recognition of continuous connected speech (speech without a pause between words) currently requires speech recognition electronics, syntactic and semantic knowledge, and a limited vocabulary or restricted language domain. At least one major vendor is currently pilot testing a voice recognition system for the entry of physicians' orders.

The ability of the computer systems to extract meaning from text or narrative, such as the history portion of the CPR, is called natural language understanding. This is a very complex topic that has only had partial success even though researchers have probed its depths for years. Narrowing the scope to a domain such as medicine is of some help, but medicine is so broad—with hundreds of thousands of terms—that even limiting research to this single domain does not solve the problem. The computer processing of natural language text is an important CPR requirement and is essential for retrieval of keywords or phrases from text or narrative that have been input into the CPR. More difficult than entering and retrieving text is text understanding. Currently, there is at least one commercially available system capable of scanning text such as a discharge summary from a patient record and extracting meaningful words or phrases to produce a list of facts derived from the narrative. These facts may then be further analyzed by the system to produce very accurate diagnosis related groups (DRGs) or additional coded output for billing and other purposes. This kind of capability seems to be significant to abstractors of CPRs and others associated with processing the record. True progress in natural language understanding requires controlled vocabularies, with appropriate synonyms, syntactic and semantic analysis, and domain knowledge. Although progress is being made in these areas, it is unlikely that, even in contextually limited domains, true language understanding will be in widespread use by 1995. Efforts to standardize lexicons, grammars, and processing tools will accelerate achievements in the field and allow sharing of resources among institutions. Systems for syntactic parsing will become more robust and commercially viable, but deep understanding will most likely remain a research topic in the 1995 time frame. The National Library of Medicine's UMLS will likely play a major role in developing knowledge sources that will greatly facilitate natural language understanding in the medical domain.

Standardization of query languages for searching and retrieving data from database systems (independent of medicine) has made gradual and consistent progress in recent years. It appears that the most uniformly agreed upon standard for searching these databases is the standard query language (SQL). There are also standard query languages, such as the common command language (CCL) developed by the National Information Standards Organization (NISO) for searching the multitude of bibliographic databases. Based on the experience of systems that have queried comprehensive clinical databases, ten universities meeting in 1989 to discuss issues related to the sharing of medical knowledge between decision support systems established the Arden syntax, which additionally modifies queries with appropriate time- and context-dependent constraints. CPR systems can now take advantage of such efforts to improve the accessibility to data elements from the CPR with industry standards that have been established or are evolving.

Comparative Strengths and Weaknesses

Text processing, storage, and retrieval technologies are adequate for the CPR. Natural language understanding will be slower in evolution because of its inherently greater complexities and slow developments of—perhaps even resistance to—efforts to encourage vocabulary control in health care. Voice recognition systems will continue to improve over the next decade. For example, a broader number of domains will be covered and difficult features such as speaker-independent, continuous speech will become common, with greater accuracy attained. Even with the advent of excellent voice recognition systems, they will not be used in all instances because of privacy and related issues.

Potential Use in Future CPR Systems

It is likely in the 1990s that text-processing systems for translating the narrative found in discharge summaries and other parts of the CPR will be in use to generate codes needed for billing. As text-processing systems improve in accuracy and performance they may be used to extract significant phrases or attributes from the CPR for matching against the terms and concepts known to the UMLS. The UMLS may then be used to lead the care provider to an array of related information sources such as searching the medical literature and other pertinent knowledge bases. By 1995 such capabilities should be demonstrable and well on their way to commercially viable attachments to CPR systems.

By the mid 1990s some small fraction of the data in the CPR will be captured via voice recognition systems attached to the CPR system. These voice recognition systems will vary in price and performance, but they should be attractive for those settings where a reasonably small controlled vocabulary (5,000 to 10,000 words) is in place and where a limited number of speakers is involved. The voice recognition systems themselves may assist in adding uniformity and consistent vocabularies to the CPR through encouraging the speaker to use clinically relevant yet consistent vocabularies.

CPR System Linkages to Knowledge, Research, and Bibliographic Databases

Description of the Technology

In recent years many clinically relevant databases have evolved that are of significant interest to health care professionals as they attempt to improve the quality of care. It is important to recognize that these collections of secondary data were abstracted from primary data in CPRs in such a way to protect the confidentiality and identity of the individual patients. Primary patient records collect all the data on all the problems for one patient. Clinical resource databases collect all the data for one problem on many patients. A few of the more notable ones include PDQ, Oncocin, and the Duke Cardiology Data Bank.

PDQ is a database provided by the National Cancer Institute (NCI) that contains detailed information about state-of-the-art treatment protocols for cancer patients. PDQ provides timely, highly relevant, and proven treatment advise to physicians treating cancer patients. Bibliographic databases, including MEDLINE, CHEM-LINE, TOXLINE, and others provided by the National Library of Medicine, represent another valuable resource when linked with the CPR. Oncocin is a knowledge base for treatment of cancer patients. Duke University's Cardiology Databank contains detailed information about patients treated for various cardiac problems and has proved to be an important resource to clinicians. Hundreds of other databases are also available or are now evolving; and some of these resources should be linked with the CPR to provide clinical decision support when needed.

Some current CPR systems already offer linkages to knowledge and research databases, although most CPR systems are lacking in this regard, mainly because of the complexity and cost of developing such linkages. Health care professionals are beginning to appreciate the synergy and support that timely access to a diverse array of external information sources could offer in enhancing their delivery of care. A 1989 study at Duke University's Medical Center compared physicians' diagnostic and prognostic outcomes with estimates from a database of the accumulated experience of many physicians over several years. Estimates from the database were more reliable (i.e., more closely corresponded to the true risk) and better able to separate patients as to estimates of clinical outcomes. Such studies indicate the potential impact on the quality of care of CPR systems effectively linked with various external information resources.

Comparative Strengths and Weaknesses

Systems that give access to knowledge and research databases support clinical decision making. Such systems provide the capability of consulting broader knowledge resources established by experts in the domain and thereby enhance user confidence levels and the quality of patient care. Analysis performed using large clinical research databases that contain populations of patients with similar initial symptoms or diagnoses improved formulating treatment plans and assessing probable patient outcomes.

Potential Use in Future CPR Systems

In order to realize the full potential for the CPR in the practice of medicine, it will be necessary to link the data from an individual patient to other sources of information that can provide clinical decision support and recommendations for diagnosis and treatment. The National Library of Medicine's UMLS, when completed, should facilitate many of the linkages envisioned here. Linkages should be in both directions, permitting relevant information contained in the CPR to be extracted for the creation of research databases while protecting patient confidentiality. For these purposes, it will be important to develop linkages that are easy to use in realtime so that feedback to the clinician occurs as part of the decision making process. Appropriate linkages should be available to bibliographic databases, large clinical databases, and decision support expert systems. These linkages will make it possible to provide feedback to physicians. In addition, they can synthesize information to provide decision support that is relevant, easily interpretable, and that can incorporate information directly relevant to a specific patient's problems. Perhaps the closest approximation to such a model, as described above, is the PDQ database from the National Cancer Institute.

It is important to emphasize that it is likely that the more successful future systems will provide access to remote bibliographic databases (e.g., miniMEDLINE, or PaperChase) under the user's control. Most physicians seem to prefer and need more targeted (information that is specific to clinical decision making for a particular patient) and more timely access to information than is typically offered by these remote databases. For example, locally accessible (perhaps via CD-ROM) databases that have been prepared in advance (updated monthly or quarterly) and tailored to the specific decision making needs of physicians are more likely to succeed. Usually only after examining these highly targeted local information resources might the care provider wish to perform more in-depth analysis. Such further analysis then might be performed by accessing the literature or other relevant information sources, which access will undoubtedly require several minutes to complete, a luxury that probably most physicians will find difficult to justify.

It will be essential to establish standard data items for CPR users in order to be able to satisfy requirements for transmitting data items to secondary databases. For policy planners, the secondary collection of relevant (nonconfidential) clinical information on large populations of patients would enable the development of policy strategies and general assessments of quality and outcomes of care. For patients, it could provide relevant information related to decisions that directly impact their own care.

Technologic Recommendations

1. The CPR with its management system (the CPR system) should be the core of the entire health care information system. All other peripheral systems (e.g., laboratory, pharmacy, accounting, etc.) should be integrated with the CPR system so that they enter data into and rely on data retrieved from the CPR.

2. The CPR system should have the capacity to provide a longitudinal, continuing record. As a *lifelong record*, the CPR must be transferable and transportable (including being capable of providing a patient-carried electronic record), so that crucial data concerning the patient is readily available for care regardless of where the patient seeks services within the health care system.

3. Database management systems and database technologies are essential for processing and storage of the CPR. However, the CPR is so complex and its data originate from so many sites that no currently available single database technology can accommodate all of its data. Accordingly, a database management system is essential to integrate data from distributed databases into a single CPR database.

4. Data acquisition and retrieval are the most crucial elements to be addressed in the future CPR systems. CPR systems should require minimal training of health professionals and should be so easy to use and unobtrusive that the total amount of time health care professionals enter and retrieve data is comparable with or less than the time used for paper-based patient records. Flexible data entry and retrieval display tailored to the specific needs of health professionals are crucial for their acceptance. CPR systems must be capable of providing all or selected parts of the patient record in any format needed by its users, such as in a problem-oriented, time-oriented, or specialty-oriented record format. Terminals and workstations will be the primary tools used by health professionals to interact directly with CPR systems. At a minimum, terminals should support text and graphics; workstations should support data selector pointers, barcode readers, flow charting, windowing, graphics, high quality images, and sound, while providing subsecond response times to most queries.

5. The CPR system should be capable of fulfilling all needed functions for all its users, who include physicians, dentists, nurses, psychologists, social workers, technologists, administrators, and others. CPR systems with an open architecture should be available in a compatible series of sizes and costs to meet the requirements for small systems in physicians' offices, medium sized systems in hospitals, and very large systems for multifacility health care programs.

6. A distributed environment with broadband, very high speed communication networks will be required in future CPR systems. The establishment of worldwide communications and connectivity standards established by the communications industry will make it possible to transmit the CPR or selected CPR data subsets across fiber optic and other high speed, high bandwidth networks—even to and from individual physicians' offices—by using, for example, ISDN technology.

7. CPR systems must support practice-linked medical education, online quality assurance, and clinical decision making. CPR systems must support clinical and health services research; they will require a two-way linkage with other relevant secondary databases, including knowledge bases and the scientific literature (e.g., MEDLINE).

8. Nationally accepted standards for CPR content are necessary for transmitting complete or partial patient records and are of prime importance to the realiza-

tion of the CPR. Significant efforts are underway to support standards development for CPR data dictionaries, for uniform coding, vocabulary, and data formatting, but much more needs to be accomplished in this area before the CPR can be shared across institutions or even within institutions.

9. Among the highest priorities in the next decade will be the development of methods to better ensure the privacy and confidentiality of patient data contained in the CPR. Much of the technology to make the CPR more secure exists. These technologies should be better deployed or embedded in CPR systems to assure data protection, security, integrity, validity, and 24-hour availability.

10. Although the health professional user's vision of an ideal CPR may not yet be completely attainable, there are no monumental or breakthrough technologies required to realize in the 1990s a CPR that can adequately satisfy all the expressed current basic requirements of health professional users. Rather, there is a need for more concerted efforts to focus existing and emerging technologies on building more effective CPR systems. Demonstrations of model CPR system and of advances in health care made possible by the CPR should be initiated to accelerate its broad realization.

15
The Computer-based Patient Record System Vendor Survey

Marion J. Ball

Hardware Vendors

Overall response from the hardware developers is limited to general comments about what is or may be available through software developers with whom they are in partnership and to general comments on the desired nature of the CPR. One hardware manufacturer states that the company is working with many partners on the development of computerized patient record systems of various types and offers no details as to the capabilities of these systems. Another offers only a limited system. A third provides information indicating that software developers with whom the company is working have many types of systems with attractive capabilities, but no detail is offered as to whether all of these capabilities are available on a single system.

Software Vendors

Overall response from the software development industry is difficult to assess. The range of responses both to the survey as a whole and to the individual items within the survey indicates a large difference in the operation and definition of the CPR within the software development industry. There is also presumed disagreement as to which items of data should be captured in a CPR. Although most of the responses indicate that it would be desirable to capture data directly into the CPR, there is general pessimism as to whether physicians and nurses can be convinced to do so. However, at least three of the vendors state they are doing so. One of these provides statistical data supporting its statement that its CPR system is already able to support a massive, flexible database in a complex hospital environment, having solved the problems of direct data entry by providers.

The surveys reflect general disagreement as to what is actually the state of the art in medical information software. This disagreement may be seen most clearly in the area of data entry. The majority of the existing CPR systems employ keyboard and barcode technology. Vendors suggest that mouse, light pen, touchscreen, and other point-and-click technology may help in implementing the CPR of the future, most notably by convincing doctors and nurses to enter data themselves. The vendor with the most impressive evidence of large-scale implementation already employs such technologies and has achieved success in convincing physicians and nurses to perform data entry directly during examinations. Other objections to the immediate implementation of a CPR in today's hospital, as opposed to the hospital of the future, include the cost of the system, the general resistance to change within the health care industry, the need for data sharing between many different kinds of systems, and the lack of a good decision support system. Forces that will propel the medical record environment into the computer age are stated more consistently. Most of the vendors speak of the need for increased access to the record at all levels. The CPR is seen as a tool that has the potential to benefit every aspect of the health care environment, if there is a way to implement a realtime record that can be flexibly adapted to changing environments. Even within these positive statements, however, there remains skepticism that the CPR can receive the broad-based, organization-wide support that will be required for the CPR to work in a hospital.

It should be noted that three of the vendors state they have implemented a full-scale electronic medical record in a hospital environment, one in a hospital of unspecified size, one in a hospital of 176 beds, and the third in a large urban teaching hospital of more than 900 beds. These vendors offer statements indicating that physicians and nurses can be convinced to use a CPR and that sufficient data can be collected to make the database meaningful, not as a future ideal but as present reality. One of these vendors presents this CPR in a totally closed environment in which the system, in order to capture the necessary data, must be used in every aspect of operations, including bedside terminals. Another of the vendors offers little detail as to the precise implementation of the described system. A third vendor offers a system that already shares data with nonproprietary systems and that has been implemented in the largest environment described, without the need for a terminal at every bedside. Two of these vendors offer decision support systems; one is described as a powerful report writing system and the other as an actual interactive decision support system, already functioning in an environment where the database has grown to contain millions of patient care documents and hundreds of millions of data items. Taken as a whole, these responses appear to indicate that the environment is right for the implementation of CPRs in hospitals, if enough of the system's beneficiaries can be convinced that such a comprehensive system is worth the trouble of implementation. There is evidence that technologies currently being spoken of as 5 to 10 years distant are in fact already being employed in workable CPR systems. There is also evidence that direct data entry by patient care practitioners is possible, resistance to change notwithstanding, provided the CPR system is user friendly enough, improves quality, and reduces costs for the hospital, clinic, or practice.

Survey Analysis

Part 1 of the Survey

Company products. Of the 12 companies that responded to the survey, including hardware and software vendors, seven responded with descriptions of products that indicate at least a claim that the package is a comprehensive CPR. One vendor responded with a software package limited to use in the obstetric area. One company responded with a system name indicative of a decision support system as well as a patient record system.

Conclusion. A close reading of the vendor survey responses leads one to some skepticism that all of the named systems meet the requirements of a comprehensive system. However, it appears that some of the systems certainly do.

Hardware requirements. With one exception, each of the vendors named a particular manufacturer of hardware on which the described CPR can run. Five different hardware vendors are named. One of the systems is apparently proprietary, since both hardware and software come from the same vendor, which is primarily a hardware vendor. Two other of the responses also come from hardware vendors.

The majority of the systems described run on minicomputers which are networked together to provide processing power which can be expanded as the needs of the hospital change. One of the systems, being UNIX based, is said to be adaptable to at least one product line of almost every hardware vendor. This feature would yield much increased flexibility in hardware selection for the customer. As might be expected, many different types of operating systems are listed as well, with no clear favorite emerging.

Given that the vendor response includes two of the largest vendors of computer hardware in the world, nearly every computer language is mentioned somewhere in the survey responses. Counting only the software vendor responses yields eight different computer languages used to write the different systems discussed in the vendor responses (some vendors offer systems in more than one language).

Responses to the peripherals listing is very general for the most part. Most vendors list terminals and printers as standard peripheral devices, but the majority do not give more detail. We can conclude from responses to the other sections of the survey, however, that most of the software vendors do not support windowing or point-and-click terminals (although one system supports both of these features). One vendor lists optical disks in this response, and one system lists laser printers specifically, although it would be expected that many of the systems would support laser printers.

Conclusion. Although hardware systems from several manufacturers are listed, the majority of systems run in multiprocessor environments, and since this configuration arises in response to the hospital's need for flexible implementation and expansion, it may be expected that this trend will continue. All systems are designed to run on the hardware of a particular vendor, except one system that is adaptable to any hardware that can use UNIX. Systems for the most part are not making use of the most advanced terminal technologies, even though these technologies are no longer new to the marketplace (the one exception to this generalization supports both windowing and point-and-click technologies and is the same vendor that is adaptable to many different types of computer hardwares).

Price of system. Because of to the different pricing structures employed by the vendors, response to the price of the systems is very difficult to assess. Some systems are offered for purchase while others are for lease. Vendors often responded cryptically to this section; two vendors offered no response, and two stated only that system price varied with the level of implementation at a given institution. However, one can conclude from the remaining responses that full implementation of these systems in hospitals, including installation costs, would range from $2 to $6 million per hospital. Another vendor responding to the cost portion of the survey listed maintenance costs in the price of the systems. Because of different methods of pricing and including maintenance, the range of this item is unclear, but the maximum listed price for maintenance is $400,000 per year for software that cost $4 million to license.

Conclusion. System costs, including installation, will likely run in the range of $2 to $6 million per medium size hospital. Maintenance costs for each system could be substantial (in the neighborhood of 10 percent of purchase or lease price per year).

Data entry and output methods. Of the 12 responses, all list data entry by keyboard, seven by barcode reader, five by light pens, three by mouse or other point-and-click devices, two by touchscreen, and none by voice input. Only three vendors support more than two varieties of input. One vendor offers a choice of three types of data input; two vendors offer users a choice of five methods of data entry. One of these vendors is primarily a hardware supplier, and thus it is uncertain that all of these data entry methods are offered under a single software package. The other vendor is a software developer and does support all of these types of data entry in its CPR package. Three of the systems described accept only keyboard input. One of these systems offers other statements that indicate it should be among the most comprehensive of the listed systems, but given the extreme importance placed on ease of data entry by virtually all responses, this limited data entry capability is extremely surprising for a truly comprehensive system.

Specialized output devices are also in the minority. Four of the systems offer high and low graphical output, and one additional vendor states that graphic output is currently in development. Five vendors support color output. Four systems offer special printer support. Four systems offer voice output. One system supports terminal windowing.

Conclusion. With the exception of a single software vendor, the industry is moving very slowly in solving the problem that is described as crucial to the future of the CPR: ease of data entry. Although devices like the mouse and the light pen are commonly used in other industrial and even in home computing, they are rarely employed in the realm of health care computing. This is notable because the only

Table 1. Automation of patient record components:
vendor response to checklist.

Orders	9 (plus 1 in development)
Laboratory results	8 (plus 1 in development)
Radiology results	9
Diagnosis	8
Nursing notes	10
Nursing care plans	10
Departmental care notes	8
Other departmental results	7 (plus 1 in development)
History and physicals	8
Operative notes	7
Patient acuity	8
Vital signs	8
Discharge summary	8

vendor to offer evidence of successfully convincing doctors and nurses to use the system is also the vendor who has exploited these technologies most fully. The same conclusion may be drawn with regard to flexible output devices. The vendor offering the most flexible data entry methods is the same vendor supporting the most varied output, including terminal windowing, and the most flexible hardware requirements.

Automated components. Eleven vendors responded to the section of the survey asking which components of the patient record have been successfully automated by the vendor's products. Table 1 summarizes the vendors' responses to the checklist items.

Five of the vendors have automated all of the listed components of the patient record. One has automated 12 of 13. One has automated ten of the 13 with the additional three components in development. Three of the remaining vendors have automated half of the record components. One has automated only four of the 13 elements for a system which relates only to obstetric patients. In addition, eight of the 11 responses list additional components of the record which have been computerized. Numbers of additional components range from 1 to 16.

Conclusion. Many of these systems do not actually constitute comprehensive CPRs because too few of the necessary patient record components have been automated.

New technology expected. Ten of 12 vendors responded to this section of the survey. Table 2 provides a rough summary of the responses, grouped into categories that appear to be similar.

In addition, there are other listings related to anticipated improvements in software itself, including the addition of decision support and flexible database management systems.

The responses to this section are skewed by the fact that one vendor already employs many of these technologies, including X-windows and point-and-click

Table 2. New technology expected within the next two to five years.

Area of improvement expected in next 2–5 years	Number of vendors anticipating
Methods of data entry:	6
Touchscreens, voice recognition, point and click devices	
Electronic storage	6
Hardware and operating systems	6
Output: Graphics, windowing	3
Networking capabilities	1

devices for data entry, and already offers networking capability, flexible database management and decision support.

Conclusion. These responses are informative about vendor attitudes toward what is state of the art, but may not be helpful in defining what is actual state of the art in CPR systems. It is surprising that, with software vendors providing the response, the emphasis should be skewed so heavily toward hardware improvements as the driving force behind improving the CPR.

Part 2 of the Survey

Few of the vendors completed all of Part 2 of the survey. Since these responses are free text and reflect the thinking of the vendors on many issues, one cannot analyze them stringently. What follows is a listing of the questions asked and summaries of the general responses.

If you believe the development direction planned for this system will allow users to automate more of their medical records, please explain why. Nine vendors responded to this question. Two of the vendors, having already developed comprehensive CPRs, stated that their systems already enable the creation of a complete online medical record. One of these vendors offered impressive database statistics from its development site in support of those statements.

The remaining vendors expressed optimism that additional components of the record can be automated if data entry methods can be improved, if price barriers are removed, and if resistance to change within the health care environment can be overcome. These issues are discussed more fully elsewhere in this report.

How do you perceive the potential of the computer-based patient record technology of 1995 to alter and improve the practice of medicine in the inpatient and ambulatory settings? Six vendors responded to this question. Two actually responded as requested, describing the changes in the inpatient and the ambulatory settings in separate responses.

The predominant theme of the response is that increased access to information will be of immense benefit to the provision of medical care in both these settings. One response stated that the availability of medical information wherever it is needed in the inpatient setting, with response time in seconds, should result in saved lives.

How do you perceive the computer-based patient record, as compared with the traditional paper-based record, improving productivity? Four vendors responded to this question. One vendor responded simply, "Improved productivity is possible in all areas." Others responded that ready access to information will improve productivity by freeing up more physician and nurse time for direct patient care.

Only two vendors actually addressed the various categories of health care personnel listed, and each addressed particular areas in which a CPR would be of increased benefit to these professions.

In your judgment, what could the market afford for a computer-based patient record system and what are the costs? Four vendors responded. One stated simply that what the market could afford depends on the benefits of the system. One vendor stated that the CPR may well enhance the revenue-collecting potential of the hospital through efficiencies in charge capture and submittal, and offered impressive numbers from its test site in support of this position.

In general, the industry showed an extreme reluctance to tackle this question.

From your perspective, what is the best that can be offered for clinical data entry and display in various settings? Five vendors responded. One wrote, "Today: bedside terminal, personal computer with graphics and mouse input. 1995: voice, graphics workstation." Another vendor stated that its system is the best that can be offered today and in 1995. This response is neither helpful nor realistic.

In general, the responses in this category reflect the uncertainty as to what is state of the art within the industry. Many of the vendors speak of improved data entry devices like the mouse, light pen, touchscreen, X-windows, and the like as if they were new technologies that must be integrated into existing systems. Two vendors are already making use of these technologies, one in a comprehensive CPR.

Please describe any technological and behavioral obstacles or barrier to widespread use of a CPR. How could we work together to overcome such barriers? Six vendors responded. Responses emphasized that, in order to implement the CPR, a demonstrable, comprehensive system must become well known. This is the necessary prerequisite to convincing the medical care profession to alter its behavior to the degree necessary for successful usage of a CPR. Included are references to improved data entry capability that have been discussed throughout this report.

How do you ensure confidentiality of the patient record now? What additional measure for confidentiality do you envision will be necessary in the future? Six vendors responded. This question elicited the most concrete response from the vendors in Part 2 of the survey.

Security measures have been considered, with vendors employing sign-on codes, passwords, dialback features, electronic cards, or some combination of the above. Looked for features include voice recognition and other computer recognition of physical features, such as retinal prints or thumbprints.

Four of the vendors have considered how to limit access within the system to discreet classes of users, and all these vendors have developed systems with the capability of allowing low level users access only to specific portions of the record system.

One response stated pessimism: "Many sites demand thorough, complex security matrices, but do not utilize them because they are maintenance nightmares." However, three vendors are using such matrices with success in actual hospital environments.

Conclusion. While no clear cut conclusions can be drawn from such sketchy and wide-ranging response to Part 2 of the survey, it is interesting to note which questions were answered and the attitudes revealed by the answers. In general, the vendors have resisted the questions that demand an imaginative response to the idea of the electronic patient record. It is perhaps that software vendors developing systems to computerize the patient record are unable to articulate any meaningful response as to what impact this system will have on the industry the system is intended to serve.

The overall response would be, in fact, somewhat discouraging, were it not for the presence of one software vendor recognizing the need for easy, friendly methods of data entry and for overall system flexibility within the hospital environment. Only one vendor has included many features in a system that are specifically designed to win hospital-wide support for its use. It already includes the majority items cited by multiple members of the Users and Usages Committee as being necessary or highly desirable. The system proves that the basic goal of the Institute of Medicine (IOM) project, a total electronic patient record created by direct provider data entry with interactive decision support, is obtainable with current technology. Only the one software vendor supports all of the following technologies: point-and-click data entry (including mouse, touchscreen, light pen, and trackball); windowing terminals (Windows); software that will function on hardware from many different vendors; interactive decision support; complete complex medical document automation; complex security criteria to the data item level; permanent online storage of all relevant patient data for clinical practice; and customization of screens, menus, output documents, and reports by the purchaser's own staff. The system is lacking in that there is no artificial intelligence time (which the Users and Uses Committee has indicated is desirable but not necessary). But this vendor has achieved concrete success in convincing physicians and nurses to enter data directly into the system, as evidenced by the fact that this system's database at its test site contains patient encounter documents from the inpatient and outpatient settings, all entered directly into the system by physician and nurse users. This vendor is proof that the general level of pessimism concerning the implementability of the CPR as demonstrated in these surveys is misplaced and that the basic goal of the IOM project is obtainable with current technology.

Section 3
The Future of the Computer-based Patient Record (CPR)

1
Future Vision and Dissemination of Computer-based Patient Records

Edward H. Shortliffe, Paul C. Tang,
Margret K. Amatayakul, Eric Cottington, Stephen F. Jencks,
Albert Martin, Robin MacDonald, Thomas Q. Morris, and
Jeremy J. Nobel

The IOM committee proposed creation of a computer-based patient record institute (CPRI) to serve as the leadership entity for establishing a national agenda to develop and adopt computer-based patient records (CPRs). An effort to motivate organizations, strategic individuals, and the public to participate in this collaborative effort requires a national, shared vision. The vision must be viewed as globally important for health care delivery nationally, as well as be of strategic importance to each participating organization in health care. The vision must portray a clear and recognizable improvement over the status quo that is well worth the costs of achieving it. It must be technically feasible and politically credible. Among other functions, computer-based patient record systems must fulfill the following:

- Provide clinicians with a readily accessible, intelligible assembly of clinical data that characterizes the condition, prior management, and current treatment plan of a patient
- Provide a clearly defined and well-organized database to permit epidemiologic assessment of patient outcomes and patterns of practice, revealing merits of management strategies in specific clinical contexts
- Provide interactive decision support tools based on information derived from critically analyzed population data
- Decrease administrative record keeping and form submission responsibilities that burden health care providers

This chapter outlines a vision, plus proposed dissemination strategies, for several important participants whose support will be crucial to the success of the CPRI. Compelling arguments and scenarios are presented that may be used to educate key decision makers (in health care, business, organized labor, and hospital administration) that computer-based patient records and information systems have become an essential technology in the management of health care quality and its costs.

The Perspective of the Physician

Vision. We envision the day when the physician's computer workstation is an integral part of the normal practice environment. Although paper records may not completely disappear, their use will become secondary to the primary electronic record to which physicians will routinely turn for current clinical data on their patients, communication with colleagues, access to the medical literature and other knowledge resources, and management of practice logistics including submission of claims to third party payers. Such workstations will adopt intuitive, graphically oriented interfaces that will allow physicians to use computer resources without obtaining extensive training or relying on constant reference to manuals. Furthermore, technologic progress in workstation development and networking will provide such environments at per physician prices that are affordable while being powerful enough to support diverse functionality. In time, the workstations will also become so compact and portable that they will be suitable for carrying under the arm like a clipboard while the physician is on rounds in the hospital or moving between examining rooms in an outpatient practice. It is likely that limited speech input to such workstations will also be available within a decade, allowing the physician to guide much of the computer interaction by voice while using pointing devices such as lightpens or trackballs for the remainder of their interactions with the machine. Integrated workstations of this type will result in legible, centralized patient records, suitable for sharing among providers, with greatly enhanced documentation of encounters and procedures, streamlined and cost-effective interactions with the health care financing system, and automatic accumulation of standardized datasets that protect patient confidentiality while supporting clinical research.

Scenario. Shortliffe and Blois (1990) present one view of the kind of integrated physician's workstation that we envision. The HyperCard (Macintosh) demonstration that was used to produce the figures in their book can also be made available for purposes of educating physicians about the concepts described here. Although the scenario document and demonstration diskette emphasize the physician's perspective in the use of such systems, the demonstration also includes materials pertinent to other health care providers such as nursing staff. Not emphasized in the scenario are the links to secondary users of the record, including the third party payers. That perspective is addressed in other sections.

Message. Past computer systems for physicians have generally focussed on single purpose, vertical applications that have had limited utility in the routine practice environment. Poor integration and clumsy interfaces have resulted in a steep learning curve and low frequency of use which have in turn made many physicians doubt that computers will ever play a role in their own practices. It is imperative that these impressions be changed through an effective educational program that identifies the reasons for problems in the past and the way in which the model we are proposing is sensitive to them and will correct them. Thus, the following key messages need to be conveyed in any educational activity for physicians on this subject:

- Extensive training of users in computer topics is not necessary if a system is well designed and intuitive. (Physicians never took a course in use of the telephone or an ATM!)
- Attention to the development of a communications infrastructure into which clinical computer systems can be introduced will help ensure the availability of workstations with such diverse functionality that the physician will find the machine useful (if not necessary) not only every day but with every patient encounter. Such an infrastructure requires planning at all levels: in the office, in the hospital, and by regional and national health planners.
- Many of the tasks and problems which physicians today find most noxious can be eliminated by well designed, easy to use, and affordable systems:
  - The problem of missing or illegible patient charts
  - Constrained, inefficient access to a patient's most recent laboratory and radiologic results
  - An overwhelming set of paper forms requiring manual interaction for everything from claims submission to adverse drug reaction reporting
  - Time consuming, inconvenient processes required in order to obtain current information on specific medical problems and their management
  - Telephone tag and the general inefficiency of communication with colleagues and with the various health agencies
- Patient data stored in computers can be effectively safeguarded with regard to both security and confidentiality.
- Computational tools need be neither a threat to the physician's autonomy nor a negative influence on the physician/patient relationship. The computer can increase the effectiveness of physicians while improving their efficiency, thus enabling them to spend more time building rapport with and educating patients.

Dissemination strategy. Traditional means for introducing physicians to new developments and attracting their interest are journal publications and presentations. There is, however, incredible competition for physicians' attention, and a strategy must be developed to assure that publications and other educational efforts attract and sustain the attention of clinicians. Several strategic points are worth emphasizing:

- We must avoid giving the impression that our recommendations are coming from futurists or from academicians who are out of touch with the reality of the current practice world. The Institute of Medicine (IOM) name will be an important asset in this regard, but we also need to be sure that the involvement of practitioners and the other groups represented on our committees is emphasized.
- Among the scientific journals, the *Journal of the American Medical Association (JAMA)* and the *New England Journal of Medicine (NEJM)* have the largest

circulations in this country, but publications in them need to be formal and peer reviewed. They must also be carefully designed if we want to ensure that readers are drawn to them when they are skimming the issue in which they appear. Nevertheless, a concise report of the committee in one of those journals (probably *JAMA*) would have a large readership and would simultaneously attract the attention of the press (which could, in turn, further disseminate the messages that we wish to convey).

- Presentations at both local and national clinical meetings will be important adjuncts to any journal publications. Although it would be ideal if every institution in the country held a grand rounds session on the subject of the committee's report, it is unrealistic to ask any single set of individuals to take an educational program on the road. It would thus seem most reasonable to emphasize national meetings (e.g., annual meetings of the AMA and the American College of Physicians) while considering the development of videotapes or packaged presentations that could be used locally around the country. However, wide distribution of presentations will be appropriate only if they are designed to convey our message in a way that is sensitive to the preexisting concerns of physicians regarding computers and the roles they could come to play in the physician's already complicated life.

- A partnership with the Association of American Medical Colleges (AAMC), which has a strong and growing interest in medical informatics topics, would help provide entree into educational programs at the nation's medical schools. This could help us reach not only academic physicians but students, house staff, and the physicians who take the continuing education courses offered by the schools.

- Hospitals are important sources of physician education. They, therefore, can serve as advocates for the notions that we are developing. To the extent that we are successful in working with hospital administrators, medical staff leaders, and the American Hospital Association, dissemination to staff physicians will be enhanced.

- Brief summaries of the committee's recommendations in the "throw-away" journals that all physicians receive are another way of attracting the attention of those physicians who are less likely to read a formal article on the subject in a scientific journal such as *JAMA* or *NEJM*. The use of eye catching pictorials will be important adjuncts.

- Finally, the IOM might consider display booths and materials for distribution at the trade shows associated with the major national medical meetings.

The Perspective of Nurses

Nurses spend an estimated 30 percent of their time documenting direct care given. The current patient record is fragmented and resides in multiple forms in multiple locations—at the patient's bedside, in various imaging departments, on a hospital computer system, on departmental computer systems, in a chart or notebook at a central nursing station, or in the medical records department. Pieces of data may be entered into the patient record several times by several different people in different forms (e.g., text, image, graphics). This redundant data entry has the potential to result in erroneous entries, misdiagnosis, or mistreatment.

Vision. The CPR offers more than just an electronic version of the record as it exists today. For nurses, the CPR offers a comprehensive view of patient data, a vehicle for collecting data once only, and the ability to look at that same data in many different ways. Other features of the system used by nurses would include decision support and knowledge based aids, (legible) communication links with other care givers and health care facilities, and tools to facilitate peer review and quality assurance. Information systems could also be used in individual patient teaching. Documenting care through a CPR would allow administrators to track and charge for actual nursing time and care given.

In all patient care settings, nurses require access to a wide range of patient data. A well-integrated and comprehensive electronic database would ensure timely, high quality care by nurses.

Scenario. The following scenario outlines some of the ways a computer-based patient record could facilitate nursing care during a hospital admission.

A patient is seen at an emergency room, complaining of abdominal pain of unknown origin and duration. The triage nurse accepts his health identification/access card. Upon accessing the patient database, the nurse determines that the patient lives nearby and has records in the hospital's clinic. He has been treated in the past for both gastric ulcers and gallbladder disease. The patient is examined by a physician and admitted for further workup and possible surgery. The clinicians update the patient's record in the system with his latest complaints, diagnostic findings, and admission.

The patient is admitted to a surgical unit, where his assigned nurse accesses the emergency room data, the patient's lifetime health summary, and the physician's admitting orders. Upon completing an admission patient assessment, the nurse formulates a nursing plan of care and nursing orders, based upon the data entered and that facility's standards of care. Decision support aids might be used to search the literature or compare the patient's profile to other patients in the database.

Also at this time, the nurse looks at the laboratory results and data gathered while the patient was awaiting admission (e.g., vital signs, physical assessment). These can be viewed in numeric, text, or graphic form, either alone or in combination with other data.

After the patient undergoes surgery, he returns to the surgical unit, where again the system communicates his care orders and treatment plan based upon the procedure he underwent and the surgeon performing it. During the patient's recovery period, he is closely monitored, and some data are automatically captured at the bedside. Data are entered at the time and place of occurrence, keeping the record current. Nursing and other clinician progress notes may be entered using free text, canned text, and/or some combination.

Upon discharge, the nurse and other health care team members generate discharge plans, specific patient instructions, and a discharge summary. Discharge orders are linked with the pharmacy for prescriptions, as well as physicians' offices and clinics for follow-up appointment scheduling.

As the scenario illustrates, CPRs provide many advantages for nursing. To sum up, CPRs do the following:

- Improve nursing care
- Provide access to a comprehensive, lifetime patient health record, in both full and summary form
- Reduce redundant data entry
- Increase legibility of the record
- Increase access to the record through:
  - Availability to multiple users at once
  - Rapid location of old and current records
  - 24-hour per day, 7-day per week online data
  - Location of terminals and workstations throughout a facility
- Provide decision support and access to knowledge and patient databases to study effects of nursing care
- Increase communications among departments, services, and care givers
- Allow linkage of nursing services with their costs
- Increase quality and uniformity of documentation through the use of standards
- Improve risk management practices of nurses, leading to fewer malpractice actions and improved peer review

Dissemination strategy. Information for nurses can be disseminated in a number of ways. One of the most effective methods is through seminars and presentations to small groups. Nurses tend to have a limited amount of time and funding to spend on continuing education. However, most are extremely interested in new, innovative technologies which aid delivery of patient care. Therefore, hands-on demonstrations of a prototype of the CPR will have the greatest impact. Nurses who have seen the benefits of such a system will not only be its greatest advocates, but they will rapidly spread the word.

Traditional educational means also can be of some use, e.g., demonstrations at national/regional meetings (ANA, AACN, NLN, AONE, etc.). Continuing education courses would provide a good opportunity for educating nurses about CPRs. The primary journals might include *American Journal of Nursing, Computers in Nursing, Nursing '90, American Association of Clinical Nursing, The New England Journal of Medicine, Hospitals,* and *Modern Health care.* Exposing nursing students at universities to CPRs may prove fruitful as well. Targeting nurse administrators as well as staff nurses will ensure support from all levels of nursing.

The Perspective of the Health Care Financing Administration

The Health Care Financing Administration (HCFA) is an important participant in anything having to do with health care delivery—witness the dramatic consequences stimulated by the October 1983 diagnostic related group (DRG) legislation. Fortunately, HCFA stands to be an important beneficiary of this project.

Scenario. HCFA could derive important benefits from:

1. Computer-based *hospital* patient records that link together all information available within the hospital could
   - Allow offsite review of almost all patient care problems
   - Accelerate review of cases by professional review organizations (PROs) while decreasing inconvenience to the hospital through a decreased rate of requests for clarification and documentation
   - Improve data for studies of effectiveness and appropriateness of care, leading to faster coverage decisions

2. Computer-based *comprehensive* patient records that link information from many places where data about the patient is stored (e.g., physician's office, insurance claims, pharmacy, outpatient physician's record, hospital record) could provide additional benefits:
   - Online authorization of services requiring authorization and expert system linkage of authorization process
   - Online generation and submission of bills with online resolution of many of the questions that currently require carrier inquiries before payment
   - Online access to previous utilization for providers, permitting them access to important medical history at minimal effort
   - Linkage of ordering, billing, and reporting for out-of-office procedures paid by Medicare
   - Realtime monitoring of care with concurrent feedback or requests for additional information and online decision support (e.g., interactions, needed tests, known data on impact of proposed therapeutic actions), moving away from the current inconsistent and highly abrasive patterns of retrospective review

The Perspective of Payers

The following discussion assumes a set of functions that places the patient record in the context of a broader system. This includes the billing and claims processing function, tools for communicating with other physicians, laboratories, pharmacies, and insurance companies for reporting and authorization of expenditures.

Vision. The payer should view the system that we are describing as an information system that facilitates a meaningful partnership between providers of care and payer through communication and shared data. Currently, providers and payers lack the information needed to understand how medical care resources are being used. The system described would allow payers more direct communication with their providers, tools for improving quality, and improved ability to manage use of resources.

Scenario. An insurance company develops an health maintenance organization (HMO) network of 500 physicians. When they join the HMO, physicians are given terminals or workstations for their office supplied by the insurance company which connects them to a central system providing several services. The physicians pay a monthly service fee for these services which eliminate much of the manual paperwork in their offices. These services greatly simplify the physician's interaction with the insurance company, providing a visible benefit to accepting patients with this type of insurance.

The system is operated by a third party separate from the insurer, a company responsible for providing these services and protecting the confidentiality of individual patient data. Individual patient data will be available only to the patient's physician and other care providers who are authorized to view it. The insurer facilitates participation in the physician network by providing expedited services to physicians who are willing to use it. Services like online patient records might be provided for any of the physician's patients, regardless of insurance coverage.

When the patient comes to the physician's office, data concerning the patient's covered benefits are immediately available online. Services requiring prior approval can be checked by sending an electronic message to the insurance company for information or prior approval. Paper insurance claim forms for this insurer would be eliminated, because billing information would be entered online and transmitted to the insurer for prompt processing and payment.

Online access to patient information allows the physician to not only access his or her data on a patient, but also retrieve other data recorded or ordered by other physicians in the network who care for that patient, avoiding duplication of effort or test ordering. A computer-based record could be semistructured to improve the completeness of patient data recorded for further aggregate analysis.

Access to other information resources like MEDLINE or consensus practice guidelines would also be provided. Guidelines would be developed by physician panels as knowledge aids or reminders for treating certain problems, and these could be made easily available on the system.

Ordering tests and issuing prescriptions could be accomplished through the system, which would be connected to a network of pharmacies and qualified testing sites approved by the insurer and known to provide good quality services. The system would also have the capability of searching the database to be sure the order is not duplicative and could check for drug allergies or drug interactions. Preventing adverse outcomes to treatment ultimately saves money for the insurer and clearly prevents morbidity for the patient. Results of the test would be reported electronically to the physician's office when complete, reducing costs associated with tracking data from multiple sources.

Consultations with other physicians on the network would be managed in a similar fashion. Referrals could be documented and, if necessary, authorized in advance. Insurers would then be able to analyze the patterns and reasons for consultation. Preferred provider lists could be drawn up based on analysis of this information.

The medical directors of the provider network could use aggregate data to analyze patterns of care for the group of physicians and later use this information to develop educational programs to improve the quality of care and cost effective use of resources. They would not be able to look at individual physician or patient information. Managers of this insurance company are enlightened and realize that using this data for punitive purposes is likely to be counterproductive, so they see the information as a constructive tool for helping physicians to improve their practice.

Message. Health care payers, particularly insurers, no longer want to passively reimburse for services as they traditionally have done. Payers are increasingly aware of the need to control costs and to understand the outcomes of care for which they are paying. They recognize they cannot do this without the help of providers. Prior attempts to control costs through regulation of payment and manipulation of benefits have been largely unsuccessful. Regulations and payment schemes have produced countermoves by providers that simply shift payment to another care sector or modality. For example, implementation of hospital DRGs led to a remarkable shift to ambulatory care and to procedures not regulated by DRGs.

Payers are interested in forging cooperative relationships with network providers in order to

- Encourage more cost-effective practices
- Reduce the administrative inefficiency of the current payment procedures
- Better monitor practice patterns and implement programs to improve quality
- Better understand the reasons for health care expenditures through more effective analysis of practice patterns

The following functions would have a valuable positive impact on payers:

- *Automated billing and claims processing.* Providers and payers suffer with the mounting costs and difficulties of processing payment for services. By tying benefits information held by the insurers to claims processing activities of the physician, claims could be processed without large numbers of clerical staff moving information back and forth. There is an opportunity to eliminate a large number of personnel in each setting, to improve cash flow to the physician and to eliminate a large amount of redundant activity related to inquiries and resubmissions.
- *Development of referral networks.* Shared information systems could greatly facilitate the development of networks of preferred consultants tied to a group of primary care providers. A shared record system would allow referring and consulting practitioners to share information about the patient, both improving quality and reducing repetition of tests and procedures. It would provide more

timely feedback to the referring physician and allow better monitoring of the referral process by encouraging the use of preferred providers, collecting data about the reasons for consultation, and documenting the pattern of use of expensive resources.

- *Decision support.* There is increasing interest in the development of guidelines for care that begin to set the parameters of good care. Written guidelines are too cumbersome and inconvenient to encourage regular usage. If a practitioner were already operating in a computer-based environment, it would be much easier for him to select and access focused information at the time it is needed.
- *Patient records.* The patient record itself serves many purposes for the provider of care that ultimately benefits the payer. First, a CPR provides an opportunity for some structuring of the collection of information so that specific elements can be captured for later analysis. By providing ready access to information about the patient and by ensuring that it is not lost, the record reduces redundant collection of information by the same and other providers, thereby reducing costs. Good records and improved documentation of the care process are known to reduce the chance of malpractice suits. Aggregate data and anonymous individual records, with suitable protection of confidentiality, are indispensable for analyzing patterns of care and the ways in which resources are being used, as well as providing information for better cost planning and underwriting decisions.
- *Quality of care measurement.* Patient records provide the only means of being able to audit and track the care process and the patterns of care for specific diseases. Recently, measures of the outcomes of care using analyses of patient functional status have received national attention. Collection of this type of information in an analyzable form is virtually impossible without a computer-based record.

Dissemination strategy. Payers of care are concerned with purchasing good services at the most reasonable price possible. To the extent that automated systems promote efficiency and provide tools for improving quality, payers are likely to be interested in them.

Education will have to be directed at the highest levels of corporate or government payers. This can probably only be done through direct presentation, since there are not publications that are likely to get information effectively disseminated at that level. Arranging conferences for large corporations or insurance companies concerned with health care costs is probably the most effective starting point. Presentations would have to include both conceptual models of how the system would work, as well as information supporting how systems of this kind could reduce costs. A video showing a patient walking through the various facets of care could effectively reinforce the message.

Because a relatively small number of insurance companies control a large portion of the health care market, the audience from the insurance side is relatively focused. Similarly, there are only a small number of government agencies that control a large portion of government-supported health care.

The Perspective of Hospital Chief Executive Officers

Vision. Chief executive officers (CEOs) of hospitals and other provider institutions have experienced and continue to address major changes in the health care delivery system. Cost control, competition, increasing regulation, measures of quality, and operating efficiency are paramount in their minds. Only by addressing all of these issues successfully can they maintain the financial viability of their institutions. Readily available accurate information concerning these issues is the most pressing need for all these executives. Questions previously considered appropriate only to the investigator are now routine if administrators guide their institutions effectively. A CPR the potential to provide efficient access to the clinical data necessary to address these issues.

Scenario. All chief executive officers are committed to and have the responsibility for providing the highest quality of care in the most efficient manner available. Consequently, any financially viable change or series of changes designed to provide more readily available, accurate data concerning patient care and resource consumption would be received enthusiastically. The advent of the prospective payment system has highlighted the need for patient- and physician-specific information so that the outcomes of care can be realistically analyzed. Further reimbursement constraints give no indication of diminishing, so the basis for clinical decision making is an area that will continue to be examined. Maximum cooperation between physicians and administrators will be essential to address this delicate interface effectively. The CPR project can be identified as a significant, if not essential, adjunct for exploring the intricacies of clinical decision making and resource consumption.

Among others, institutional administrators have the responsibility to

- Meet requirements of voluntary accreditation standards set by the Joint Commission on Accreditation of Health care Organizations (JCAHO)
- Conform to government regulations, both federal and state
- Compile physician experience
- Organize a risk management program to reduce the liabilities of the institution
- Create an internal organization that constructively engages all types and levels of staff in achieving organizational objectives
- Assure the presence of the human, information, and technologic infrastructures necessary for an organization to be successful

All of these functions can clearly be performed more effectively and efficiently with access to computer-based information.

Message. Institutional administrators are well acquainted with the benefits and burdens of information systems. Most institutions and large physician groups have for many years been required to gather and store financial data electronically. This experience has clearly demonstrated the efficacy of handling large amounts of complicated information expeditiously. In many settings, financial data is also accompanied by significant demographic and diagnostic data. Consequently, institutional administrators are familiar with not only the challenges and positive aspects of developing such systems but also the cost.

Efforts to develop financial systems were largely mandated by the government or other third party payers. Growth of other computer-based information systems, however, have been made possible by philanthropy, grants, or allocation of institutional resources. The growth of laboratory information systems and pathology and radiology reporting are clearly the outcome of choices made by institutional administrators in concert with their medical staffs. In the process they have helped to guide behavioral change, particularly among the physicians and nurses. Institutional executives should be recognized for their past accomplishments and called upon to help assure the success of developing a computer-based patient record.

In order to motivate and mobilize CEOs, the plan for development of the computer-based record must be realistic. Of first importance is the availability of adequate funding to support the endeavor. With shrinking hospital margins throughout the country, there is no doubt that special funding mechanisms must be identified to make the investment possible. Savings in both clinical and administrative functions may be envisioned for the future, but immediate resources must be identified for the period of implementation. The national scope of the effort presupposes support at the federal level. Second, recognition of the need to phase the project over a sufficient period of time must be clearly apparent. Finally, issues of standards and confidentiality must be clearly addressed so that institutions will not have to redirect their energies once the effort is underway.

Dissemination strategy. The most effective approach to other CEOs is through a peer who has lived through the experience, although this may not be entirely possible. Significant efforts by some CEOs to develop a computer-based patient record are underway; their experiences should be shared. The challenges and hurdles involved should be made very clear.

Reaching CEOs can frequently be accomplished through state and regional hospital associations. Broader though less focused presentations will also be productive through such avenues as journals (e.g., *Modern Health care*, *HFMA Trustee*, *Hospitals*), national organizations (e.g., American Hospital Association, American Management Association, Group Health Association of America), videotapes, and regulatory agencies. There is no doubt, however, that a whole new avenue for institutional consulting will emerge as the endeavor progresses.

If the CPR project is realistic, it will certainly rivet the attention of CEOs. Consequently, the following strategic considerations should be kept in mind:

- *Articles.* Introductory presentations should be no longer than one page if possible. Flow charts are useful as are titles with before and after problems and benefits orientation. Articles written by peers and respected individuals in the health care industry, physicians, and corporate health care administrators should be sought.
- *Videos.* Presentations should be no longer than 5 minutes as an introduction, 15

minutes as a detailed description of ideas and benefits to be realized. A lead-in after the 5 minute introduction will certainly keep the viewer interested.

- *Meetings.* Peer group meetings and seminars are the best network method for people and ideas. Suggested meetings include but are not limited to: HFMA meetings, health executive conferences, vendor/user group meetings, American Hospital Association meetings, and state and regional hospital associations. Activities at these meetings could be presented in several ways, including

  - CEO presentation to other CEOs in a formal auditorium setting
  - Slide presentation in a group discussion format
  - IOM booth with audiovisual materials running, descriptive literature available, and reprints available upon request
  - Vendor exhibits

The Perspectives of Business and Labor

This section describes the potential value of CPRs for decision makers within the business and organized labor communities. In the last few years, the major health care concerns of these groups have turned towards the impact of skyrocketing costs on company profitability. On the business side, this relates to the ability of a company to operate or expand, particularly in markets where foreign competitors are less heavily burdened with the cost of providing health care to their employees. On the labor side, there is concern for jobs and compensation, both of which are tied to corporate profitability.

The following paragraphs specifically describe the current crisis in health care as it is perceived by the business and organized labor communities. Beginning with a general overview, we discuss the emerging focus on quality and, in particular, the concept of continuous quality improvement. The potential role of guidelines and protocols in influencing care delivery is summarized, and change of physician behavior is targeted as a policy goal. Use of information systems to directly reduce the overhead-related costs of care delivery by improving hospital operating efficiency and enabling effective medical malpractice risk management is discussed. The final section is a brief overview on message development, and how best to communicate these points to thoughtful leaders in business and organized labor.

Although cost worries may be of paramount importance, concern for quality is linked directly. Savvy leaders in the private sectors are quite aware that their future success depends on a healthy and productive work force. Stripping away access to quality care in no way serves their interests. On the labor side, pressure to maintain access to what is perceived to be quality care is growing from both currently employed and retired union members. Current systems for delivering and financing care were not designed with mechanisms for measuring the effectiveness of that care, or for facilitating improvements in the delivery of care. Instead, what is prevalent in the United States today are various rules for defining access, linked to a complex series of reimbursement mechanisms including fee for service, health maintenance organizations (HMOs), preferred provider organizations (PPOs), Medicare, Medicaid, and veterans' health care. The attractiveness of a CPR to business and labor rests in the opportunity it presents to begin a process of measurement, assessment, and systemic design, thereby opening the door to health care delivery with documentable effectiveness, administrative efficiencies, and continuous improvability.

Scenario. Any scenario that would be compelling to business and labor leaders must focus on those features of a CPR that will provide an ability to improve the quality of the health care delivered and simultaneously allow for a rigorous process of assessing cost and value. It is also important to stress the administrative benefits inherent in automation, as it has been documented that these clerical and administrative costs are the most rapidly rising fraction of those related to health care delivery and at least twice and possibly ten times those experienced by several other countries, including Canada and the United Kingdom. Work by Eli Finsberg and others suggests that these costs may represent as much as 20 percent of the total health care bill and, as such, represent a reasonable target for intervention.

In constructing the scenario for the IOM subcommittee, it was not deemed necessary to focus exhaustively on the clinical details, because those particulars are not key concerns. Rather, we must focus on the transaction benefits of automation that include improved record keeping, high quality editing and auditing, retrospective reviewability, opportunity for provider feedback and behavior change, and dramatically reduced costs from administrative efficiencies. We should anticipate concern about confidentiality by noting that computer-based systems provide even greater safeguards in this respect than conventional paper charts. The communication challenge will be to show the business and labor communities that these features provide a platform for addressing their key concerns relating to cost and quality without introducing new and unresolvable problems.

Business and labor leaders, stunned by rising costs and concerns as to what these dollars are actually purchasing in the health care markets, are asking themselves the following questions:

- Why is it that the rate of certain surgeries are dramatically different in, say, New Haven as compared to Boston?
- Why is it that variation in rates seem to correlate well with the number of specialists and subspecialists available?
- Why is it that studies performed by the Rand Corporation and others seem to indicate that a large number of highly invasive and risky surgical procedures may be unnecessary? Why is it that costs for procedures seem to vary widely even in fixed geographical regions?
- Why is it that new technologies are being introduced despite the absence of rigorous studies documenting that they represent an improvement over conventional technologies?

This list of questions goes on and on, representing a growing distrust that the medical community is attentive to these concerns and is instead largely motivated by professional and personal self-interest.

In the business community and among organized labor as well, the question of quality is now being discussed in the terms of recent innovations in industrial quality control as manifested in the work of Deming, Crosby, Juran, and others. A core tenet of the industrial quality control philosophies is that quality is a process with certain distinctions, including mechanisms for setting goals and assessing progress toward those goals. In comparison with this emerging style, the management of quality in the delivery of health care seems woefully inadequate, lacking both vision and commitment to grapple with difficult allocation and process issues. It is a fundamental belief of modern managers that what cannot be measured cannot be managed. The current health care delivery system is lacking even the most fundamental capability to monitor the services delivered in terms of incidence, cost intensity, and resource utilization—or even to perform the simplest outcome correlations to document that the medical procedures were worth doing in the first place. The ability of CPRs to provide a platform for systematic data collection starts to make the process for continuous improvement a realizable possibility in an industry that currently consumes almost 12 percent of our gross national product at a cost approaching $600 billion.

Recent months have witnessed an increased interest on the part of many payers, including the government in exploring the possibility of designing protocols and guidelines for channeling the delivery of care. Even the American Medical Association has come out in favor of this general approach, although there are the expected differences of opinion as to the format and scope of these mechanisms. Fundamentally, though, payers endorse the view that, for a vast array of clinical scenarios, patients may be grouped into certain categories, and their care channeled along certain pathways. The expectation is that guided care will be managed care and that quality benefits will accrue if care is delivered with more systematic and rigorous attention as to the criteria that warrant the delivery of that care. The basis for these guidelines must at first arise from the general clinical knowledge base; however, if care delivery is coupled to the measurement of outcome (another growing payer and popular interest), it is conceivable that data collected in the delivery of managed care can be used CPR to improve the appropriateness and, by definition, the value of the care. Again, the role of a CPR here is to collect accurate data for developing protocols and, perhaps more intriguingly, to act as the decision making platform from which various decision rules can be fired or specific knowledge bases brought to bear to guide clinical decision making.

Since many of the extrinsic administrative efforts designed in the last decade to manage care delivery's quality and cost parameters (e.g., precertification review and second surgical opinion) have done little to stem the tide of skyrocketing costs, greater attention is now being focused on the physician as the decision maker. In addition to specific guidelines, there are other mechanisms being explored to guide decisions that are less explicit. Attempts to influence physician behavior are not new (drug companies have been succeeding at this for years), but now they are directed toward shifting the nature of clinical decision making by feeding back to the clinician aggregate results of clinical outcomes relative to the those decisions, with the expectation that decision making criteria will shift toward generating favorable outcomes. There is already some evidence to show that this approach works and, more importantly, that it works best if physicians can be confronted with results of their own decisions as opposed to national data. The message here for the CPR is clear. Only with the precision and accuracy inherent in this approach is it feasible to collect, store, analyze, and feedback data of suitable clinical quality to begin to influence behavior. One can visualize having aggregate historic data available as a knowledge base which can in itself be used as a resource for guiding decision making.

Another and more politically charged use of physician-specific data would be to use it as a basis for including or excluding specific physicians from a care delivery network or even structuring compensation such that physicians' pay is adjusted for adherence to quality and cost-effectiveness parameters, modified by patient outcomes. The identification of outlier physicians' practice patterns has already become standard practice in certain managed care settings. A precise record keeping system will allow this process to case adjust for severity of illness and other factors, avoiding the inequity of penalizing physicians who treat the sickest patients and thus risk being discriminated against if only simple screening tools are used to assess their performance.

Message. Compelling messages can be constructed to demonstrate that the CPR, linked to appropriate knowledge bases and communications gateways, opens up new possibilities in the systematic delivery of high quality, cost-effective care. Emerging industrial quality models that feature measurement, goal setting, criteria specification, outcome measurement, and information feedback should be heavily emphasized.

Information systems have already proven themselves in the business community as cost effective in the management of both simple and complex administrative activities. One would only have to pass around an example of a paper medical record, complete with scrawled progress notes, unreadable discharge plans, and incomplete entries to demonstrate the obvious advantages of an electronic chart. In addition to these straightforward problems, electronic charting offers the possibility for direct submission of claims to third party payers, online utilization review and quality control, and transmission of documents electronically to other clinical entities involved in a patient's care after discharge (e.g., home health care agencies, nursing homes, and medical consultants). These messages could be interwoven in a video interview with a hospital administrator or simply provided in written form as a testimonial from a notable thought leader in the field.

A CPR can also be used as a platform to drive hospital operating efficiencies. This message would be quite compelling since it is an attribute of computerization with which business leaders are familiar and to which they subscribe. With accurate, aggregate patient care data, the tasks of materials management, human resource and staffing support, and other organizational requirements can be coordinated to maximize internal operating efficiencies, thus maintaining quality care at lower overhead costs. This clearly benefits the payer for health care services. It is hard to argue with the point that any technology that can improve operating efficiencies, eliminate waste, streamline the production process of delivering care, and at the same time improve quality, is worth investing in from the ultimate payer's perspective.

Related to the topic of reducible overhead is the issue of hospital and professional risk management. It has been estimated that perhaps as much as $50 billion a year is spent on defensive medicine, often in the form of unnecessary and duplicative diagnostic procedures. Adding to this is the difficulty of successfully defending suits when documentation in the chart is poor and there is no socially accepted standard for optimal care. The CPR, supported by appropriate guidelines and protocols, addresses both these issues. The message related to medical malpractice risk management should be compelling to both labor and industry since these issues are familiar as a standard business concern. In fact, a recent decision in Massachusetts has led to a reduction in medical malpractice rates of 20 percent among emergency room physicians who provide a summary of the clinical visit in machine-readable format to a chart review agency that screens for completeness. It is difficult to argue against a technology that reduces lawsuits by providing systematic guidelines for quality clinical care in a documentable format.

Dissemination strategy. Given the current climate of interest in the labor and business communities relating to health care cost and quality, it will not be hard to get a suitable audience. Care must be taken as to the crafting of the message. A dazzling computer-driven display might intimidate more than it informs. Since our message is straightforward and compelling on the surface, there is no real utility here in overwhelming the audience with technical complexities.

Appropriate groups to address would include the executive committees of some of the larger trade organizations and labor councils. The National Association of Manufacturers, the Washington Business Group on Health, and the Business Roundtable would be good groups to begin with. On the organized labor side one could start with the AFL-CIO and spread out to the social security departments of the UAW, CWA, and USW. On a more intimate level, this message fits very nicely as a one-on-one CEO sell, whenever we can identify a highly visible leader known to be a spokesperson able to face colleagues in a particular business community.

Almost all major trade and labor groups have annual conferences where health care is a major topic. Currently, these meetings are given over in large part to examining the current problem in excruciating detail with little light being presented at the end of the tunnel. There seems to be a thought and policy vacuum where any reasonable suggestions would be eagerly entertained and carried by media follow-up to the meeting as one of the "hot" topics in health care. This could be stimulated by strategically placed press releases and interviews.

The bottom line is that our health care delivery system is in trouble. Skyrocketing costs are threatening the well being of employers and employees. The CPR system is a core-constitutive element of a health information system that could efficiently network both hospital and nonhospital-based providers. This network would establish a platform for the delivery of high quality, cost-effective care that could be continuously assessed for outcomes in the domains of clinical parameters, functional patient status, quality of life, and satisfaction with care. We as a society are likely to evolve toward a health care delivery system with centralized control mechanisms, continuous micromanagement, and explicit and implicit rationing. We cannot afford to further delay the development of the critical tools necessary to manage this process equitably and effectively. Business and labor will be attentive to this message, particularly considering the alternative option of the status quo.

The Perspective of Patients

Patients should not be viewed as passive in either the deliberations or the design and implementation phases. As part of the coordination, education, and promotion charter of a proposed CPR institute, patients' interests and concerns should be adequately represented in an organized way.

Message. Patients have three major concerns which must be addressed by the CPR. Stated briefly, they want health information

- To be complete, accurate, and accessible for care purposes
- To be held confidential and secure
- To permit them to make informed health care choices, including information about quality and cost of care

A concern that may not be visible to the average patient but is related to the quality and cost of care is that aggregate health information must also be available for education and research to continually improve patient care and constrain costs.

The general public should be made aware both of the pitfalls of current record keeping in health care and the potential benefits (and pitfalls) of CPRs. The advantages of using CPRs in everyday care of patients as well as the potential utility of using population data to advance the understanding of diseases and the effects of our interventions should both be clearly presented to the public through scenarios, demonstrations, and selected examples of public good derived from their use. Examples from the Centers for Disease Control (CDC), including the discovery process of AIDS as a transmissible disease, would help demonstrate the usefulness of population databases. Projected increases in the efficiency and turnaround time of evaluating and approving new drugs would help clarify potential benefits to the population and individual patients. Individual patient scenarios showing how timely access to patient data and medical information can improve care while decreasing its costs (to the patient) would have the most general appeal.

Dissemination strategy. The general public is probably most reachable through public media. Informative articles and news releases directing people's attention to the issues and ongoing activities would be powerful methods for informing and engaging the public. These educational efforts must be carefully planned and formulated. The proposed institute would have a central role in this responsibility. Ongoing public forums for education and communication could keep the public aware and engaged in this substantial undertaking.

Patient representative groups and other organized patients' advocates (e.g., American Association of Retired Persons) should be involved to render advice to the institute as patient advocates and to help provide qualified opinions to the public.

The Perspective of the Researcher

The goal of clinical research is to understand the determinants and consequences of clinical decisions. It relies heavily on clinical data related to diagnosis, treatment, and outcome. Consequently, the efficiency and effectiveness of clinical research are directly related to the accessibility, validity, and completeness of necessary clinical data.

A CPR holds great potential for clinical research. Foremost is its capacity to save time. Without a CPR, researchers interested in cross-sectional or retrospective (e.g., case control) must spend an inordinate amount of time identifying patients eligible to be studied, manually abstracting information from the medical record, and manually entering data into a computer for analysis. With the ideal CPR system, the clinical researcher should be able to identify quickly a study population of records that meet certain eligibility criteria (e.g., closed head injury patients admitted in 1990), isolate the pertinent clinical data needed to test a research hypothesis, and statistically analyze this data.

Another advantage of a CPR system is that it can facilitate more valid and precise research because a larger sample of patient records with more data can be studied. Because the manual collection of clinical research data can be so time consuming, these studies have often been small and less comprehensive. CPR systems permit analysis of a large sample of records that have accumulated over time; as a result, the precision of the study estimates is improved. By providing a wealth of data on which to conduct multivariate analyses, CPR systems can also enhance the validity of such studies.

Nevertheless, the use of a CPR system is not without concerns. These concerns relate to the ease of use, completeness and accuracy of data, generalizability of results, data confidentiality, and system security. Presently, many clinical researchers are not very computer literate, although this may change in the next few years as the younger generation of physicians who grew up with computers begin clinical research activities. Thus, current efforts to develop CPR systems should focus on the human interface such that the system responds quickly and is as easy to use as possible.

The use of the CPRs depends on completeness of the data. Many hospitals currently house computer-based patient registries (e.g., trauma, tumor), which are used for clinical research. Nevertheless, these systems, although very efficient at isolating a subset of patients of interest, often lack certain data elements, such as laboratory results or follow-up information related to outcomes that are needed to conduct the study. Thus, the clinical researcher must continue to resort to some manual abstraction of information to complete the data collection phase of the study. Although it is unreasonable to expect that a CPR should be all things to all researchers, it should be designed to include a comprehensive collection of data elements of value in clinical research. These elements should include patient demographic and risk factor information, diagnostic data (including laboratory and other test results), procedure and treatment data, discharge diagnoses, and follow-up information (clinical endpoints, functional status, well-being, satisfaction with care). All of these elements need not reside in a single database, but access (e.g., through a network of databases) should be provided.

Clinical researchers using a CPR system will also be concerned about the accuracy of the data, particularly if it requires coding. It is important that standard and well-accepted methods of coding clinical data are employed by well-trained individuals. Data entry mechanisms that use error checking algorithms can improve data accuracy. Periodic surveillance of the system to evaluate the accuracy of the data should also be required.

Another concern for researchers is the generalizability of clinical research results from a hospital-based CPR system. Depending on the goals of the research, the analysis of data from a single hospital may produce results that are either biased or of limited generalizability. This situation occurs most frequently with clinical research projects that attempt to estimate the occurrence of particular outcomes in a patient population that may be highly skewed in terms of disease severity (e.g., patients from a tertiary care facility). CPR systems that allow patients to be segregated by whether they are primary or referral or that are regional or national rather than hospital based may reduce the likelihood of these biases for certain types of clinical research.

Finally, in using a CPR system, clinical researchers would be concerned about two related issues, data confidentiality and system security. Because clinical research involves the analysis of patient information, there are obvious concerns about who has access to the data, the type of data that is available (e.g., patient name and address) and how it is distributed. To ensure the confidentiality of patient data, specific system security measures should be implemented. These could include written access request forms that would need to be approved, password requirements to access the system, patient identifying information inaccessibility measures, and the ongoing monitoring of system usage.

Access to a CPR system should be multifaceted. Advances in network technology argue for the system to be on a network and available to investigators from their microcomputers. Thus, decentralized access is desirable. However, given the lack of computer literacy among clinical researchers, more centralized access should also be available. Centralized access could be provided by a shared biostatistics and computational laboratory that would provide the data retrieval and statistical analysis services to busy clinicians who also have an interest in research. In sum, the system should be structured in such a way that it can accommodate the various needs and skills of the clinical researcher.

Reference

Shortliffe, E.H., and M.S. Blois. 1990. The computer meets medicine: Emergence of a discipline. In *Medical informatics: Computer applications in health care*, ed. E.H. Shortliffe, L.E. Perreault, G. Wiederhold, and L.M. Fagan. Reading, MA: Addison-Wesley, 3–36.

2
A Bold Vision: The Computer-based Patient Record Institute

Richard Dick

During the deliberations of the Institute of Medicine's (IOM) committee for improving the patient record, it became apparent that a sustained, coordinated, and concentrated effort will be required to establish the widespread use of computer-based patient records (CPRs) and CPR systems. Therefore, the committee recommended the establishment of a public/private initiative which they called the Computer-Based Patient Record Institute (CPRI). Simply stated, the mission of the CPRI will be to initiate and coordinate activities facilitating and promoting the routine use of the CPRs throughout health care.

Of the seven recommendations made by the IOM, the keystone recommendation was to establish the CPRI. Consistent with their standard practice, the IOM will refrain from involvement in implementation processes. With the release of the report, the work of the IOM was completed. During the early summer of 1991, leaders in both the public and private sectors joined in a coalition to begin implementation. They acknowledged that no single organization acting alone could equal the impact of the proposed CPRI.

The urgency of forming the CPRI to establish the routine use of CPRs throughout health care is underscored by the remarks of a physician who had just read the IOM report for the first time:

> The routine use of the CPR holds the potential to simultaneously and effectively address more core issues in health care than any other single thing that might be undertaken at this time.

Although some might wonder at such a statement, consider for a moment that we lack the evidence to make more informed decisions in health care today across the spectrum from the bedside up the formulation of national health care policy. Most of the evidence needed to make more informed decisions remains embedded in fragmented, irretrievable, and often illegible paper-based patient records. Therefore, the widespread use of CPRs will make available substantial clinical data in machine readable form. Clinical data (with patient and provider identifiers removed or encrypted) pooled in regional and national databases and made available through networks will constitute a vast information resource upon which to base health care policy, clinical studies of effectiveness and appropriateness, equitable reimbursement policies, and scientific hypothesis for further research.

Mission of the CPRI

The mission of the Computer-Based Patient Record Institute (CPRI) as recommended by the Committee on Improving the Patient Record in the Institute of Medicine Report, *The Computer-Based Patient Record: An Essential Technology for Health Care*, will be

> To initiate all necessary and essential activities which will establish the routine use of computer-based patient records (CPRs) in virtually all health care settings in the U.S. as soon as possible, but preferably within a decade (by 2001).

Thus, activities must be designed which

- Support the effective, efficient use of computer-based patient information in patient care, health care policy making, clinical research, health care financing, and continuous quality improvement.
- Educate change agents and stakeholders (including the general public and health professionals) about the value of CPRs in improving health patient care.
- Foster the CPR as the primary vehicle for collecting patient data.
- Promote the development and use of standards for CPR security, data content, structures, and vocabulary (Institute of Medicine 1991).*

The CPRI Structure

Leaders from the public and private sectors met throughout the summer of 1991 to explore issues pertinent to the creation of the CPRI. Joining in the coalition to create the CPRI were representatives from the U.S. Chamber of Commerce, the American Medical Association (AMA), American Nurses Association (ANA), American Medical Record Association (AMRA), and the Agency for Health Care Policy and Research (AHCPR of the HHS). Representatives from vendors, government, and third party payers began attending the meetings and making commitments to this effort.

As noted in the IOM report, there are many organizations that have a great deal at stake in the transition to the widespread use of CPRs. Those stakeholders would be able to influence how the transition to CPRs evolves over the next decade. The CPRI's governance structure, using a board of governors, is vital to its success. In

---

*Used with permission. Taken from Institute of Medicine, *The Computer-Based Patient Record: An Essential Technology for Health Care*, Richard S. Dick and Elaine B. Steen, editors. © 1991 National Academy Press, Washington, D.C.

addition, appropriate structuring of the committees and subcommittees, where the real work occurs, will be crucial to the CPRI's success. Below is one of the views being considered for governance of the CPRI. Representatives from the following categories might have a seat on the board of governors of the CPRI:

Medicine (3 Seats)
Nursing (2 Seats)
Dentistry
Record administrators
Other health care professionals
Hospitals
Managed care
Third party payers
Congress (Senate and House staffers)
Government agencies (e.g., Departments of Defense and Veterans Affairs)
Employers
Labor
Citizens
Health education and training organizations
Professional societies
Vendors of CPR related health care technologies
Foundations and other philanthropic organizations
Regulatory agencies, public (e.g., FDA) and private (e.g., JCAHO)

Examples might include organizations such as the American Medical Association (AMA), the U.S. Chamber of Commerce, the American Nurses Association, the American Medical Records Association, the American Dental Association, the American Association of Retired Persons, the American Federation of Labor-Congress of Industrial Organizations (AFL-CIO). Generally, a rotating board is envisioned for the CPRI. For example, the Robert Wood Johnson Foundation might provide a representative on the board of governors (representing foundations and philanthropic organizations) for a period of time (perhaps 2–3 years) and later the John A. Hartford Foundation might be elected from within their category to serve the next term on the board of governors. The CPRI has recently been conceived as having two official organizations so that a full range of activities including lobbying can be explored. As of summer 1991, legal documents to formalize both entities of the institute were in the process of being drafted by the Epstein, Becker and Green law firm.

Committees and Subcommittees

The coalition to create the CPRI has been exploring the establishment of several committees and subcommittees. The committees have been grouped into two categories: Essential or core committees and other committees. Below is a brief description of the committees and subcommittees being established as of mid-summer 1991.

Core committees

Legal, Confidentiality, and Privacy Committee. This committee will be responsible for examining the state of legislation currently and for creating a more favorable environment for the deployment of CPRs and CPR systems. It will formulate statements on ethical, legal, privacy, and confidentiality issues that may become official positions of the CPRI. These position statements should help to guide legislative activities initiated by the CPRI or its members. This committee will initiate legislative language for consideration by the board of governors of the CPRI and subsequent submission to federal and state legislative bodies. In addition, it will respond to other legal issues and questions that may arise from time to time.

Health Data Standards Committee. This committee will work with existing health data standards efforts and complement their work and encourage more rapid development of health data standards. It will have several subcommittees as seen below. In addition, this committee will plan and prepare for the establishment of a composite clinical data dictionary (CCDD or C^2D^2), which will be developed and perpetually maintained by the CPRI as a national resource for encouraging standards. This C^2D^2 will be vital to and facilitate all health data standards development efforts. This committee, primarily through its subcommittees, will focus on the following areas of interest:

- *Health Data Transmission Standards.* Once an appropriate set of data elements from the C^2D^2 has been selected which are determined to be relevant for a specific purpose, the transmission of those data between disparate systems will be actually carried out by an appropriate health data transmission standard such as HL7, Medix etc.
- *CPR System Security Standards.* CPR systems themselves are in need of significantly greater security measures to deter unauthorized access to sensitive information on patients and providers. Standards need to be developed, tested, and deployed for the CPR industry. Care must be taken that there is appropriate balance between security and reasonable access to those authorized to use CPR systems.
- *CPR System Framework Standards.* There are no commonly understood and widely agreed upon definitions of CPR systems. The IOM report lays out in general terms the attributes of robust CPR systems which should assist the committee in establishing guides for future developments in CPR systems. This will undoubtedly be one of the most controversial activities for the CPRI.
- *Composite Clinical Data Dictionary.* The C^2D^2 is a high priority item for the CPRI and the coalition to address. It will facilitate the entire standards efforts and help build confidence in coalition's efforts.
- *Standards Dissemination.* The rapid dissemination and enforcement of health data standards will be essential to the deployment of CPR systems. This subcommittee will be responsible for the development of effective means of deploying the standards which the other subcommittees will develop or foster.

Demonstration Projects Committee. This committee will submit proposals for consideration by the board of governors for demonstration projects which will lead to establishing confidence in the CPR and its ability to address substantive issues facing health care. Demonstration projects should address issues that the public and key decision makers such as Congress can easily understand and appreciate.

CPR Systems Financing Committee. Today there are no generally accepted mechanisms that give provider institutions the incentive to procure and operate CPR systems. This committee will be responsible for establishing creative and innovative mechanisms for the procurement and maintenance of CPR systems in the near future. Only appropriate viable mechanisms can seriously be considered. They must be acceptable to government agencies, employers, third party payers, practitioners, provider institutions, CPR technology vendors, and patients.

The CPRI will need strong and sustained financial support for its programs and operations. The CPRI will have a life span of more than a decade and may be in existence for a considerable period of time. Membership fees will help to sustain the CPRI, but additional substantial support should come from foundations, employers, payers, and government. This committee is responsible for exploring short-term, and long-term financing for the CPRI so that it may accelerate the realization of the CPR throughout health care.

Professional Education Committee. It is important that educational institutions become more conversant with the CPRs and CPR systems. Therefore, this committee will be responsible for encouraging educational societies, and institutions to begin educating faculty, and students regarding the CPR. It is important that the nation begin "filling the pipeline" with students that are properly trained in the use of these new technologies. This committee will focus on all issues related to educational matters concerning the CPR and CPR systems.

CPR Implementation Committee. This committee will be responsible for addressing the strategies for deploying the CPR and CPR systems in all health care environments as quickly as possible. This committee will in large part set the agenda and raise issues for consideration by many of the committees within the CPRI. It will propose specific coordinated strategies for overcoming identifiable barriers to the CPR and explain clearly how such strategies may impact all associated with health care. It will focus first on those strategies which have a high potential as a *win/win* for all members of the CPRI. The AMA and the U.S. Chamber of Commerce should be the primary or lead organizations in forming and guiding this committee.

Other committees

Publicity and Communications Committee. If established, this committee will be responsible for establishing policy statements and other important media related releases which will be approved by the executive committee or by the coalition, depending upon the significance of the topic. It will be responsible for publicizing the coalition's efforts and will continue on after the CPRI is fully functional.

Grant Applications and Proposals Committee. Once fully formed, the CPRI will be able to receive funding from many sources for research relevant to the CPRs deployment such as standards setting activities and demonstration projects. This committee will work to submit grant applications to various government and private agencies with an interest in CPRI related activities. This committee will enable the CPRI to marshall grant support early on.

Advisory Council

Members of the coalition felt that it is essential that an advisory council be formed which might consist of IOM committee members, a few current and former IOM staff, and key executives from the Department of Health and Human Services (HHS). Two or three additional individuals may also be included because they offer special skills and insights which will be helpful. Advisory council members will be offered a standing invitation to attend virtually all meetings of the coalition and schedules of such meetings will be regularly distributed. Members of the advisory council will be expected to allocate approximately one to two hours per month to fulfill their duties. The coalition will from time to time (e.g., once every 3–6 weeks) arrange a conference call to advisory council members to solicit their advice regarding certain issues. Advisory council will not have veto or voting powers concerning programs or policy for the CPRI. This arrangement will permit certain funding agencies (e.g., HHS) to maintain an appropriate level of involvement while avoiding any potential conflict of interest. The coalition for creating the CPRI has asked Dr. Don E. Detmer, who served as chair of the IOM committee, to act as chair of the advisory council.

Priorities for the CPRI Agenda

There are many potential items for the agenda of the CPRI as outlined in the IOM report. Some will have more immediate impact; others will have a larger pay off in the long run. It is imperative that the CPRI demonstrate some early wins or successes; and the likelihood of having such can be enhanced by activities to be started during the formation phase of the CPRI. The following high priority items are being organized even while the CPRI is still being formed. Doing so ensures that the CPRI can "hit the ground running" once it comes fully online. The logic behind why the following are high priority CPRI agenda items may be self-evident, but a brief explanation is provided to put things in context.

Funding CPR Systems

It is one thing to say that hospitals and other health care institutions should migrate toward the routine use of the CPR as soon as possible, but unless the CPRI can address the need for providing appropriate financial mechanisms that encourage such a migration, progress will remain at a snail's pace.

With many hospitals now finding it difficult to make payroll, it is ludicrous to suggest that they invest a few million dollars in a CPR system without substantial incentives and means for doing so. Therefore, it is important that high priority be given to exploring and establishing appropriate funding mechanisms (including cost sharing) for enabling the procurement of CPRI systems. This is the recommendation of the IOM report. Such funding mechanisms should be addressed from three perspectives: the immediate future (next 12–24 months), intermediate (two to five years), and long range (five to 15 years).

The CPR Systems Financing Committee is to be formed consisting of individuals from the U.S. Congress (staffers for the Hill), Office of Management and Budget (OMB), Executive Office of the President (EOP), Health Care Financing Agency (HCFA), third-party payers, U.S. Chamber of Commerce, American business (employers), American Hospital Association (AHA), Group Health Association (GHA) and other managed care organizations, health practitioners as represented by professional associations (e.g., AMA, AMRA, ANA, and ADA), CPR system vendors, and others. The committee will begin by exploring funding issues and problems in the hopes of identifying alternative means for acquiring, installing, and maintaining CPR systems. The coalition for creating the CPRI has requested that a key person from the AHA chair this committee.

Health Data Standards

Health data standards are now developing, but not as rapidly as the situation demands. The lack of standards prevents the aggregation of significant quantities of clinical data. Today, we do have a few sources of significant clinical data but cannot easily pool them for analysis. The lack of health data standards remains a major barrier to achieving many significant milestones in health care and broad deployment of CPRs and CPR systems. The following are high priority areas for standards development by the CPRI.

Health Data Transmission Standards. There are no internationally accepted data transmission standards for health care data in 1991. Those now being proposed greatly need fostering. This activity will have a very high pay-off and should be encouraged.

CPR System Security Standards. There are no commercially viable CPR systems in 1991 that utilize significant state of the art security mechanisms to protect patient data, provider information, and other confidential information. Coordinated efforts need to be launched to address these deficiencies.

CPR System Framework Standards. There are no commonly understood and accepted definitions of a CPR system in the health care community. The IOM report identifies the characteristics which need to be defined so that potential users can compare CPR systems.

Composite Clinical Data Dictionary (CCDD) Standards. The IOM report suggests that a critical missing ingredient is the Composite Clinical Data Dictionary (CCDD), which will become increasingly important to standards efforts. The CPRI should commence efforts to create and maintain the CCDD. Such efforts may actually help to bring the synergy between the various partners in the coalition created in this phase.

Making the CPR Legal and Protecting Confidentiality

Because some states have laws discouraging or prohibiting CPRs, the CPRI must develop model legislation that will encourage and foster the adoption of CPRs and CPR systems in all practice settings. In addition, more attention needs to be paid to ensuring and protecting confidentiality of primary and secondary patient records.

The primary record is the patient's record used by members of the health care team to provide actual care. The secondary record is a derived or subset record from the primary record which is devoid of patient and practitioner identifiers (or such identifiers may be encrypted and stored in other generally inaccessible computers). Secondary records can be aggregated into local and regional databases for use by researchers and others interested in health care issues.

Demonstration Projects

Demonstrations of the benefits of the CPR and CPR systems need to be brought before the public and the U.S. Congress to stimulate escalating support for the deployment of CPRs. Demonstrations may focus on such aspects as

- *CPR Enabling Technologies*
  - Automated speech recognition (ASR) systems
  - Automated text processing and coding systems
  - National high speed networking for health care
- *Benefits of CPRs*
  - Productivity gains for all members of the health care team
  - Liability reductions in such areas of emergency care

Demonstrations may resort to showing the benefits of existing clinical databases to show what can be done with even limited clinical data. Activities and plans in these and other areas should be developed during CPRI formation.

CPRI Telecast

At the time of this writing, the U.S. Chamber of Commerce was planning a major television broadcast to highlight the need for the CPR. Topics to be covered may include the following: where we are today and the contribution of the traditional paper-based record to the current state of affairs; an overview of the IOM committee's work and report; exploration of the CPR's potential as a powerful tool for health care reform; the need to create a friendlier environment for the CPR; the need to create more appropriate mechanisms for procuring and maintaining CPR systems; the state of the art for today's CPR systems; emerging technologies and their potential to enhance the CPR systems of the future; a view of the future CPR system and what it will be capable of providing; the CPRI as a catalyst for the deployment of CPRs and CPR systems throughout health care; a view of how the CPRI works and its agenda for change; a call for action on supporting the CPRI's activities, thereby accelerating substantive health care reform.

Plans called for a full day telecast with satellite downlinks to many organizations interested in health care. Arrangements with a professional broadcasting organization for this program were in progress as of mid-summer 1991; tentative scheduling called for the program to be aired in late fall 1991.

Potential of the CPRI

Some have suggested that the role of the CPRI is so large and far reaching that it might be likened to the U.S. "moonshot" of the 1960s. Although the CPRI's goals are difficult to achieve, they are not comparable to the technical challenges of the moonshot. Clearly, the principal challenges are behavioral and sociopolitical rather than technical. Today health care lacks leadership and a clearly articulated goal and plan for emerging from the current state of affairs. The IOM report articulates a goal and suggests an appropriate leadership mechanism for achieving the goal. The CPRI has the opportunity to coalesce leadership into a structure that can have far reaching impact on health care at a particularly critical time. The CPRI can provide

- Leadership and structure for a major new initiative in health care
- Clearly articulated goals which can significantly improve health care
- A coherent and compelling plan for implementing the recommendations of the IOM report

We hope that the diverse organizations coming together in the CPRI to take a leadership role will have a positive impact on the future of health care. The CPRI can create a more favorable environment for the widespread use of CPRs. Those of us who served on the IOM committee are convinced that CPRs will enable caregivers and policymakers alike to respond to the most challenging issues facing health care today.

Reference

Institute of Medicine. 1991. *The Computer-based Patient Record: An Essential Technology for Health Care*, ed. R.S. Dick and E.B. Steen. Washington, D.C.: National Academy Press, p. 139.

Index